Diabetes & Carb Counting

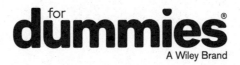
A Wiley Brand

Diabetes & Carb Counting

by Sherri Shafer, RD, CDE

Diabetes educator

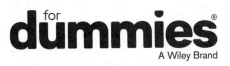
for dummies®
A Wiley Brand

Diabetes & Carb Counting For Dummies®

Published by: **John Wiley & Sons, Inc.**, 111 River Street, Hoboken, NJ 07030-5774, www.wiley.com

Copyright © 2017 by John Wiley & Sons, Inc., Hoboken, New Jersey

Published simultaneously in Canada

For general information on our other products and services, please contact our Customer Care Department within the U.S. at 877-762-2974, outside the U.S. at 317-572-3993, or fax 317-572-4002. For technical support, please visit https://hub.wiley.com/community/support/dummies.

Wiley publishes in a variety of print and electronic formats and by print-on-demand. Some material included with standard print versions of this book may not be included in e-books or in print-on-demand. If this book refers to media such as a CD or DVD that is not included in the version you purchased, you may download this material at http://booksupport.wiley.com. For more information about Wiley products, visit www.wiley.com.

Library of Congress Control Number: 2017933632

ISBN 978-1-119-31564-3 (pbk); ISBN 978-1-119-31572-8 (ebk); ISBN 978-1-119-31570-4 (ebk)

Manufactured in the United States of America

10 9 8 7 6 5 4 3 2 1

Contents at a Glance

Introduction 1

Part 1: Getting Started with Carb Counting and Diabetes Management 5

CHAPTER 1: Delving into Diabetes and Carb Counting 7
CHAPTER 2: Exploring the Diabetes-Carb Connection 25
CHAPTER 3: Calling All Carbs: Recognizing Carbs in the Foods You Eat 39
CHAPTER 4: Tracking Carbs through the Body 53
CHAPTER 5: Finding Your Sweet Spot: The Right Amount of Carbs for You 67
CHAPTER 6: Timing Your Carb Consumption 79

Part 2: Carb Counting: From Basic to Advanced 95

CHAPTER 7: First Things First: Reading and Deciphering Food Labels 97
CHAPTER 8: Mastering Carb Counting and Portioning Fundamentals 117
CHAPTER 9: Adding Tools for Carb-Counting Ease and Accuracy 137

Part 3: Going Beyond Counting Carbs 143

CHAPTER 10: Accounting for Variations in Digestion and Absorption Rates 145
CHAPTER 11: Rethink That Drink 159
CHAPTER 12: Let Me Call You Sweetie: Sugars and Substitutes 175

Part 4: Embracing Whole Health and Happiness 189

CHAPTER 13: Eating for Health and Happiness 191
CHAPTER 14: Reaping the Rewards of Fitness 207
CHAPTER 15: Getting a Handle on Hypoglycemia 227
CHAPTER 16: Keeping the Beat with a Healthy Heart 251
CHAPTER 17: Living with Diabetes throughout the Life Cycle 267
CHAPTER 18: Going Gluten-Free (Or Not): Does the Batter Matter? 283

Part 5: Sampling Menus Complete with Carb Counts 297

CHAPTER 19: Beginning with Breakfast Menus 299
CHAPTER 20: Looking for Lunch Menus 305
CHAPTER 21: Delving into Dinner Menus 313
CHAPTER 22: Surveying Snack Ideas 319

Part 6: The Part of Tens 327

CHAPTER 23: Ten Tips for Monitoring Your Blood Glucose 329

CHAPTER 24: Ten Tips for Controlling Carbs 337

CHAPTER 25: Ten Worthwhile Websites to Help You Manage Diabetes 343

Part 7: Appendixes 349

APPENDIX A: Diabetes Exchange Lists 351

APPENDIX B: Conversion Guide 365

Index 367

Table of Contents

INTRODUCTION 1

About This Book. 2
Foolish Assumptions 3
Icons Used in This Book 3
Beyond the Book 4
Where to Go from Here 4

PART 1: GETTING STARTED WITH CARB COUNTING AND DIABETES MANAGEMENT 5

CHAPTER 1: Delving into Diabetes and Carb Counting 7
Getting Up to Speed on Diabetes Basics 8
Checking out concerning trends in the diabetes epidemic 8
Improving outcomes and preventing complications 8
Building your diabetes team 9
Staying up to date with advances in diabetes care 10
Examining the Carb-Glucose Connection 11
Getting Acquainted with Carbs 12
Introducing the so-called simple carbs 13
Catching up on complex carbs 13
Noting the nutrition in carb food groups. 13
Acknowledging that staying healthy isn't just about carbs 14
Making the Case for Carb Counting: To Count or Not to Count? 15
Counting carbs with type 1 diabetes: An essential tool 15
Gaining tighter control over blood-glucose levels with
type 2 diabetes. 15
Sticking with consistent carb counts when you're on
set insulin doses 16
Managing weight with carb counting and portion precision 17
Regulating Carb Intakes 18
Figuring out how much carb you need. 18
Timing your carb intake 18
Counting Carbs Successfully 19
Looking at the label lingo 19
Gathering carb-counting resources 19
Increasing carb-counting accuracy 20
Living Well with Diabetes: The Seven Pillars of Diabetes
Management 20
Eating a healthy diet 20
Staying fit with exercise 21
Taking your medication 22

       Monitoring your blood-glucose levels 22
       Managing stress. 23
       Discovering how to problem-solve 23
       Reducing risk with healthy behaviors and
       regular medical checkups 24

CHAPTER 2: Exploring the Diabetes-Carb Connection. 25
   Wrapping Your Brain around Diabetes and Related Conditions 26
       Seeing how the body is supposed to process carbs. 26
       Discovering what causes diabetes 27
       Noticing the symptoms of diabetes 28
       Distinguishing the types of diabetes 29
   Recognizing Diabetes Risk Factors and Getting Diagnosed 32
       Type 1 diabetes risk factors. 32
       Type 2 diabetes risk factors. 33
       Diagnosing diabetes 34
   Moving Forward with Managing Diabetes. 35
       Knowing that diet matters 36
       Keeping in touch with your diabetes team 36
       Embracing your central role in your own self-care. 37

**CHAPTER 3: Calling All Carbs: Recognizing Carbs
in the Foods You Eat** 39
   Looking at the Chemical Structure of Carbohydrates 40
   Introducing the So-Called Simple Carbohydrates. 42
       Going au naturel with glucose, fructose, and lactose 43
       Finding other forms of sugar: Sucrose, maltose,
       honey, and syrups. 44
       Spotting simple carbs in the grocery aisles 45
   Checking Out the Complex Carbohydrates. 45
       Identifying the starches 45
       Focusing on fiber. 46
       Spotting complex carbs in the grocery aisles 48
   Recognizing Carb-Free Counterparts 49
       Pumping up with proteins: Meat, fish, and other sources 49
       Finding the healthiest fats and oils. 50
       Exploring the role of noncarb foods in diabetes management. . . .51

CHAPTER 4: Tracking Carbs through the Body. 53
   Filling Your Tank and Fueling Your Cells 54
       Settling in your stomach. 54
       Extracting glucose via digestion 55
       Pumping through your bloodstream 56
       Fueling your cells. 56

Saving Some for Later: Glycogen, the Storage Form of Glucose 57
    Making a layover in the liver 57
    Maintaining the muscles' glucose reserves 58
Noting What Happens When Glucose Levels Remain Elevated 58
    Spilling glucose into the urine 58
    Sticking glucose where it doesn't belong: Glycosylation 60
Recognizing the Risks of Undereating Carbs. 62
    Depleting glucose reserves and dealing with hypoglycemia 62
    Making glucose but losing lean body mass 63
    Producing ketones. 64

CHAPTER 5: Finding Your Sweet Spot: The Right Amount of Carbs for You 67
Checking Out the Official Diet Guidelines 68
    Advice from the American Diabetes Association 68
    The 2015–2020 Dietary Guidelines for Americans 68
    Intakes and allowances from the National Academy of Sciences 69
Figuring Out Calorie and Carbohydrate Intake Targets. 69
    Estimating your caloric needs 69
    Adjusting calories for your weight target. 71
    Deciding on carb intake targets. 72
    Distributing carb intake 74
    Leaving room on your plate for protein and fat 74
Tweaking Your Carb Intake Target When Conditions Change 75
    Changing needs throughout the life cycle 75
    Altering intake to account for activity. 76
    Adjusting portions when blood glucose is out of control 76
    Managing sick days 76

CHAPTER 6: Timing Your Carb Consumption 79
Distributing Your Daily Carb Intake 80
    Striving to eat three meals per day. 80
    Opting for smaller meals with controlled snacks 81
Stabilizing Blood-Glucose Levels at Breakfast and Dinner 82
    Breaking your fast: The importance of breakfast 83
    Considering the merits of an earlier dinner 83
Understanding Insulin Action 84
    Comparing insulin options. 85
    Checking out concentrated insulins 85
    Looking at blended insulin preparations. 86
    Pumping and inhaling insulin 87

Coordinating Insulin Action with Meals 88
    Enjoying the flexibility of insulin-to-carb ratios 89
    Keeping carbs consistent when using sliding-scale
    insulin dosing 90
    Basing injection timing on pre-meal blood-glucose levels 91
    Being regimented if you use 70/30 insulin 91
Managing Carbs on Oral Diabetes Meds 93
    Keeping the carbs appropriate 93
    Knowing your limits 94

**PART 2: CARB COUNTING: FROM BASIC
TO ADVANCED** 95

CHAPTER 7: **First Things First: Reading and
Deciphering Food Labels** 97
Finding Your Way around Food Labels 98
    Paying particular attention to amounts 98
    Viewing versions of traditional labels 100
    Taking a sneak peek at newfangled food labels 101
Scrutinizing the Nutrition Facts 104
    Sorting out serving sizes and servings per container 105
    Calling out calories 105
    Finding the fat 105
    Noting the cholesterol content 106
    Surveying the sodium 107
    Focusing on total carbohydrate 107
    Pinpointing the protein 110
    Taking note of other valuable nutrients 111
    Investigating the ingredients 111
    Identifying allergens 111
Heading to the Grocery Store 112
    Being skeptical about label claims 112
    Preparing your carbohydrate cheat sheet 115
    Developing supermarket savvy 115

CHAPTER 8: **Mastering Carb Counting and Portioning
Fundamentals** 117
Estimating Carb Counts for Foods without Labels 118
    Relying on food composition lists 118
    Solving carb-counting conundrums in mixed dishes
    and ethnic foods 124
    Calculating carbs in your favorite recipes 126
    Preparing your carbohydrate cheat sheet 126

Sizing Up Servings with Measures and Weights 127
    Measuring with standardized cups and spoons 127
    Weighing in on whether to weigh foods 128
Dealing with Special Cases 132
    Controlling carb intake when eating out 132
    Keeping track of the carbs you drink 133
Guesstimating: When Carb Counts Aren't Critical 133
    Balancing your plate with the plate model 134
    Handling portions with the hand model 136

CHAPTER 9: Adding Tools for Carb-Counting Ease and Accuracy 137
Reviewing the Printed Resources 137
    Reading the fine print for carb counts 138
    Looking at labeling regulations for chain restaurants 138
Tapping into Online Resources 139
    Digging up chain restaurant food facts 139
    Foraging through Internet food databases 140
    Using your search engine to count carbs 140
Enlisting the Assistance of Apps: One More Reason to
Love Your Smartphone 140
    Finding useful diabetes apps 141
    Integrating apps and a food scale 142

PART 3: GOING BEYOND COUNTING CARBS 143

CHAPTER 10: Accounting for Variations in Digestion and Absorption Rates 145
Comparing Digestion Speeds for Fluids and Foods 146
    Looking at liquid carbs 146
    Singling out sugars 147
    Figuring out fruit 147
    Focusing on complex carbs and fiber .148
    Recognizing the fat factor 149
    Considering other variables 149
Gauging the Glycemic Index and Glycemic Load 150
Reducing Blood-Glucose Fluctuations: Tips and Tricks 152
    Controlling portion sizes of foods that pack a
    blood-glucose punch 152
    Adding activity for extra carbs 153
    Combining foods to reduce glycemic effect 153
    Altering the order in which you eat the components of
    your meal 154

Aligning Insulin and Digestion Rates 154
    Optimizing mealtime insulin coverage. 155
    Using your insulin pump's fine features .156

CHAPTER 11: **Rethink That Drink** 159
Noting the Importance of Hydration and Low-Carb Drinks 159
Exploring the Pros and Cons of Different Drinks 161
    Giving water a special place in your life .162
    Sipping and swigging low-carb beverages. 162
    Mentioning the merits of milk and nondairy
    milk substitutes 163
    Facing the facts about fruit juice 165
It's Not Just the Carbs — It's the Calories Too 167
Last Call for Alcohol: What's the Verdict? 169
    Being informed about the risks. 169
    Going behind the scenes: How alcohol affects the body. 170
    Looking at liquor's carbs and calories .171
    Drinking safely 173

CHAPTER 12: **Let Me Call You Sweetie: Sugars
and Substitutes** 175
Comparing Sugars: The Sugar Showdown. .176
    Introducing the heavyweights: Sugar, honey, syrup,
    and other notables 178
    Pointing out the qualities of natural fructose and
    agave nectar. 180
Examining Sugar Alcohols 182
Opting for Alternatives: The Sugar Substitutes. 184
    Digging into the differences of the substitutes
    on the market. 186
    Exploring sugar-substitute safety records. 186
    Using substitutes in cooking and baking 188

PART 4: EMBRACING WHOLE HEALTH
AND HAPPINESS 189

CHAPTER 13: **Eating for Health and Happiness** 191
Eating a Rainbow of Fruits and Vegetables .191
Loading Up on Whole Grains. 193
    Identifying best-bet grains 193
    Increasing your options and trying new grains. 194
Leaning Toward Leaner Proteins 194
    Choosing the healthiest options 195
    Fishing for reasons to eat more seafood. 196
    Vegging out with meatless proteins 197

Daring to Do Dairy 197
    Watching the fat content 198
    Packing in more protein 198
    Boning up on calcium 198
    Checking out nondairy substitutes 199
Focusing on Healthy Fats 200
Having Diabetes and Dessert, Too 201
    Making your own treats 201
    Dressing up healthy fruits 202
    Enjoying dessert while controlling the carbs 202
Trying Cooking and Serving Tips that Support Health
and Weight Goals 203
    Opting for lower-fat cooking methods 204
    Controlling portion sizes 205

CHAPTER 14: **Reaping the Rewards of Fitness** 207
Exercising Safely 208
    Getting the green light from your doctor 208
    Being prepared: What to keep handy .210
Encouraging Exercise for Everyone 211
    Developing an exercise plan 211
    Enjoying the benefits 214
    Being mindful of medical limitations .215
Clarifying What's Going On Behind the Scenes
When You Exercise 217
    Controlling blood glucose: How hormones are supposed
    to do it automatically 217
    Identifying how diabetes alters fuel use 218
    Sustaining exercise by tapping into fuels 219
    Understanding hypoglycemia 219
Exercising with Type 1: Staying Safe While Having Fun 220
    Monitoring matters 221
    Fueling up or dialing down: Fine-tuning carbs and insulin 221
    Knowing when to postpone activity: Too high or too low,
    don't go 223
Exercising with Type 2: Why It's Right for You 223
    Improving glycemic control 224
    Reducing cardiovascular risks 224
    Supporting weight-control efforts 225

CHAPTER 15: **Getting a Handle on Hypoglycemia** 227
Understanding Hypoglycemia 228
    Defining a low blood-glucose level 229
    Identifying causes of hypoglycemia 229
    Recognizing the symptoms of hypoglycemia 235
    Losing symptoms of lows: Hypoglycemia unawareness 236

Treating Hypoglycemia 237
    Choosing quick-acting carbs 237
    Taking the right amount of carb 237
    Rechecking your blood-glucose level 239
    Watching out for rebounds 240
    Requiring assistance: Severe lows and glucagon 240
Strategizing for Common Hypoglycemia Scenarios 242
    Managing mealtime lows 242
    Sleeping safely after a bedtime low 244
    Considering insulin action when treating hypoglycemia 244
Preventing Hypoglycemia 246
    Being prepared 246
    Looking for patterns and problem-solving 246
    Reflecting on prior exercise 247
    Remembering your carb intake 247
Enlisting Your Doctor's Help 247
    Keeping and reviewing blood-glucose logs 248
    Sharing your data with your doctor 249

CHAPTER 16: **Keeping the Beat with a Healthy Heart** 251
Eating Smart for Your Heart 251
    Getting the facts on cholesterol and fats .252
    Acquainting yourself with types of fats 253
    Choosing fats wisely 254
    Adding soluble fiber to your healthy heart regimen 257
    Creating a heart-healthy grocery list 258
    Cooking your foods the heart-healthy way 259
Handling the (Blood) Pressure 260
    Taking a look at the DASH diet 260
    Shaking the salt habit and opting for alternate seasonings 261
    Identifying hidden sodium suspects 262
    Deciphering label claims related to sodium 263
Embracing Heart-Healthy Habits 263
    Managing stress 264
    Avoiding tobacco and secondhand smoke 264
    Staying active 264
    Controlling weight 265

CHAPTER 17: **Living with Diabetes throughout the Life Cycle** 267
Raising a Child with Diabetes 267
    Beginning with basic pointers 268
    Addressing type 2 diabetes in youth 271

Managing Diabetes in Pregnancy 273
    Planning for pregnancy when you have type 1 or
    type 2 diabetes. 273
    Developing gestational diabetes. 274
    Understanding blood-glucose targets and fluctuations
    in pregnancy. 275
    Employing eating tips for diabetes during pregnancy 277
Keeping the Golden Years Golden When You Have Diabetes 279
    Evaluating seniors' dietary concerns 279
    Keeping physically fit. 281

**CHAPTER 18: Going Gluten-Free (Or Not): Does the
Batter Matter?** 283
Weighing In on the Gluten-Free Debate: Fad or Fact? 284
    Avoiding gluten fastidiously when you have celiac disease 284
    Forgoing gluten if you are allergic or have an intolerance 286
    Choosing to go gluten-free for personal reasons. 287
Against the Grain: Beginning a Gluten-Free Diet 288
    Avoiding grains that contain gluten 288
    Eliminating gluten-containing foods. 290
    Finding hidden gluten. 291
    Avoiding cross-contamination. 292
Staying Gluten-Free Without Nutrient Deficiencies 293
    Embracing foods naturally free of gluten 293
    Incorporating gluten-free grains. 294
    Watching out for nutrient deficiencies. .295

**PART 5: SAMPLING MENUS COMPLETE
WITH CARB COUNTS** 297

CHAPTER 19: Beginning with Breakfast Menus 299
Starting Your Day Right with Breakfast 299
Personalizing Your Breakfast Meal Plan 303

CHAPTER 20: Looking for Lunch Menus 305
Loving Your Lunch Options 305
Personalizing Your Lunch Meal Plan. 310

CHAPTER 21: Delving into Dinner Menus 313
Determining What's for Dinner 313
Personalizing Your Dinner Meal Plan. 317

CHAPTER 22: Surveying Snack Ideas 319
Choosing Carb-Controlled Snacks. 320
Picking Packaged Snacks 325

PART 6: THE PART OF TENS 327

CHAPTER 23: Ten Tips for Monitoring Your Blood Glucose 329
Picking a Meter for Your Needs...............................329
Safely Obtaining a Blood Sample 330
Acknowledging Error Issues...................................331
Assuring as Much Accuracy as Possible 331
Disposing of Lancets and Needles Properly 332
Varying Your Test Times.....................................332
Knowing Your Blood-Glucose Targets 333
Keeping a Log and Reviewing Your Data 333
Getting Your A1C Done Regularly 334
Considering Continuous Glucose Monitoring...................336

CHAPTER 24: Ten Tips for Controlling Carbs 337
Saving a Step with a Measuring Cup..........................337
Weighing Fruits in Advance 338
Having a Carb-Counting Contest..............................339
Making Better Breakfast Choices 339
Packing Your Own Lunch 340
Choosing Wisely at the Deli 340
Considering the Condiments..................................341
Fitting in a Favorite Dessert 341
Planning and Portioning Snacks 342
Curbing Late-Night Snacking 342

CHAPTER 25: Ten Worthwhile Websites to Help You Manage Diabetes 343
American Diabetes Association...............................343
American Association of Diabetes Educators 344
Academy of Nutrition and Dietetics 344
U.S. Food and Drug Administration 345
American Heart Association..................................345
UCSF Diabetes Education Online 346
Mayo Clinic...346
Joslin Diabetes Center......................................346
U.S. Department of Agriculture Food Composition Databases 347
WebMD 347

PART 7: APPENDIXES 349

APPENDIX A: **Diabetes Exchange Lists** 351

Starches 352
Fruits 354
Milk and Yogurt 356
Nonstarchy Vegetables 357
Meats and Meat Substitutes 358
    Lean meats and meat substitutes 359
    Medium-fat meats and meat substitutes 360
    High-fat meats and meat substitutes 360
Fats 361
Free Foods 363

APPENDIX B: **Conversion Guide** 365

Index 367

Introduction

O nce upon a time, the diet advice for people with diabetes was fairly concise, and it went something like this — "Don't eat sugar!" Well, guess what? That strategy didn't seem to cure anybody. Strike one. Next up was an attempt at the one-size-fits-all, handy-dandy, pre-printed tear-off diet sheet that directed you to follow your 1,800-calorie diabetes diet plan (or whatever calorie level you were assigned to). Not that many people were thrilled with being told to eat the exact same tedious diet pattern day after day for the rest of their lives. Strike two. Most recently, health experts have come to the conclusion that dietary interventions for people with diabetes should be individualized. That's a home run, finally!

From here on out, when I use the word "diet" I'm referring to your overall food choices and pattern of eating. I don't mean diet in terms of a temporary fix or in the sense of dieting for weight loss (although that can be built into the plan). When I say "diet," I'm referring to the way you eat or aim to eat most of the time.

The management of diabetes has a dietary component. What you eat, how much, and when you eat it directly affects your blood glucose and overall health. Diabetes and diet principles are inseparable. Now throw in a few more variables such as exercise, stress, body weight, concurrent health problems, and medications. It isn't uncommon to feel like you're a juggler trying to keep six balls in the air without ever slipping up. If you can relax and focus on one variable at a time, diabetes self-management becomes doable. Instead of thinking about juggling, imagine that each aspect of diabetes management is a piece of a larger puzzle. *Diabetes & Carb Counting For Dummies* is designed to help you put those pieces together.

The current diabetes trend lines are alarming. It's impossible to keep up with the statistics because they change so fast, but the 2016 tally has the count at 29 million Americans with diabetes and 86 million more with prediabetes. That's one out of every three American adults on the path to diabetes — unless action is taken. Studies conclusively show that diet and exercise are the most effective strategies for slowing or reversing that trend. I'm writing this book to reach as many people with diabetes and prediabetes as possible. This book provides an overview on diabetes and looks at dietary strategies and diabetes self-management principles. The nutrition information is geared for overall health; in other words, even people without diabetes will find worthwhile content.

About This Book

It's impossible to approach diabetes management without focusing on food. Finding out more about diet, especially carbohydrates, gets to the very core of diabetes treatment. Sure, medications are important, but you can't just slap on a medication and ignore diet because you can out-eat any medication. Managing your diet doesn't have to mean giving up all of your favorite foods. On the contrary, you should be able to eat most foods. It's a matter of balancing carbohydrate intake with exercise and medications (if you take them). While there is room for individual preference, the diet you choose to follow should support overall health, provide a variety of nutrient-dense foods in appropriate portions to promote a healthy body weight, and assist in reaching treatment targets for blood glucose, lipids, and blood pressure.

This book has a focus on understanding and managing carbohydrate, but it addresses all aspects of diet with diabetes. As each topic is covered:

>> You're provided with clear, understandable information that thoroughly explains each concept.

>> You know why the recommendations are being made and what the payoffs are.

>> You're made aware of potential consequences should you opt out of the advice.

Diabetes self-management takes some effort, but you're worth it. Taking care of your diabetes improves health and reduces risks. The rewards may be a little less tangible than saving up for a flat-screen TV, but health and quality of life are far more important than material things. Remember: *The best things in life aren't "things" at all.*

A few more comments and clarifications about this book:

>> I've chosen to use the term *blood glucose* because glucose is the type of sugar streaming through your blood vessels, but it is equally acceptable to call it *blood sugar*. In the United States, blood glucose is measured in milligrams per deciliter (mg/dl). If you're accustomed to millimoles per liter (mmol/L), simply divide mg/dl by 18.

>> Occasionally, I include sidebars, shown in shaded boxes. Some, but not all, of the sidebars provide personal stories that uncover solutions to common diabetes management issues. Feel free to skip sidebars or anything with the Technical Stuff icon, which highlights information that's interesting but not essential to understanding carb counting and diabetes.

>> Diabetes doesn't define you, so you will never hear me call you a diabetic. You are a person who has been dealt the diabetes card, but the deck is not stacked against you. Play your cards wisely and chances are you'll have a winning hand.

>> Within this book, you may note that some web addresses break across two lines of text. If you're reading this book in print and want to visit one of these web pages, simply key in the web address exactly as it's noted in the text, pretending as though the line break doesn't exist. If you're reading this as an e-book, you've got it easy — just click the web address to be taken directly to the web page.

Foolish Assumptions

When planning the content for this book, I thought critically about who my potential readers would be. I assumed there would be diversity because, for starters, there's more than one kind of diabetes. Additionally, many people with diabetes are simultaneously trying to manage weight, cholesterol, or blood pressure.

I've made the following assumptions about who you might be:

>> You have diabetes: type 1 diabetes, type 2 diabetes, or any other form of glucose dysregulation. You may have been recently diagnosed or you may have had diabetes for years (or decades) and are looking for up-to-date, accurate, and tangible information.

>> You've heard that diet, weight control, and exercise are foundational strategies for managing diabetes or preventing prediabetes from progressing to type 2.

>> You may have developed gestational diabetes or be a woman with pre-existing type 1 or type 2 diabetes who is committed to having a safe pregnancy and a healthy baby.

>> You may be a parent of a child with diabetes or have a family member or other loved one with diabetes, and you want to know how you can help.

Icons Used in This Book

The four icons used throughout this book identify different kinds of information.

TIP

A tip may save you time, simplify a concept, improve health, or present you with your "aha" moment of the day.

This icon identifies essential information, a take-home message worth sharing with family and friends. This symbol also identifies concepts that you should discuss further with your healthcare provider, such as medication dosing adjustments.

Don't skim over or ignore any warnings. This icon is there to protect you from harm.

Text marked with this icon provides details that are not essential to the book's main theme — for example, an interesting scientific explanation, background details on a study, or information pertaining to a subset of readers who use medical devices.

Beyond the Book

In addition to the content in this book, you can access free companion materials online. Simply navigate to www.dummies.com and search for "Diabetes & Carb Counting For Dummies Cheat Sheet." From there you'll be able to read or print several useful articles about choosing carbs wisely, making better food choices, and more.

Where to Go from Here

Please feel free to read this book's chapters in any order. *For Dummies* books are not linear, meaning content doesn't build sequentially. Each chapter develops a core concept and provides usable information that stands alone yet ultimately dovetails with other pieces of the diabetes puzzle. Review the table of contents and see whether any particular chapter is calling your name.

If you aren't sure where to begin, Chapter 1 provides a glimpse of the key content in the book and directs you to the appropriate chapters where you can find more details on each topic. Chapter 2 is a great place to get an overview on diabetes.

Be sure to read Chapter 4 sooner rather than later. Chapter 4 has concepts and illustrations that are integral to much of the rest of this book. It explains what happens to food after you eat it — how the body processes carbohydrates and then uses, stores, and even creates glucose. It also explains what happens when glucose levels rise too high or fall too low.

1

Getting Started with Carb Counting and Diabetes Management

Understand how diet and diabetes are intimately connected.

Explore why glucose is essential to fuel the brain and body.

Find out how much carb you really need and discover how to balance carb intake with medication doses.

Get a handle on how your food choices affect blood-glucose response.

Take note of the nutrients in carbohydrate foods.

Build your diabetes team and embrace your role in self-care.

Chapter **1**

Delving into Diabetes and Carb Counting

D iabetes is a disorder that is largely *self-managed.* You are the one making the daily decisions that affect your health outcomes. That's a significant responsibility! The thought of taking on diabetes may seem overwhelming, but you can do it.

There's a learning curve, of course. Being successful at any skill, sport, task, or job takes effort, training, patience, and support. Think about a preschool child who picks up his parent's paperback novel and stares blankly at the foreign squiggles on the page, wondering how anyone could possibly read it. We've each been that child and faced that same challenge. We still encounter words that we don't recognize from time to time, but we can look them up.

Learning about diabetes is similar. First you tackle the basics, and then you build on that foundation. Learning to manage your own diabetes requires diabetes self-management education. This book is designed to be your companion text in the learning process. The goal is to build knowledge (especially about counting carbs) and foster the skills needed for successful self-management. This chapter introduces you to the world of diabetes and carb counting.

Getting Up to Speed on Diabetes Basics

Diabetes is a condition of abnormal blood-glucose regulation. Lack of insulin (type 1 diabetes) or ineffective insulin (type 2 diabetes) both lead to elevated blood-glucose levels and a diagnosis of diabetes.

Diabetes and diet are intimately intertwined. It's impossible to talk about managing diabetes without discussing food in great detail. Blood-glucose levels are influenced by what you eat, how much you eat, and when you eat. The goal is to eat healthy foods, properly portioned, at appropriate times. The following sections introduce the basics of managing diabetes.

Checking out concerning trends in the diabetes epidemic

Nearly 30 million Americans are living with diabetes. Type 2 diabetes accounts for roughly 95 percent of cases. Over 86 million American adults have *prediabetes,* a condition where blood-glucose levels are above normal but not yet high enough to be classified as diabetes.

The best way to turn that trend around is to improve dietary choices, lose weight if you are overweight, and exercise regularly. Prediabetes can progress to type 2 diabetes, but lifestyle changes cut the risk by up to 58 percent. If you already have diabetes, eating right and exercising comprise the foundation of treatment.

Improving outcomes and preventing complications

I don't plan to list scary statistics on how many people with diabetes have developed complications. Fear isn't a good motivator. Hope is. In this book, I focus on how to better manage diabetes to help prevent complications. Keep in mind that when people developed diabetes many years ago, they simply did not have the resources, knowledge, tools, medications, and technologies needed to adequately manage their disease. Those tools are available now: blood-glucose monitors, insulin and other medications, insulin-delivery options, and knowledge. The roles of diet and exercise in managing diabetes are understood. Multiple studies from around the globe provide a hopeful message, which is taking care of your diabetes has a big payoff: your improved health.

WARNING

While the onset of type 1 diabetes is more obvious, type 2 diabetes can go undiagnosed for many years. Screening is critically important and may alert you to your risk long before diabetes develops. Chapter 2 sorts through the types of diabetes, delineates risk factors, and explains diagnostic criteria.

You should take diabetes seriously. Uncontrolled diabetes may lead to complications. For example, elevated blood-glucose levels over time can damage blood vessels and tissues. People with diabetes are twice as likely to suffer a heart attack or stroke. Your eyes, kidneys, feet, and nerves are all vulnerable to the damages inflicted by persistently elevated glucose levels.

REMEMBER

If you currently have complications, talk to your diabetes specialist for appropriate treatment. Request a referral to a registered dietitian if treating your complication has a dietary component. Two examples: Kidney disease may impose restrictions on dietary sodium, potassium, phosphorus, fluid, and possibly protein. Treating *gastroparesis* (nerve damage that alters the digestive system) involves dietary modifications to improve digestion and absorption of food. When diet becomes part of the treatment for a disease, it's referred to as *medical nutrition therapy*. A registered dietitian is a trained medical professional who can help you learn to make dietary changes that support the treatment of diabetes, heart disease, lipid problems, hypertension, and more.

TECHNICAL STUFF

A landmark study called the Diabetes Control and Complication Trial (DCCT 1983–1993) followed 1,441 people with type 1 diabetes for ten years. Results showed definitively that *improving blood-glucose control reduces the risks of developing complications.* The results were astounding: 76 percent reduction in eye disease, 50 percent reduction in kidney disease, and 60 percent reduction in nerve disease. The United Kingdom Prospective Diabetes Study (UKPDS 1977–1997) focused on people with type 2 diabetes. With 5,102 study participants, it was shown conclusively that both *blood-glucose control* and *blood-pressure control* are important in reducing complications.

Building your diabetes team

Your diabetes team starts with you. You are the team captain, and you get to pick who will be there to assist you on your diabetes management journey:

>> Your primary care provider manages your overall healthcare needs. Look for one who has experience with diabetes.

>> If you have type 1 diabetes or your type 2 diabetes is not under adequate control, your general practitioner may refer you to an endocrinologist, a doctor who specializes in diabetes.

>> You may also benefit from the expertise of a diabetes nurse educator (RN or NP), who can teach you how to monitor your glucose levels, keep and review blood-glucose records, properly administer insulin, handle travel and sick days, and more. In addition, a registered dietitian (RD or RDN) can help you plan balanced meals, teach you to read Nutrition Facts labels and count carbs, and provide dietary advice to help you achieve weight goals, manage blood pressure, improve cardiovascular health, understand the impact of alcohol, treat hypoglycemia, and more.

>> A certified diabetes educator (CDE) is a healthcare provider who has advanced training in diabetes management and has passed a comprehensive national exam. To maintain the CDE status, the healthcare professional must complete 75 hours of continuing education in the field of diabetes every five years.

>> Also on the roster to join your team are an eye doctor (either an ophthalmologist or an optometrist), a dentist, and a pharmacist.

>> At times you may choose to see a mental-health specialist: a counselor, social worker, psychologist, or psychiatrist.

>> Should you need them, a podiatrist is available for foot care and an exercise physiologist or physical therapist can guide your physical fitness plan.

REMEMBER

>> Don't forget your loved ones, family, and friends. Enlist the support and help of the important people in your life. People want to help; just let them know how best to assist you.

Staying up to date with advances in diabetes care

Diabetes specialists (like those listed in the preceding section) stay up to date on the latest advancements in the field of diabetes. Capitalize on their knowledge; stay up to date with your medical appointments and healthcare screenings. Having a few reputable diabetes management books (like this one!) on your home bookshelf is also helpful. Read and reread the sections most pertinent to you.

TIP

Keep in mind that not everything you read online is factual. Chapter 25 links you to reputable websites for gathering sound information.

Examining the Carb-Glucose Connection

This book offers in-depth info about the nutrients in food and how nutrients are used in the body. Carbohydrates, proteins, and fats are *macronutrients*. We need them in relatively large amounts as compared to *micronutrients*, such as vitamins and minerals, which are required in smaller amounts. Here's what they do:

>> Carbohydrates provide glucose, the body's primary fuel.

>> Proteins contribute amino acids for building and repairing tissues and cells.

>> Fats provide fatty acids, assist in the absorption of fat-soluble vitamins and, along with glucose, are used for energy.

>> Vitamins and minerals are essential nutrients required for hundreds of jobs throughout the body. To obtain the full complement of vitamins and minerals needed for health, choose a wide variety of wholesome foods.

Chapter 4 focuses on carbohydrates because carbs have the most profound effect on blood glucose, also known as blood sugar. There, you get a behind-the-scenes tour of carbs' journey through the body. You find out how carbohydrate foods are digested, turn into glucose, and are absorbed into the bloodstream. You also track the glucose through the system and discover why insulin, "the key to the cell," is required for proper fuel usage.

Glucose is so critical for human function that the body stockpiles glucose in the muscles and the liver. The storage form of glucose is *glycogen*. Glycogen reserves can be tapped into when the body is running low on glucose. If glycogen reserves become depleted, the liver will make glucose from scratch (but it may cost you a little muscle tissue . . . because you can't make something from nothing).

Diabetes interrupts the delicate balance of glucose regulation. Managing dietary carbohydrate intake is one of the most important lessons when learning to self-manage your diabetes. It's not only the amount and timing of the carbohydrate (see Chapters 6 and 8); it's also the quality of the carbohydrate and what it's mixed with (see Chapters 10, 11, and 12). In the bigger picture, carbs must be balanced with medications and exercise. Table 1-1 lists the most significant variables affecting blood-glucose levels for people with diabetes.

TABLE 1-1   **Variables Affecting Blood-Glucose Regulation**

Hyperglycemia (High Glucose Levels)	Hypoglycemia (Low Glucose Levels)
Too much carbohydrate	Not enough carbohydrate
Concentrated sweets, soda, juice	Alcohol
Mismatched timing of meds and meals	Mismatched timing of meds and meals
Illness, stress, hormonal surges	Skipping a meal
Lack of insulin or insulin resistance	Too much insulin or too many diabetes pills
Medication dosing errors	Medication dosing errors
Lack of physical activity	Strenuous or unplanned activity
Certain medications, steroids	Certain medications

REMEMBER

Diabetes imposes the need to understand how to juggle carbs, exercise, and medications, but it can be done, as you find out in Chapters 6 and 14. No one has perfect blood-glucose control, so set realistic expectations. Use a blood-glucose monitor (see Chapter 23) and have A1C levels checked regularly. You and your healthcare team can use glucose data to make adjustments to your self-care regimen. If your medications put you at risk for low blood glucose, find out more about preventing, recognizing, and treating hypoglycemia in Chapter 15.

Nutritional needs and diabetes management strategies change and evolve through all ages and stages of life. Chapter 17 provides specific tips for managing diabetes in childhood, during pregnancy, and into the golden years.

Getting Acquainted with Carbs

Carbs have been getting a bad rap lately. Many people are swept up in the notion that carbs are fattening or carbs are bad. Perhaps the pendulum has swung too far, causing some diets to be too low in carbs and excessive in protein or fat. The human body has basic needs, and glucose is one of them. Carbohydrates provide glucose, which is the preferred fuel source for the brain, nervous system, and muscles. For the sake of your health, it's important to find a happy medium . . . a little carb equilibrium.

What all carbs have in common is their chemical make-up. Simple carbohydrates and complex carbohydrates are made out of the same basic building blocks: sugar molecules. Chapter 3 boils it down into super simple chemistry concepts; a preview is just ahead. In this section I also talk about the nutrients in carbs and other food groups.

Carbohydrate foods do more than just contribute simple or complex carbs; they provide vitamins, minerals, and good taste too!

Introducing the so-called simple carbs

Imagine a pile of Legos. Lego blocks can exist separately or be snapped together in pairs. Those would represent the "simple" carbohydrates, which are single or double sugar molecules. The sugars in fruit are single sugars, while lactose, the sugar in milk, is a double sugar molecule. White sugar, brown sugar, honey, and syrups are simple carbohydrates too, but they don't offer the same health benefits as fruit, milk, and yogurt. Spoon for spoon, most sugars and syrups have similar amounts of carb. Agave nectar is a natural carb-containing sweetener that has less impact on blood-glucose levels if used in moderation.

Desserts that contain sugar alcohol can claim to be "sugar free," but they typically have as many carbs and calories as their sugar-containing counterparts. Chapter 12 sorts through the many sugars and alternative sweetening agents, and separates fact from fiction when it comes to carb-free sugar substitutes.

Catching up on complex carbs

Consider again the Lego analogy introduced in the preceding section. If you connect many Lego pieces together, you can build complicated structures. The same thing is true of starches; starches are complex carbs that are made out of many sugar molecules. Fiber is also considered a complex carb, but it doesn't digest. Chapters 3 and 16 fill you in further on fiber facts.

Noting the nutrition in carb food groups

Carbohydrates are found in many healthy, nutrient-packed foods, including grains, legumes, whole-grain breads, starches, milk, yogurt, fruits, and vegetables. Beware of sweets and desserts, though. They are usually high in sugar (and oftentimes fat) and don't offer much in terms of nutrition. Desserts and processed snack foods can contribute to weight gain and health problems if eaten in excess. Chapter 13 shows best-bet options in all food groups and even helps you figure out how to have a little dessert when you have diabetes; the key is moderation.

The term "carb" encompasses many foods, and not all carb foods are alike. Healthy carbs shouldn't be condemned like junk-food carbs. Guilt by association isn't fair. Give carbs a break and enjoy wholesome carb-containing foods in appropriate portions. Chapter 5 reviews carb-intake targets and reflects on established dietary guidelines.

Fruit is packed with nutrition, but you can't ignore that it's a simple sugar and that too much of a good thing isn't good anymore. Fruits should be enjoyed in smaller serving sizes and one portion at a time. Chapter 11 specifically addresses fruit juice and sugary soft drinks and makes a convincing case against consuming your carbs in liquid form.

A balanced diet includes an appropriate amount of carbohydrate, protein, and fat and adequate intakes of all key vitamins and minerals. Some vitamins and minerals are found across a wide array of food choices, while other nutrients are unique to specific foods. Cutting out entire food groups cuts the nutrition in those groups. For example, vegetarians need to focus on getting adequate intakes of protein and iron. In addition, vegans must seek out vitamin B12 and calcium. When people try to avoid carbs, all kinds of nutrition red flags go up.

While focusing on carbohydrate is important, don't lose track of the overall quality of your diet. Learn to make choices that are good for your heart, weight, and health. Check out Chapter 13 for more information about eating for health and happiness.

Acknowledging that staying healthy isn't just about carbs

Diabetes requires that you control carbohydrates, but that isn't the whole story. Keeping healthy means eating smart for your weight and heart (see Chapter 16); learning to identify the perfect proteins and the heart-healthiest fats and oils (see Chapter 13); and putting together balanced meals (see Chapter 8 and Part 5). A balanced diet not only assures nutritional needs are met, but blood glucose is also easier to control when meals have appropriate amounts of carbohydrate, protein, and fat.

Physical fitness plays an essential role in overall health. While exercise is encouraged for everyone, there are diabetes-related considerations and safety tips to be aware of (check out Chapter 14).

Making the Case for Carb Counting: To Count or Not to Count?

Whether you loosely manage your carbs or strictly count them depends on your situation. Carb counting is the gold standard if you have type 1 diabetes, but people with type 2 diabetes also stand to benefit from knowing how to count carbs. Establishing carb budgets and adhering to those budgets is one method of managing blood-glucose levels while simultaneously controlling calories and managing weight.

Counting carbs with type 1 diabetes: An essential tool

When you count carbs accurately, you know exactly how much glucose is going to end up in your bloodstream. Insulin doses can be adjusted to cover that amount of carb. People with type 1 diabetes don't make any of their own insulin. If insulin doses are based on carbohydrate intakes, counting carbs as precisely as possible is really important. It takes a little extra time initially, but with experience it gets easier and quicker. Label reading and carb-counting fundamentals are covered in Chapters 7 and 8. See Chapter 9 to add Internet tools to your carb-counting tool chest. For a deeper understanding of the dietary variables that affect blood-glucose readings, check out Chapter 10, and to find out how to line up insulin timing with digestion timing, see Chapter 6.

Gaining tighter control over blood-glucose levels with type 2 diabetes

Type 2 diabetes is characterized by insulin resistance. The body has insulin, but the insulin doesn't work as well as it should. For better blood-glucose control, strive to spread carbohydrate intake between three meals and perhaps one or two small snacks per day. Chapter 22 offers snack ideas.

TIP

People who skip breakfast or lunch often end up eating too much in the evening. Big meals with lots of carbohydrate can derail glucose control. There are several ways to set portion limits. The plate model puts perspective on portioning and is a simple visual tool. The carb portioning and counting fundamentals covered in Chapter 8 aren't reserved for people on insulin. Carb counting is an option for anyone who wants to accurately control carb portions.

THE EFFECTS OF CARB COUNTING WITH TYPE 1 DIABETES

Coral took one unit of rapid-acting insulin for every 15 grams of carbohydrate. She hadn't been completely satisfied with the results. Sometimes her blood-glucose levels were higher or lower than expected. Upon close inspection we identified several issues:

- She was putting in effort but had gaps in her accuracy. She never counted the carbs in nonstarchy vegetables, such as green beans and broccoli. Coral was diagnosed at age 9, and at that time she didn't really eat many vegetables, so her diabetes team told her family that vegetables were "free."

- Another issue: No one had ever told her to subtract the fiber from the total carbohydrate when reading food labels. She's now 28 years old and eating lots of vegetables and whole grains. After nearly 20 years of diabetes, she felt a measuring cup wasn't needed. What she had been calling "one cup" of rice had gradually grown in size. She was easily having 1⅓ to 1½ cups, thinking it was just a cup. Inaccuracies in carb counting meant she wasn't getting the right doses of insulin.

After our visit she went home, implemented the tips, and returned for follow-up three months later. Her blood-glucose levels had improved and were more predictable, so she felt safer and more confident. We explored how to further hone accuracy with a food scale, and we identified apps and online resources to count the carbs in mixed dishes and ethnic foods.

Sticking with consistent carb counts when you're on set insulin doses

Do you check your blood-glucose level at mealtime and then refer to an insulin chart to determine what your dose should be? That insulin dosing method is called *sliding-scale insulin.* The dose goes up incrementally for higher blood-glucose readings. Some individuals are on *set insulin doses* at mealtimes. In other words, the dose of insulin is the same from one day to the next regardless of blood-glucose levels.

WARNING

The problem with sliding-scale insulin dosing and set insulin dosing is that they don't take into consideration what you are planning to eat. The carbs in the pending meal will determine how much more glucose enters the bloodstream. Consider a low-carb salad for lunch one day and a burrito the next day. The two meals contain very different amounts of carbohydrate, but sliding-scale or set insulin dosing doesn't take that carb variability into consideration. These insulin dosing plans require mealtime carb intakes to be consistent from one day to the next.

EXPLORING THE GLYCEMIC INDEX

The glycemic index (GI) is a tool to measure how individual foods are expected to impact blood-glucose levels. The basic concept may be used in addition to carb counting and other carb management strategies. It's true that not all carb foods affect blood glucose in the same manner, which is why pizza isn't used to treat hypoglycemia. Liquids move through the stomach quickly, so the sugars in juice and soda show up in the blood-stream in a matter of minutes. That's just what you need if you're trying to treat hypo-glycemia. Juice isn't what you need if blood-glucose levels are already running high.

Instead of deferring to a chart to choose from low, medium, or high GI foods, it pays to get to the bottom of why foods behave the way they do (check out Chapter 10). With a solid grasp of the concepts, you can make food choices work in your favor. For example, whole grains and legumes have fiber and a lower glycemic index than white refined grains and breads. Meals that contain fiber and balanced amounts of carbohydrate, protein, and fat produce a blunter blood-glucose rise and more stability in blood-glucose levels.

Establish mealtime carb targets (with the help of Chapters 5 and 6). You can vary your food choices daily but keep the carb amounts consistent. Sample menus for breakfast, lunch, and dinner with set carb amounts are found in Chapters 19, 20, and 21.

REMEMBER

Set insulin dosing and sliding-scale insulin dosing aren't ideal for type 1 diabetes but may suffice for some people with type 2 diabetes. Talk to your healthcare providers to determine a safe and effective insulin dosing plan for you.

Managing weight with carb counting and portion precision

Counting carbs and eating appropriate amounts at meals and snacks helps with weight control. When you adhere to budgeted amounts of carbs at mealtimes and snacks, you are automatically putting a cap on portion sizes for fruit, bread, grains, starches, cereals, milk, yogurt, sweets, and many other items. Controlling carb portions helps with blood-glucose control and weight management. Here are some pointers:

>> Use the Exchange Lists in Appendix A to choose lean proteins and limit mealtime protein portions to the size of the palm of your hand.

>> Choose lower-fat cooking methods and limit added fats.

>> Eat plenty of vegetables and salads.

REMEMBER

The benefits are cumulative. Controlling portions helps with weight loss; losing weight improves insulin action; better-working insulin improves blood-glucose control; and controlling diabetes and weight lowers your risk of heart disease! For more tips on eating smart for your weight and heart, see Chapter 16.

Regulating Carb Intakes

The human body relies on glucose to fuel many functions. The biggest user of this essential fuel is the brain. The minimum recommended intake for carbohydrate is 130 grams of carb per day, whether you are 1, 10, or 100 years old. Who says and why? The National Institutes of Health establish nutrient intake guidelines. The guidelines on carbohydrate intake assure adequacy for vital functions and baseline needs. Actual intake should be assessed individually, as discussed in the following sections.

Figuring out how much carb you need

Glucose is an important fuel for the human body. You can't live without it. The brain requires a steady supply of glucose around the clock and lifelong. Glucose is the preferred fuel source for muscles and other tissues. Foods supply glucose and other nutrients.

REMEMBER

Carbohydrate requirements depend on age, gender, height, weight, and level of physical activity. Use Chapter 5 to assess your body mass index (BMI) and weight status. Estimate your daily caloric needs. Choose a daily carbohydrate budget based on calorie goals and personal preference.

Timing your carb intake

There's something to be said about proper meal spacing. If meals are too close together, blood-glucose levels can climb. If meals are too far apart, appetite can overtake willpower and make portion control difficult. Going to bed on a full stomach can lead to elevated glucose levels overnight and into the next day. Try having dinner at least three hours before going to bed. Eat three main meals four to six hours apart. Tuck in a snack if needed to curb appetite or to supply energy for exercise. Determine how to divvy up the carbs among meals and snacks to regulate appetite and blood-glucose levels in Chapter 6.

Matching insulin timing to digestion timing takes a bit more finesse. It's critical to understand onset, peak, and duration profiles for the insulins you use. Chapter 6 reviews insulin action times. Chapter 10 looks at the variables that affect digestion timing. Some foods digest quickly (liquids, simple sugars, and refined grains), while others digest more slowly (whole grains, foods with fiber, and meals higher in protein and fat).

Counting Carbs Successfully

Make use of the many carb-counting resources available to you. The following sections introduce food labels, food lists, menus, brochures, apps, websites, and more.

Looking at the label lingo

Nutrition details are clearly marked on packaged foods. Look for the Nutrition Facts food label. First, identify the serving size. The calories, total carbohydrate, fiber, and everything else on the label refers to "one serving," not necessarily the whole package. Did you know that fiber isn't digestible so you can subtract it from the total carbohydrates to get a more accurate carb count?

Tune in to Chapter 7 to sharpen your supermarket savvy and find out all about food labels. You can even take a sneak peek at the new look; the food label is undergoing a makeover.

Gathering carb-counting resources

Some of the most nutritious foods are harvested, not manufactured. Don't let the lack of a label keep you from reaching for wholesome foods. You can still closely estimate carbohydrate counts in fruits, vegetables, legumes, and grains with food composition lists (see Chapter 8 and Appendix A). The Exchange List concept groups foods by macronutrient composition; the items on a list have similar amounts of carbohydrate, protein, and fat. Every item on the fruit list, for example, identifies a portion size that equals 15 grams of carbohydrate: A small apple or orange, 17 grapes, 1 cup of cantaloupe or raspberries, or ½ banana all provide the same amount of carbohydrate. Variety isn't only the spice of life; it's also a great way to assure you get a wide array of important nutrients.

Measuring cups are essential for accuracy. Cooking from scratch? No problem! Chapter 8 also walks you through figuring out how to calculate carbs in your homemade recipes. Add tools to your carb-counting tool chest by tapping into online resources (flip to Chapter 9).

Increasing carb-counting accuracy

With type 1 diabetes, insulin doses must be carefully matched to carbohydrate intakes. Once you've mastered carb counting 101 (food labels and carb-counting lists), you're ready for more advanced carb-counting strategies.

A food scale can verify exact carb counts on numerous foods, including fruits. By weighing foods occasionally, you'll hone your ability to accurately estimate carbs in the future. Chapter 8 provides a list identifying the number of grams of carb per ounce of fruit. Weighing nails the carb counts in baked potatoes or a chunk of French bread.

Apps and web-based food databases offer nutrition facts on ethnic foods and combination foods, including pizza and lasagna. Chapter 9 describes how to combine the technologies: your food scale and a food database or app. Weigh your food item — a tamale, for example — and then plug the weight of your tamale into the food database to get an exact carb count on the item you're about to eat. There is no need to do this for every food every time, but it sure helps to improve your ability to guestimate more accurately in the future.

Living Well with Diabetes: The Seven Pillars of Diabetes Management

Eating for health and happiness and reaping the rewards of fitness should be a lifelong commitment through all ages and stages of life. The following sections cover these and the other pillars of diabetes management.

REMEMBER

We are all responsible for what we think, what we say, and what we do.

Eating a healthy diet

Food should be a positive part of creating and maintaining health, and it should be something to enjoy and savor too! Chapter 13 provides pointers for choosing the foods that promote health and wellness: colorful fruits and vegetables, whole grains, legumes, nuts, lean proteins, fish, vegetarian protein alternatives, heart-healthy fats, and dairy foods (or nondairy substitutes).

REMEMBER

If you eat wholesome foods in appropriate portions, you'll have the right recipe for health. This book provides you with a deeper understanding of how food choices affect your diabetes, weight, blood pressure, cholesterol, and cardiovascular health.

If you have celiac disease or gluten intolerance, it's time to go gluten-free all the way. Chapter 18 provides details.

Staying fit with exercise

Exercise has long been recognized as a foundation therapy in the treatment of type 2 diabetes. If you have prediabetes, exercise coupled with moderate weight loss has been shown to prevent or delay the onset of type 2 diabetes.

Everyone can cash in on multiple health benefits related to physical fitness. Exercise helps with weight control, improves blood pressure and cholesterol, strengthens bones and improves circulation, relieves stress, and improves sleep. No one comes back from an exercise session saying, "I wish I hadn't done that!" On the contrary, most people feel better and actually think, "I'm so glad I did that! I'll have to do that more often!"

TIP

If you aren't currently engaged in regular exercise, start by building more activity into your usual day. Don't sit for hours on end. Get up and move around. You can decide whether you move for one minute or for ten minutes. The first step is simply taking the first step. Walk while talking on your mobile phone. Do leg lifts and use hand weights while watching television. Put on some music and dance in your living room. Join an exercise class or a water aerobics group. Chapter 14 can help you get off on the right foot with fitness. The chapter also provides guidelines for building a safe exercise regimen.

Taking your medication

REMEMBER

People with type 1 diabetes rely on insulin *for life.* Prior to 1921 when insulin was first discovered and made available for use, type 1 diabetes was a fatal disease. Insulin is essential for transporting glucose (fuel) into cells. Chapter 6 explains the importance of matching insulin doses with carbohydrate intakes. Take all insulin doses as prescribed. Insulin omission can lead to diabetic ketoacidosis, which is a potentially life-threatening condition. Look at the physiology behind the process in Chapter 4.

Insulin isn't just for treating type 1 diabetes; many people with type 2 diabetes use insulin to manage their diabetes. Type 2 diabetes is a state of insulin resistance and oftentimes a concurrent deficiency in insulin production. When diet and exercise fail to adequately control glucose levels, medications are required. There are several classes of diabetes medications. Some stimulate insulin production, while others improve the way insulin works. Medications can decrease the amount of glucose released by the liver, increase the amount of glucose excreted in the urine, or delay the digestion of glucose. Whether it takes one medication or multiple medications, the goal is blood-glucose control because that's how you prevent complications.

Some people struggle with medication adherence. It may be due to the number of medications prescribed or the dosing schedule. Pill caddies that separate morning and evening doses assist with remembering meds. Another reason for missing meds is simply a lack of perceived benefit. Many people with diabetes feel fine. Feeling good is important, but knowing your ABCs is important. That means know your **A**1C, **B**lood pressure, and **C**holesterol results. Those numbers are a window into what is happening in your body.

REMEMBER

There is no denying that well-controlled diabetes and cardiovascular health have big payoffs. If you wait until you feel bad before you decide to adhere to the medication regimen prescribed, you might wait too long. Discuss any side effects with your provider. Your doctor can decide whether a different dose or a different medication would be more appropriate.

Monitoring your blood-glucose levels

Home blood-glucose monitors are amazing little machines. Apply a tiny droplet of blood, and within five seconds, you know the result. Glucose meters have been available for home use only since the 1980s. In the scope of things, that's a relatively short period of time. Prior to glucose monitoring, people with diabetes checked their urine glucose levels, which was a grossly inaccurate way to attempt to evaluate blood-glucose levels. Back in the diabetes "dark ages," people didn't have the tools and technologies to safely manage diabetes, so some people developed complications.

REMEMBER

Monitoring your blood glucose and knowing how to respond to those numbers can greatly reduce the risks of diabetes-related complications. Ask your healthcare provider how often you should check and what your targets are. Keep records and share the results with your diabetes team. Diabetes management decisions are based on glucose results. When your numbers aren't in target ranges, don't get discouraged. There's no such thing as good numbers or bad numbers. All numbers are useful. Managing diabetes is somewhat like solving a puzzle; each and every piece of the puzzle is important.

Chapter 23 provides tips on glucose monitoring and takes a look at another glucose measurement, A1C, which provides information on your average glucose control for the previous three-month period.

Managing stress

Most people encounter stressful situations from time to time. Finding healthy ways to cope with stress before small problems fester, grow, and get out of hand is important. If stress goes unchecked, it can contribute to anxiety, low mood, a feeling of hopelessness, or depression. Chronic conditions such as diabetes can contribute to stress and may have an additive effect to life's other challenges. Talking about it helps. Confide in friends, family, support groups, and your diabetes healthcare team.

Physical activity is a wonderful outlet. Exercise increases natural chemicals that improve mood. Hobbies, arts, crafts, volunteer work, and faith-based gatherings are other positive ways to relieve pressure and boost mood. When you're feeling blue, think about some of your favorite people and your best memories. Keep the self-talk in your head positive. Don't focus on your shortcomings; recount your successes instead.

REMEMBER

If you can't shake the funk and the stress is preventing you from taking care of yourself, seek the help of a mental-health specialist.

Discovering how to problem-solve

Part of diabetes self-management is understanding how to assess a situation and decide the best course of action. Understanding cause and effect allows you to make adjustments to steer outcomes in the direction you desire. When something goes awry, reflect carefully on the chain of events that led up to the issue. If you can decipher the cause, you can formulate a solution. Over time you gain experience, which makes it easier to predict outcomes and make adjustments to your diabetes care. Your diabetes team can help you learn how to make informed decisions. There will still be things that happen unexpectedly from time to time because that's just how life is. You can't plan for all scenarios, but you can be prepared for most.

REMEMBER

Problem-solving means reflecting and trying to figure out why things didn't go as planned. Formulate a new plan or make adjustments to the old plan. Execute your plan, pay attention, and see whether things improve.

Reducing risk with healthy behaviors and regular medical checkups

Taking care of your diabetes is an investment in your future health and quality of life. Diabetes complications are preventable. Follow these guidelines:

>> Eat right and exercise.

>> Don't smoke. Smokers are more likely to develop serious diabetes-related complications.

>> Limit alcohol. Alcohol can cause profound hypoglycemia for some people with diabetes (see Chapter 11).

>> Stay up to date on medical visits and health screenings.

>> Get a handle on hypertension. High blood pressure increases the risk of health problems because it can damage small and large blood vessels.

>> Have the necessary bloodwork needed to monitor diabetes, heart health, and other medical conditions.

>> See your doctor regularly (every three months or as your doctor advises).

>> Get your flu shot and have your eyes and kidneys checked annually.

>> Keeping healthy will keep you happy, so show your smile to your dentist at least every six months.

Chapter **2**

Exploring the Diabetes-Carb Connection

Twenty-nine million Americans have diabetes. About 90–95 percent have type 2 diabetes, while 5–10 percent have type 1 diabetes. A couple other forms of diabetes make up a smaller percentage of cases. Eighty-six million American adults — over one-third of the population — have prediabetes, a condition of elevated glucose levels but not yet a diagnosis of diabetes.

If you rewind the clock by 50 to 100 years, diabetes was not nearly as prevalent as it is today. The societal trend is that Americans are now heavier and less active than our ancestors were a few generations ago. Being overweight and physically inactive are key risk factors for developing prediabetes and type 2 diabetes. It is now predicted that by the year 2050, one out of every three adults will have diabetes. It's time to turn those trend lines around.

The Centers for Disease Control and Prevention (CDC) say, "Obesity-related conditions including heart disease, stroke, and type 2 diabetes are among the leading causes of *preventable* death." Very convincing studies from all around the globe show that lifestyle interventions can delay or prevent diabetes. Those lifestyle interventions are also at the core of treating diabetes and are focused on improving dietary patterns, exercise habits, and weight management.

Diabetes can go undetected for many years, so screening is critically important. The CDC estimates that 25 percent of people with blood-glucose levels in the diabetes range remain undiagnosed, and an alarming 90 percent of people in the prediabetes range don't realize that their glucose levels are elevated. This chapter identifies the risk factors and potential symptoms of diabetes, the diagnostic and classification criteria, and where to go next if you're diagnosed.

Wrapping Your Brain around Diabetes and Related Conditions

We rely on foods to provide our bodies with energy, vitamins, minerals, and essential nutrients. On the most basic level, food and water are required for survival, but food is so much more than just a way to survive. We savor and enjoy food. We have cultural traditions, family recipes, and memories associated with food. Friends and relatives socialize around dinner tables and celebrate holidays and special occasions over meals.

When you're diagnosed with diabetes, the focus on food shifts, and the next thing you know you are being asked to read food labels and break out the measuring cups. Your vocabulary expands to include the words "pancreas," "insulin," "carbohydrate," and "blood glucose." The good news is diabetes is manageable, now more than ever before. The first step in successfully managing your diabetes is to understand how the body is supposed to work and what has gone awry if you've developed diabetes. The following sections cover these topics.

Seeing how the body is supposed to process carbs

Human bodies need fuel to function. Glucose is the primary fuel source for the brain and red blood cells. It is also the preferred fuel source for muscles. Carbohydrate-containing foods provide glucose through the process of digestion and absorption. Glucose travels throughout the body via the bloodstream to all awaiting organs, tissues, and cells. For more on that process, see Chapter 4.

When all systems are working properly, a hormone called *insulin* helps the glucose move from the bloodstream into the cells where it's burned for energy. The *pancreas* is the organ that makes and secretes insulin. Think of insulin as a "key" that has to unlock the cells to allow the glucose in. Insulin is supposed to bind to an insulin receptor on the surface of the cell. Once the insulin and the receptor are coupled, then the glucose may enter the cell. See Figure 2-1.

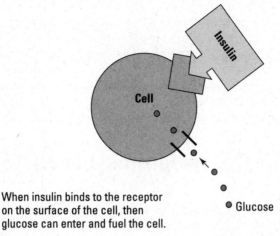

FIGURE 2-1:
Insulin allows
glucose to enter
the cell.

When insulin binds to the receptor
on the surface of the cell, then
glucose can enter and fuel the cell.

© John Wiley & Sons, Inc.

If you have diabetes, it means either you don't make enough insulin, or the insulin you make simply doesn't work effectively. The next section elaborates further.

Discovering what causes diabetes

The surface of the pancreas has insulin-producing cells called *beta-cells* or *islet cells.* In the case of type 1 diabetes, the beta-cells are destroyed so they are no longer able to produce insulin. Without insulin, glucose cannot properly nourish the body.

TECHNICAL STUFF

Prior to 1921 when insulin was first discovered, people with type 1 diabetes didn't survive very long. Initially insulin was harvested from cattle and pig pancreases and injected into humans. It wasn't perfect and it caused allergic reactions, but people lived. In the 1970s genetically "human" insulin was produced in the lab and became widely available. Fast forward to today: There are numerous types of insulin and advanced technologies for administering them. Researchers around the globe continue to make progress in leaps and bounds, and they likely won't stop until they find a cure.

Type 2 diabetes is a state of "insulin resistance." People with type 2 are able to make insulin, but the insulin isn't fully effective. It's similar to having a key made for your front door, but when you attempt to use it, you are frustrated to find out that it doesn't work smoothly. The key is there, the lock is there, but it takes persistence and jiggling and coaxing until finally the door opens. That's the case with type 2 diabetes. The insulin is there and the insulin receptor is there, but the cell isn't responding properly. Glucose uptake is delayed due to insulin resistance, so blood-glucose levels rise.

Insulin resistance precedes the onset of type 2 diabetes. Long before the diagnosis, the pancreas responds to rising blood-glucose levels by working harder to produce extra insulin. The pancreas works overtime because insulin levels have to rise higher than normal in order to manage glucose levels. Eventually the pancreas tires out and the beta-cells can no longer keep up the pace, so blood-glucose levels rise into diabetic ranges. (When glucose levels rise high enough, you may have symptoms, but not always. Symptoms are explained in the next section.)

Noticing the symptoms of diabetes

With insufficient amounts of insulin or insulin that doesn't work properly, glucose can't effectively get into the cells. Instead, the glucose accumulates in the bloodstream. Blood is filtered through the kidneys. Kidneys dispose of some of the excess glucose by removing it from the blood and dumping it into the urine. The bladder fills more quickly, which leads to frequent urination. Because the calories from glucose are flushed down the toilet, the cells aren't fed as much and weight loss may occur.

TECHNICAL STUFF

There's an interesting history behind the naming of the disease. The Greeks called it Diabetes Mellitus. *Diabetes* means "a siphon," which refers to the excessive urination associated with the disease. *Mellitus* means "like honey," which refers to the sweet smell and taste of the urine. Doctors in ancient Greece relied on their sense of taste and smell to make the diagnosis.

WARNING

Symptoms are associated with uncontrolled diabetes. However, some people are asymptomatic, so diabetes can brew undetected for many years. In fact, some people are diagnosed with diabetes *after* developing a complication associated with uncontrolled, long-duration diabetes. It is important to have standard screening protocols for those at risk. Identifying risk factors and screening criteria are addressed later in this chapter.

The common symptoms associated with elevated blood glucose include

>> **Increased urination:** This occurs because the kidneys are dumping some of the excess glucose into the urine.

>> **Thirst:** Frequent urination can lead to dehydration, which triggers thirst.

>> **Hunger:** The result is hunger as glucose is lost in the urine instead of being available to feed the cells and tissues. Additionally, when cells aren't fed, muscles and body fat break down to provide an alternate fuel source. The body can break itself down to feed itself, which can lead to weight loss.

>> **Additional symptoms:** These may include fatigue, blurred vision, tingling or numbness in feet and hands, yeast and fungal infections, and wounds that are slow to heal.

- When glucose isn't used properly, the body lacks its main energy supply, which may result in fatigue or weakness.

- Blurry vision is usually temporary. It's caused by glucose accumulating in the lens of the eye, which in turn causes fluid retention and swelling of the lens. Once glucose levels are controlled, the lens goes back to its usual shape and vision should improve.

TIP

  Do not buy a new pair of glasses when your blood glucose is out of control. The lens of the eye may be temporarily misshapen due to concentrated glucose levels, and that can alter vision. Your eye specialist should evaluate your baseline vision once your glucose levels have stabilized in the near normal range.

- Uncontrolled diabetes can lead to nerve damage. Peripheral neuropathy, which refers to the nerves farthest from the brain and spinal cord, can cause tingling, burning, pain, or numbness in the feet or hands.

- High blood glucose means more sugar is available for yeast and bacteria to thrive on, so infections can fester.

- Healing may be impaired because the body's immune system is compromised when glucose is out of control.

REMEMBER

The symptoms associated with diabetes are not diagnostic and are sometimes related to other medical conditions. Discuss all medical concerns with your healthcare providers. Diabetes screening protocols are based on risk factors including weight and age and are clarified later in the chapter.

Distinguishing the types of diabetes

There are several types of diabetes. The suggested treatment depends upon the type. The vast majority of people have type 2 diabetes. Some people with type 2 diabetes can achieve control through diet and exercise modifications, while others need to add one or more oral medications. Everyone with type 1 diabetes and some people with type 2 diabetes require insulin.

Type 1 diabetes

Type 1 diabetes is an autoimmune disease. The body's immune system, which is supposed to fight off bacteria, mistakenly destroys the insulin-producing beta-cells of the pancreas. People with type 1 diabetes no longer make insulin, so they must take insulin to live.

In the past this form of diabetes was called juvenile diabetes, insulin-dependent diabetes, or IDDM (short for insulin-dependent diabetes mellitus). The preferred term is type 1 diabetes, which may be abbreviated T1DM or T1D. The old terms don't hold true for all cases. Not all kids with diabetes have type 1; there are many adolescents with type 2 diabetes. Insulin is used to treat other forms of diabetes, not just type 1. While it is true that type 1 diabetes is most often diagnosed when a person is below the age of 20, some adults are diagnosed with type 1 diabetes in their 20s, 30s, 40s, and even later.

Blood tests can determine whether the diagnosis is type 1 diabetes by detecting autoimmune markers in the blood. Another lab test called *C-peptide* estimates the amount of insulin being produced. (Find out more about diagnosing diabetes later in this chapter.)

Type 2 diabetes

Type 2 diabetes is due to insulin resistance. People with type 2 diabetes make insulin, but the insulin doesn't work very well. Their own cells are *resistant* to the action of their insulin. Type 2 diabetes is due to a progressive insulin deficiency imposed on top of the initial insulin resistance.

Previously it was called adult-onset, non-insulin-dependent diabetes, or NIDDM (non-insulin-dependent diabetes mellitus). The current standard is to call it type 2 diabetes, which can be abbreviated T2DM or T2D. Unfortunately, type 2 diabetes often occurs alongside of high blood pressure and dyslipidemia (abnormal blood fats). A major shift must take place in the lifestyle of Americans to turn this trend around.

Prediabetes

Prediabetes is when blood-glucose levels are above normal but not yet in the range of diabetes. One in three American adults has blood-glucose levels in the prediabetes range. Up to 90 percent of them don't know it. Prediabetes can lead to type 2 diabetes within five to ten years. The good news is that studies clearly show that progressing to type 2 diabetes isn't inevitable. Weight loss of roughly 5–10 percent of starting weight coupled with moderate exercise of at least 150 minutes per week reduces the risk by up to 58 percent. Early detection and intervention may return blood-glucose levels to near normal ranges.

Gestational diabetes

Gestational diabetes is typically diagnosed in the second or third trimester of pregnancy. Pregnancy hormones interfere with the way insulin works by inducing a state of insulin resistance. As the pregnancy progresses, the mother's pancreas has to work harder to make enough insulin to keep blood-glucose levels controlled. Some women simply can't keep up with the demand, and they get diabetes during pregnancy, which resolves after delivery. Gestational diabetes is abbreviated as GDM (gestational diabetes mellitus). Women should be screened for GDM at 24 to 28 weeks of pregnancy. GDM also indicates a risk for developing type 2 diabetes in the future. (See Chapter 17 and the nearby sidebar "Diabetes and pregnancy" for more information.)

Other forms of diabetes

Other forms of diabetes make up only a small fraction of the cases of diabetes. These forms include the following:

>> **Neonatal diabetes** occurs within the first six months of life and can be transient or permanent. Genetic testing is needed to clarify the defect, because some babies are best treated with oral medications while others require insulin.

>> **Cystic fibrosis–related diabetes** (CFRD) can affect as many as half of the adults and 20 percent of the children who have cystic fibrosis. Insulin is the therapy of choice for CFRD.

>> **Maturity-onset diabetes of the young** (MODY) is inherited and caused by any number of different chromosomal mutations. Treatment depends upon the specific genetic defect, so testing is required to clarify the diagnosis.

DIABETES AND PREGNANCY

Diabetes during pregnancy is considered a high-risk pregnancy. It is imperative for women with type 1 and type 2 diabetes to have tightly controlled blood-glucose levels prior to becoming pregnant. Uncontrolled diabetes can have devastating consequences. When maternal glucose levels are elevated, the extra glucose readily passes to the baby and that can cause big problems. High blood glucose in the first trimester increases the risk of birth defects and miscarriage. Gestational diabetes doesn't develop until later in the pregnancy, so birth defects aren't a concern with GDM.

There are late-pregnancy risks that apply to women with type 1, type 2, and gestational diabetes. High glucose in the second half of the pregnancy can cause the baby to grow too big, which makes for a riskier delivery for both baby and mom. Uncontrolled glucose levels also increase the risk of preeclampsia and stillbirth. Stringent glucose control throughout the entire pregnancy is critical. Women with diabetes who are of childbearing age should have preconception counseling. Some medications are not safe for the baby and thus must be discontinued prior to conception, including meds used to treat hypertension and cholesterol. Have a discussion with your healthcare provider. For more information on managing diabetes during pregnancy, see Chapter 17.

Recognizing Diabetes Risk Factors and Getting Diagnosed

The onset of type 1 diabetes tends to be sudden and come as a complete surprise. Prediabetes and type 2 diabetes can go undetected for years. Early diagnosis and intervention improve outcomes. I address screening protocols and diagnostic testing in the following sections.

Type 1 diabetes risk factors

The risk factors for type 1 diabetes are still being researched but may include the following:

>> **Family history and genetics:** Caucasians have the highest risk of developing type 1 diabetes. The risk is increased if you have a parent, sibling, or child with type 1. If a mother has type 1 diabetes, her child has a 2–3 percent chance of developing it. If the father has type 1, the chance is a little higher: about 6–8 percent. If a child in the family has type 1 diabetes, the chance that a sibling will develop it is close to 4 percent. Family members can be screened with a lab test that identifies markers in the blood. Often, however, a person with type 1 diabetes has no relatives with the condition.

TECHNICAL
STUFF

TrialNet is a network of clinical centers dedicated to the study of type 1 diabetes. They have numerous ongoing clinical trials aimed at finding better ways to prevent, diagnose, and treat type 1 diabetes. If someone in the family has type 1 diabetes, then the parents, children, and siblings can be screened to see whether they have markers in the blood that indicate the risk of developing diabetes. For more information, visit www.diabetestrialnet.org.

>> **Geography:** Interestingly, the incidence of type 1 diabetes increases the farther you travel north away from the equator. Northern European countries have a high prevalence, with Finland being the highest. In general the colder climates have a higher prevalence of type 1 diabetes.

>> **Viral triggers:** Exposure to the following viral infections is being investigated: Epstein-Barr, Coxsackie, mumps, and cytomegalovirus. However, none have yet to be proved causal.

>> **Early infant feeding practices:** These factors are being explored to see whether what babies are fed matters; breastfeeding seems to decrease the risk of type 1.

Screening for T1DM in asymptomatic low-risk individuals is not cost-effective or recommended. If you have an immediate family member with T1DM, you can be screened for auto-antibodies. These markers in the blood indicate risk but do not mean that you will develop the disease.

Type 2 diabetes risk factors

Diabetes is often linked with other health issues in what is referred to as *metabolic syndrome.* Body fat accumulated around the waistline is linked to developing diabetes more so than having extra pounds in the hips and thighs. High blood pressure and lipid issues also seem to go hand in hand with type 2 diabetes.

REMEMBER

Many of the risk factors for developing diabetes are modifiable. Food choices and eating habits affect overall health. The right food choices can promote health and healing, while poor eating habits can hinder health and increase the risk of chronic diseases. Diabetes, weight, blood pressure, blood fats, and heart health all respond to improvements in eating habits.

The following risk factors are associated with developing type 2 diabetes and indicate the need for screening:

>> **Inheriting the risk:** Type 2 diabetes runs in families. Having the risk doesn't mean a certain diagnosis. Eating healthfully, controlling weight, and being more physically active can reduce the risk of developing diabetes. If you have diabetes, your children are at increased risk, so it's important to teach them healthy habits. All overweight children with risk factors associated with type 2 diabetes should be screened every three years starting at age 10 or puberty. Early detection and treatment improves outcomes.

>> **Being from a high-risk ethnic group:** Certain ethnicities have a stronger risk of developing type 2 diabetes: African Americans, American Indians, Pacific Islanders, Asian Americans, Hispanics, and Latinos. However, anyone can develop type 2 diabetes.

>> **Getting older:** Aging increases the risk of developing type 2 diabetes. Being above 45 years old is considered a risk factor and is the recommended age to begin screening. Having other risk factors means you should be screened earlier. If screening results are negative, you should be rescreened at least every three years.

>> **Being overweight:** Obesity tends to run in families. There is a genetic component to weight, but families also tend to share similar eating and exercise habits. Modest weight loss reduces the risk of developing diabetes; studies show that weight loss and exercise are the most effective strategies to prevent prediabetes from progressing to type 2.

>> **Living a sedentary lifestyle:** Exercise lowers the risk of developing diabetes in several ways. Exercise improves the way insulin works and how muscles burn glucose. Exercise reduces the risk of developing diabetes because it helps with weight management and preserves muscle mass. (See Chapter 14 for more about fitness.)

>> **Struggling with insulin resistance or impaired glucose tolerance:** If you've had borderline or high glucose levels at any point in your life, it may indicate an underlying issue with the way your insulin works.

>> **Having lipid issues:** People with diabetes may have high LDL (the bad cholesterol), but they most commonly have low HDL (the good cholesterol) and high triglycerides (blood fats).

>> **Battling high blood pressure:** Hypertension is a common co-morbidity. High blood pressure should be managed aggressively as it can increase the risk that a person with diabetes will develop long-term complications to blood vessels in the eyes, kidneys, and even the heart.

>> **Contending with cardiovascular disease:** If you have a history of cardiovascular disease, your risk of having diabetes increases.

>> **Being a woman under some circumstances:** Women who had gestational diabetes (GDM), delivered a baby that weighed over 9 pounds, or have polycystic ovarian syndrome (PCOS) are also at an increased risk of developing type 2 diabetes. Gestational diabetes indicates a struggle to manage blood glucose when faced with insulin resistance caused by pregnancy hormones. Future variables such as aging, weight gain, or inactivity could push you again into a situation where your insulin cannot keep up with the demand. PCOS has a component of insulin resistance.

>> **Having acanthosis nigricans:** Dark, thick patches that may occur on the back of the neck and in the armpits are called *acanthosis,* which is an indicator of insulin resistance.

REMEMBER

Anyone who is overweight and has one or more of the preceding risk factors associated with type 2 diabetes should be screened at a lab. If results come back normal, testing should be repeated at a minimum of every three years. All adults should begin screening at age 45 regardless of other risk factors because aging is a risk factor. Overweight children should begin screening at puberty or age 10.

Diagnosing diabetes

Diabetes is diagnosed using one or more of the three blood tests shown in Table 2-1.

>> Fasting blood glucose requires an eight-hour fast.

>> The oral glucose tolerance test (OGTT) test checks blood-glucose response two hours after drinking 75 grams of glucose.

>> The A1C test is reflective of a three-month average, so you do not need to be fasting to have this lab test.

TECHNICAL STUFF

The A1C test measures the amount of glucose attached to a specific protein known as *hemoglobin A protein,* located on the surfaces of red blood cells (RBCs). Glucose binds to proteins in a process known as glycosylation. A1C is reflective of glycosylation throughout the body, so it's also used to assess blood-glucose control and risk for complications. Glycosylation can damage delicate tissues such as the retina of the eye, nerves, kidneys, and blood vessels. See Chapter 23 for more on glucose monitoring and A1C.

If just one of the lab tests comes back abnormal it should be repeated to confirm the diagnosis. If two lab tests are done and both are abnormal, that confirms diagnosis.

TABLE 2-1 **Screening Tests and Diagnostic Criteria**

Screening Test	Normal	Prediabetes	Diabetes
Fasting blood glucose	Under 100	100–125	126 or more
Oral glucose tolerance test (OGTT)	Under 140	140–199	200 or more
A1C	Under 5.7	5.7–6.4	6.5 or more

The screening tests in Table 2-1 diagnose prediabetes and diabetes but don't differentiate between type 1 diabetes and type 2 diabetes. A definitive diagnosis of type 1 diabetes requires additional blood work to identify autoimmune markers.

Moving Forward with Managing Diabetes

Healthy lifestyle behaviors can prevent or delay the development of type 2 diabetes. If you already have diabetes (either type 1 or type 2), then nutrition and exercise are foundation management strategies. Blood–glucose control is essential because poorly controlled diabetes increases the risks of heart disease, stroke, and serious complications including blindness, cataracts, glaucoma, kidney damage, blood vessel and nerve damage, impotence, altered digestion, infections, and lower limb amputations.

Take a breath and listen to this important message: *Well-controlled diabetes is the leading cause of nothing!* That's right. Complications aren't an automatic inevitability. They are preventable. What you eat affects your health. You need to eat carbohydrates, but it is important to understand how to manage carbs in order to manage diabetes, and that's what this section and this book are all about.

Knowing that diet matters

Carbs are an important part of a balanced diet. This book focuses on learning to eat the right carbs, in the right amounts, at the right time. Diabetes management means controlling your blood-glucose levels, which ultimately requires knowing how to manage carb choices. It doesn't mean divorcing carbs.

Think about the big picture. Weight control, blood-pressure control, lipid control, and overall health and happiness are also influenced by dietary choices. That means paying attention to more than just the carbs. If you make the right food choices most of the time, you should see a payoff in terms of your health and quality of life. See Chapter 13 for more on healthy eating.

Keeping in touch with your diabetes team

Many variables affect diabetes control and outcomes. Managing diabetes is a bit like solving a puzzle. You have to figure out how diet, exercise, glucose monitoring, and medications all fit together. It's pretty tough to figure it all out on your own. Try the following:

>> Build your diabetes team. Ask your doctor to refer you to a diabetes self-management class or make appointments to see a nurse and a registered dietitian (RD or RDN). Choose professionals who are well-versed in diabetes management, such as Certified Diabetes Educators, if available.

   Note: The abbreviations RD (registered dietitian) and RDN (registered dietitian nutritionist) are synonymous and indicate a trained medical professional who is credentialed by the Commission on Dietetic Registration. RDs and RDNs have a college degree, have passed a stringent national exam, and participate in ongoing continuing education to maintain their credential. Be aware that anyone can call himself a *nutritionist* regardless of training or experience because that term isn't regulated.

>> Sometimes life just gets in the way and it's hard to prioritize diabetes self-management. If diabetes is altering your mood and you're feeling depressed or just plain "stuck," then you may benefit from counseling with a mental-health specialist familiar with the issues associated with chronic illness.

>> Keep in mind that diabetes management strategies may need to be tweaked along the way. Over time what used to work may no longer be effective. Things change. Have diabetes evaluations and tune-ups by meeting with your diabetes experts on a regular basis.

TIP

If you search for health information online, be sure to access reputable resources. See Chapter 25 for a list of worthwhile websites.

Embracing your central role in your own self-care

REMEMBER

You are the most important person in your healthcare team. In the course of a month, year, or lifetime, you spend only a small fraction of time face to face with the medical providers. Enlist the support of your family and friends, but ultimately remember that it is up to you to integrate diabetes management into your daily routine. Check your blood-glucose levels and know how to interpret the results. Let your medical providers know if your blood glucose isn't being well-controlled. Medication regimens may need to be adjusted or intensified with long-standing diabetes. Advocate for yourself. Don't settle for sub-optimal control. You are in it for the long haul, and you're worth it.

Chapter **3**

Calling All Carbs: Recognizing Carbs in the Foods You Eat

Managing diabetes hinges on managing carbs. The first step is being able to identify which foods have carbohydrate. Carbohydrate is considered a macronutrient, rather than a micronutrient:

» **Macronutrients:** Dietary components that are required in relatively large amounts are known as *macronutrients*. There are three main macronutrients in the foods we eat: carbohydrate, protein, and fat.

» **Micronutrients:** Vitamins and minerals are essential but needed in relatively small amounts, so they are considered *micronutrients*.

Macronutrients are measured in grams, and most micronutrients are measured in micrograms or milligrams. To put that in perspective, there are 1,000 micrograms in one milligram, and 1,000 milligrams in one gram. Carbs are counted in grams.

Each macronutrient group is important, but for different reasons. Carbohydrates, proteins, and fats have critical roles in human nutrition:

>> **Carbohydrates:** Carbs are the powerhouses; they provide energy in the form of glucose to the tissues, organs, and cells. Each gram of carbohydrate provides 4 calories of energy.

>> **Proteins:** Dietary proteins are made out of amino acids, which are the very building blocks that we use to create and repair cells, tissues, and muscles.

>> **Fats:** Fats are concentrated sources of energy and are needed to transport fat-soluble vitamins.

Most of the foods that we eat are a combination of macronutrients laced with various micronutrients. For example, meats contain both protein and fat. Legumes have both protein and carb. Even grains and vegetables have a little protein along with the carbs. This chapter identifies the key members in the family of carbohydrates and discusses the role of the noncarb counterparts.

Looking at the Chemical Structure of Carbohydrates

All carbohydrates have something in common: They are built out of sugar molecules. Sugar molecules can exist separately as single units, or they can join together in pairs to form double sugars. The scientific term for a single sugar is *monosaccharide.* The double-sugar units are known as *disaccharides.* Many sugar molecules can join together in long chains, and those are called *polysaccharides.* Starch and fiber are examples of polysaccharides.

Monosaccharides (single sugars) and disaccharides (double sugars) are also known as *simple carbohydrates.* Polysaccharides (many sugars linked together) are referred to as *complex carbohydrates.* See Figure 3-1 for a closer look at the chemical structure of carbohydrates. Note that both starch and fiber are considered polysaccharides (complex carbohydrates) made out of chains of glucose molecules. The key difference is that starches are digestible and fiber is not. Digestive enzymes in the intestine easily cut the bonds that link the glucose molecules in starch. The enzymes can't cut through the stronger bonds that link the glucose chains in fiber.

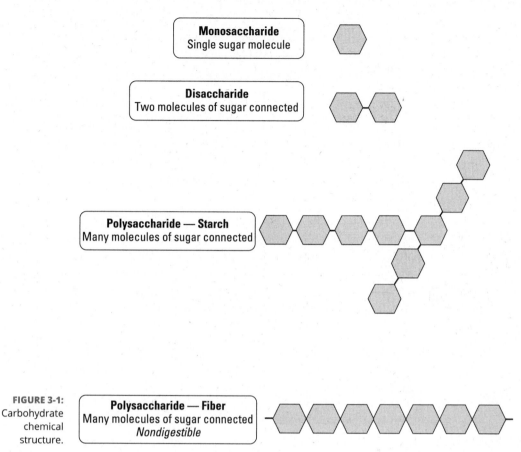

FIGURE 3-1:
Carbohydrate
chemical
structure.

A common question I hear is "If carbs digest and turn into glucose, why not skip the carbs and just eat proteins and fats?" The flaw with that approach is that we need the nutrients found in healthy carb foods. Health experts warn against over-consumption of artery-clogging saturated fats. Plant foods are naturally low in saturated fat, while animal foods (such as meats, cheese, and butter) often have significant amounts of saturated fat, depending on which cuts of meat you choose. Plant foods such as whole grains, fruits, and vegetables offer fiber, while meat, cheese, eggs, and fat do not have any fiber. Every food group offers health benefits if you choose foods wisely. The best diets provide a variety of nutritious foods, from all food groups, as long as they're consumed in appropriate serving sizes.

REMEMBER

Not all carbs are created equal when it comes to good nutrition, though. Whole grains, legumes, fruits, and vegetables are filled with the nutrients we need for health. Refined grains, desserts, sodas, and the seemingly endless supply of junk foods don't offer much in terms of healthy nutrition. Unhealthy food choices dump in carbs and calories and do more harm than good. Healthy, natural carbohydrate-containing food groups provide a diverse array of critical nutrients:

>> **Whole grains** provide fiber, B vitamins, magnesium, phosphorus, manganese, iron, and vitamin E.

>> **Fruits and vegetables** contribute fiber and are rich in vitamin A, vitamin C, potassium, folic acid, bioflavonoids, and antioxidants, just to name a few.

>> **Milk and yogurt** provide protein, calcium, vitamin D, vitamin B12, phosphorus, and more.

>> **Legumes** are not only high in fiber, but they also pack in the protein and offer several B vitamins, as well as magnesium, zinc, and iron.

REMEMBER

We simply must have glucose traveling through our bloodstream at all times. Glucose is the preferred fuel for the brain, the central nervous system, and red blood cells. Glucose also provides fuel to muscles. You can also burn fat for energy, but you need to burn glucose and fat in the proper fuel mix to keep metabolism on an even keel. An appropriate amount of carb is needed to properly fuel your body. You can't drive a car without fuel, and you can't operate a human body without glucose in your bloodstream. (I realize we have electric cars now, but we don't have electric bodies, so I stand by my statement!) To find out just how much carb you need, see Chapter 5. For more information on how glucose is utilized as fuel for the human body, see Chapter 4.

Introducing the So-Called Simple Carbohydrates

The monosaccharides and disaccharides illustrated in Figure 3-1 are considered simple carbohydrates (sugars). There are naturally occurring sugars in many foods. Fruits, milk, and yogurt are examples of foods that contain natural sugars.

Take a closer look at the carbohydrate building blocks, the single sugars. Sugar molecules are made out of carbon, hydrogen, and oxygen, which can be assembled to form glucose, fructose, or galactose. Those are the three monosaccharide single sugars. The single sugars can decide to partner up with each other, form a loving bond, and become disaccharides. See Figure 3-2 to meet the happy couples. The following sections go into more detail on all the simple carbohydrates.

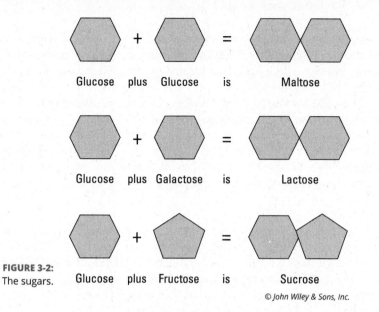

© John Wiley & Sons, Inc.

FIGURE 3-2:
The sugars.

Going au naturel with glucose, fructose, and lactose

All fruits have natural sugar. Fruits contain both glucose and fructose. In fact, fruit is 100 percent sugar. There's no protein or fat in fruit. Avocados and tomatoes are considered fruits if you ask a botanist. However, when considering the actual composition of those foods in terms of calories, carbs, and the effect on blood sugar, tomatoes get shipped off to the "vegetable" group and avocados are relegated to the "fat" group because they are more similar in composition to the items in those respective food groups. Vegetables also contain glucose and fructose, but in lower amounts than fruit.

WARNING

While fructose is a natural sugar, high-fructose corn syrup is not. The latter is made in mass quantities and added to foods during manufacturing. Fruit has positive nutritional benefits and is part of a balanced diet. High-fructose corn syrup does not offer any nutritional benefits. For more information about sugars and various alternative sweeteners, see Chapter 12.

Lactose is the natural sugar in milk. It is a disaccharide, or double sugar. Lactose is digested in the intestine as lactase enzymes clip apart the double sugar into its two single sugars, glucose and galactose (refer to Figure 3-2). Only single units of sugar are absorbed into the bloodstream.

TIP

Some people do not have enough of the enzyme to properly break down lactose. If you are unable to digest milk, then you are likely lactose intolerant. People who are lactose intolerant feel gassy and bloated or crampy (or have diarrhea) after consuming milk (and sometimes other dairy products). One solution is to buy lactose-free milk. Lactose-free milk has the enzyme pre-added to the milk. The double sugar, lactose, breaks down into the individual sugars, glucose and galactose, before you even drink it. The carton will say 100 percent lactose-free milk, but keep in mind the actual amount of sugar is exactly the same as normal milk — it just contains single sugars instead of the double sugar. Another work-around on lactose intolerance is to use a nondairy milk substitute. For more tips, see Chapter 11.

TIP

If you are lactose intolerant, you may still be able to tolerate cheese. That's because cheese is basically carbohydrate-free. Cheese is made from the protein and the fat from milk, but it has no (or only trace amounts of) lactose. Some people who are lactose intolerant seem to tolerate yogurt fairly well too. The lactase enzyme needed to digest lactose sugar is also available in tablets and liquid drops, so you can take it as needed when you have a serving of dairy.

Finding other forms of sugar: Sucrose, maltose, honey, and syrups

Sucrose is the fancy name for white sugar. It is a disaccharide (double sugar) that is made from glucose paired with fructose (refer to Figure 3-2). When you digest it, which occurs in the intestine, the two sugars break apart and are individually absorbed into the bloodstream.

Maltose consists of two glucose molecules joined together (refer to Figure 3-2). Maltose results when starches are being broken down into sugars. The maltose can quickly split into individual glucose sugars. Maltose and malted grains are used for making alcoholic beverages. Maltose and other sugars can be converted to alcohol by yeast during the fermentation process.

Honey is composed of fructose, glucose, several oligosaccharides, and water. *Oligosaccharides* are chains of three to nine monosaccharide sugars, whereas polysaccharides have ten or more sugar molecules in the chain. The bees add enzymes to the honey when they produce it, so most of the sugars exist in monosaccharide form. Honey is slightly sweeter tasting than sugar, so you may achieve the same sweetness when using a smaller portion.

Syrups may be of the naturally occurring variety, such as pure maple syrup. Many other types of syrups are manufactured, often out of high-fructose corn syrup. Maple syrup is high in natural sucrose but also has traces of fructose and glucose.

Spotting simple carbs in the grocery aisles

When looking at Nutrition Facts food labels, the grams of sugar are indented and listed under the total carbohydrates. All the sugars discussed thus far in this chapter are lumped together and called "sugar." That means the natural sugars in fruit and milk get counted as sugar on the food label. It's more informative when carb counting to look at the total grams of carbohydrate on Nutrition Facts labels. The sugars are already included in the total carbs. If you've been looking only at the grams of sugar, you've been missing the big picture. The starches eventually break down into simple sugars during digestion, so keep your eye on the total carbohydrate counts. For more information on label reading, see Chapter 7.

REMEMBER

Look to the perimeter once you're inside the supermarket, as that is where you typically find the healthy foods that contain natural sugars. Fresh fruits and vegetables and reduced-fat dairy products such as milk and yogurt are considered to be part of a well-balanced and healthy diet. Those are real foods with real nutrition. Fruits, vegetables, and reduced-fat dairy products contain important vitamins and minerals and offer health benefits.

WARNING

On the other hand, many not-so-healthy foods are loaded with added sugars in the form of sweets and treats, such as cookies, pastries, ice creams, and candy. Use caution when steering your grocery cart down those aisles. Excessive intake of desserts can end up piling on the carbs and the calories. Use caution at the checkout stand too, as the store is making one last attempt to sell you candy.

Checking Out the Complex Carbohydrates

Complex carbs are made out of many glucose molecules linked together. Starch and fiber (refer to Figure 3-1) are both considered complex carbohydrates. Starches digest and eventually break down into individual glucose molecules. Fiber, on the other hand, does not turn into glucose. Fiber is the nondigestible part of whole grains and other plant foods. The following sections give you the full scoop on complex carbs.

Identifying the starches

Grains, breads, bagels, tortillas, cereals, oats, grits, rice, quinoa, barley, farro, millet, bulgur, and pasta are all examples of complex carbs. When counting carbs, foods are grouped according to the amount of carbohydrate they contain. Some vegetables have carb counts similar to grains and breads, so those particular vegetables are lumped together in the "starch" group. Examples of starchy vegetables include potatoes, corn, hominy, parsnips, peas, yams, yucca, pumpkin, and the family of legumes. Legumes include the split pea and dried bean family, pinto beans, black beans, kidney beans, lentils, red beans, navy beans, and garbanzo beans (also known as chickpeas). For a more complete list of starches, see Appendix A.

Focusing on fiber

Fiber is found only in plant foods. You find fiber in whole grains, legumes, nuts, fruits, and vegetables. Refined grains, such as white bread and white rice, are stripped of their natural fibers during processing.

Fiber is made out of glucose molecules, so it fits the definition of a carbohydrate. The glucose molecules are all linked together tightly in long chains. The bonds that hold the glucose molecules together are strong, and our digestive enzymes are unable to cleave them apart. Fiber is not digested or absorbed, so when counting grams of carbohydrate, fiber grams can be subtracted from the total grams of carbohydrate. For more tips on identifying total carbohydrate and fiber counts on packaged foods, see Chapter 7.

In the following sections, I describe the health benefits and types of fiber, and I explain how to set your fiber intake goal.

Highlighting fiber's health benefits

Fiber has numerous health benefits. For example:

>> Fiber is vitally important to the digestive system. Fiber keeps the food moving through the intestinal tract. In so doing, fiber promotes intestinal health.

>> Fiber, the soluble variety, is heart-healthy because it helps reduce blood cholesterol levels. See Chapter 16 for more details.

TECHNICAL STUFF

A whole grain has three main components: the bran, the endosperm, and the germ. The bran is the fiber-rich outer layer. The inner part of the grain contains the endosperm and the germ. The endosperm is the starchy part but also contains some protein. The germ is the actual seed for a new plant, and it contains vitamins, minerals, and healthy oils. Refining grains removes the bran and the germ. Many nutrients are lost in the refining process, so grains are often fortified. Fortification is an attempt to put back some of the vitamins that were removed by refining, but the fiber is not replaced.

Giving a nod to the two fibers: Soluble and insoluble

There are two main types of fiber: soluble (absorbs water) and insoluble (does not absorb water). Both types of fiber have health-promoting qualities. Soluble fiber is heart healthy because it can naturally help to lower your blood cholesterol levels. Insoluble fiber can improve intestinal health. Many plant foods contain both types of fiber. For example, legumes are high in both soluble and insoluble fiber.

Soluble fiber absorbs water and swells. Oatmeal has soluble fiber, and when you add water and cook it, the grain swells and gets sticky. The dried-bean family is also rich in soluble fiber. For a more in-depth discussion on how soluble fiber performs its cholesterol-lowering feat, see Chapter 16. That's also where you find a more complete list of foods that contain soluble fiber.

Insoluble fiber does not absorb water. You could sprinkle bran into a glass of water and it would float on top all day. As insoluble fiber moves through the intestinal tract, it pushes the food through and helps prevent constipation. Insoluble fiber gently rubs the intestinal walls as it moves past, and that helps keep the intestine and colon healthy. Fiber in the diet may reduce the risk of developing hemorrhoids and diverticular disease. Foods that contain insoluble fiber include whole grains, legumes, nuts, seeds, fruits, and vegetables. The skins of fruits and vegetables are particularly high in insoluble fiber.

REMEMBER

When it comes to having diabetes, a diet higher in fiber offers additional benefits. Refined grains such as white rice and white bread digest quickly, which can cause higher post-meal blood-glucose spikes (which are not good). Whole grains and legumes take more time to digest, so the glucose from the meal enters the bloodstream gradually and the blood-glucose level may not peak as sharply (which is good). Additionally, since a meal with more fiber takes longer to digest, you may feel satisfied for a longer period of time. That could reduce between-meal snacking and help with weight control.

Setting your personal fiber intake goal

The National Academies of Sciences, Engineering, and Medicine provide Dietary Reference Intake guidelines for nutrients including fiber. Their suggested intake targets for fiber are in Table 3-1.

TABLE 3-1   **Daily Fiber Recommendations for Adults**

Gender	Ages 19 to 50	Ages 51 and Older
Women	25 grams	21 grams
Men	38 grams	30 grams

REMEMBER

If your diet is typically low in fiber, it is best to increase your intake gradually over a period of a few weeks to give your body a chance to adjust. Increasing fiber intake too rapidly could lead to gassiness and bloating. Be sure to drink plenty of water too. Fiber keeps things moving along, but only if you stay well hydrated.

WARNING

If you have a diabetes complication known as gastroparesis, you should not be eating much fiber at all. *Gastroparesis* is a type of neuropathy that affects the intestinal tract. The nerves that stimulate peristalsis no longer function properly; therefore, foods end up transiting very slowly and unpredictably, which makes it difficult to predict blood-glucose levels and insulin dosing. Gastroparesis can lead to nausea, vomiting, and constipation. The diet recommended for gastroparesis is a low-fat and low-fiber diet, with smaller, more frequent meals. Those recommended dietary modifications help foods digest more quickly and predictably. Given the complexities of the condition and treatment, seek advice from your healthcare provider and discuss nutritional interventions with a registered dietitian.

Spotting complex carbs in the grocery aisles

Try the following tips as you shop for complex carbs at the grocery store:

» The produce section offers complex carbs in potatoes, yams, sweet potatoes, yucca, corn, peas, and an array of winter squashes (butternut, acorn, Hubbard, and pumpkin, to name a few.)

» In the canned-food section or the dried-goods section, you can choose from any of the dried beans, split peas, and lentils.

» As you head down the cereal aisle, look for whole-grain breakfast cereals with little or no added sugars.

» As for snacks, choose whole-grain crackers and pretzels, or popcorn (opt for microwave lite or pop your own to control the fat).

» Look for the words "whole grain" or "whole wheat" when picking breads, bagels, or tortillas. There are even pastas that are made with whole grains. Seek out whole grains to cook and serve with lunches and dinners. Skip the boxes of flavored (usually high sodium) rice mixes and try unprocessed whole grains such as brown rice, quinoa, farro, teff, millet, amaranth, barley, and bulgur. They are all easy to prepare.

For more information on identifying whole-grain products in packaged foods, see Chapter 7.

Recognizing Carb-Free Counterparts

Many foods do not contain any carbohydrate, as you find out in this section. Protein and fat are the two macronutrients that don't directly raise blood–sugar levels because they are not made out of glucose molecules:

>> **Proteins** are made out of building blocks called *amino acids.* The body uses dietary proteins to obtain the amino-acid building blocks needed to create and repair its tissues, cells, organs, and muscles.

>> **Fats** are made from fatty acids. Dietary fats add flavor and also help transport fat-soluble vitamins. A certain amount of dietary fat is essential, but that budget is easily met, and often exceeded, so it pays to be mindful about how much fat is being consumed. It's also important to choose the heart-healthier fats.

Pumping up with proteins: Meat, fish, and other sources

If it once flew, swam, or roamed the earth and now it's on your dinner plate, then it's a protein food and does not contain carbs. It pays to choose lean meats, because meat fats tend to be saturated, and that kind of fat is not healthy for your blood vessels (as I explain later in this chapter). Look for meats that are not marbled. Take the skin off poultry before eating. Fish, on the other hand, contains one of the heart–healthiest kinds of fat: omega–3 fatty acids.

Other carb-free protein sources include eggs and cheese. Egg whites contain quality protein, and egg yolks contains cholesterol and fat. (Chapter 16 brings you up to date on the cholesterol debate; current recommendations may surprise you.) Cheese doesn't have carbs even though it is made from milk. To make cheese, enzymes are added to whole milk. The enzymes cause the protein and the fat from the milk to come together and form a solid curd. The liquid that remains behind contains the carb. Cottage cheese is mostly protein and is very low in carb because not that much liquid is retained in packaging the cottage cheese.

Vegetarian meat replacements vary, but most are low- or no-carb. Check labels on vegetarian hot dogs, burgers, or other faux meats for the product's nutrition information, and check out Chapter 7 if you need help with reading labels.

Finding the healthiest fats and oils

Fats and oils do not contain carbohydrate. They add flavor to foods and come in many forms. Some fats are solid at room temperature, such as butter, while others are liquid at room temperature, such as oil. Some fats come from animals, which include the fats found in meats and dairy products. Other fats come from vegetable sources, such as nuts, oils, and avocados. All fats are calorically dense. For example, a single tablespoon of oil has about 135 calories, and ¼ cup of nuts is close to 200 calories. It pays to pick your dietary fats wisely and to savor them in reasonable portions.

Sampling the good stuff: Unsaturated fats

The heart-healthiest fats are unsaturated. Unsaturated oils tend to be liquid at room temperature. Two types of unsaturated fats exist:

» **Monounsaturated fats** are some of the best when it comes to heart health. They are found in olive oil, canola oil, peanut oil, avocados, and nuts.

» **Polyunsaturated fats** are found in many oils, including corn, cottonseed, flaxseed, grape seed, safflower, sesame, soybean, and sunflower oils. Mayonnaise and margarine also contain polyunsaturated fats.

Unsaturated fats should be enjoyed in reasonable portion sizes. See Chapter 16 for more on choosing fats wisely and zeroing in on the Nutrition Facts food label sections related to fat and heart health.

Trimming your intake of saturated fats

Saturated fats are linked to blood-vessel diseases such as heart disease. Saturated fats can increase LDL cholesterol levels. LDL is the artery-clogging, bad kind of cholesterol. Saturated fats are more likely to be solid at room temperature. Examples include marbled meats, bacon, lard, and full-fat dairy products including butter, cream cheese, sour cream, cream, and whipped cream.

TIP

To trim back on saturated fats, choose nonfat or reduced-fat dairy products, pick lean meats, and use smaller amounts of butter. Replace saturated fats with unsaturated fats when possible, such as sautéing in olive oil instead of butter.

Steering clear of trans fats

Trans fats are public enemy number one, if you ask heart-health experts. Eating trans fats increases your risk of developing heart disease and stroke. They raise LDL cholesterol levels (the *artery-clogging*, bad kind) just like saturated fats do.

However, trans fats hit you with a double whammy because they also lower your HDL cholesterol (the *artery-cleaning*, good kind).

Animal products contain traces of naturally occurring trans fats, but the vast majority of dietary trans fats are formed during a food manufacturing process known as *hydrogenation*. When hydrogen atoms are forced into liquid vegetable oils, the chemical structure of the oil changes and the oils begin to solidify. Hydrogenated oils are solid or semi-solid at room temperature. The word "trans" refers to the orientation of the hydrogen atoms as they bond to the carbon atoms in the fatty acid.

Hydrogenated fats have a long shelf life. Restaurants, especially the fast-food industry, use hydrogenated fat in the fryer because it can be used over and over again before changing the oil. You can minimize your intake of trans fats by avoiding fried foods when dining out.

Vegetable shortening is another source of trans fat. Beware; many baked goods are made with shortening, so limit commercially produced pastries and baked goods. Your best-bet margarines are the liquid or tub varieties instead of the stick versions.

REMEMBER

Food labels are allowed to say 0 grams of trans fat as long as there is less than 0.5 grams of trans fat *per serving*. If you eat multiple servings, they potentially could add up to a significant amount of trans fat. That's why you should read ingredients lists and simply avoid products with hydrogenated or partially hydrogenated oils. For packaged foods, read the Nutrition Facts food labels and look for "0 g trans fat." Read the ingredients list too and make sure there are no hydrogenated or partially hydrogenated oils listed. See Chapter 7 for more info on reading food labels.

Exploring the role of noncarb foods in diabetes management

Protein foods and heart-healthy fats and oils provide key nutrients, and they also add variety and pleasure to eating. For tips on choosing foods wisely as you manage diabetes, see Chapter 13; the following sections give you an introduction.

Satisfying your appetite

Have you ever had a light lunch, such as fruit and nonfat yogurt, and then been hungry again in an hour? Or have you been uncomfortably stuffed for several hours after a heavy, high-fat meal? A balanced, mixed meal takes roughly four hours to fully digest. *Mixed meal* refers to a meal that has a balanced amount of carbohydrate, protein, and fat. Fat tends to delay digestion, and it increases satiety (gratification and satisfaction). Even lean proteins have some fat, so no need to go out of your way to add too much fat. People generally feel satisfied for a longer period of time if they eat balanced meals.

TIP

The plate model is a good tool for striking the right balance in meal planning. Chapter 8 provides more information about using the plate model. To get some ideas on meal planning, check out the sample menu plans for breakfast, lunch, and dinner ideas in Chapters 19, 20, and 21.

Smoothing out your numbers

When carb foods digest too rapidly, the glucose from the meal ends up in the bloodstream very quickly. For example, fruit juice or sugary beverages take only about 15 minutes to get digested and absorbed. The rapid rush of glucose into the bloodstream can wreak havoc with blood-glucose control efforts. To minimize blood-glucose spikes, it makes sense to limit liquid concentrated carbs. (For more info on the pitfalls of sugary beverages, see Chapter 11.) Beyond that, careful meal planning can help to minimize blood-glucose variability.

REMEMBER

Choose foods wisely and control portion sizes. Strike a balance between carbs, proteins, and fats. Pick lean proteins and aim for a portion about the size of the palm of your hand. Choose higher-fiber grains and keep the portion to about the size of your fist. For more information on the mealtime variables that influence post-meal blood-glucose levels, see Chapter 10.

Chapter **4**

Tracking Carbs through the Body

The human body is absolutely amazing. It consists of complex systems that function independently yet are intricately interconnected. The nervous system, respiratory system, and circulatory system work behind the scenes around the clock. When functioning properly, the human body's systems are more or less on autopilot. It's easy to take these functions for granted. Our bodies do require some upkeep, though. For starters we need food, fluids, and fitness. For optimal health our bodies require specific amounts of vitamins, minerals, and other key nutrients.

It does sound a little repetitive, but we really do need a balanced and complete diet. Eating is how we provide the critical nutrients that our cells, organs, and tissues require. Our bodies must have carbohydrate, protein, fat, and a wide array of vitamins and minerals. The digestive system breaks food down into its basic building blocks. In the intestine, carbohydrates turn into glucose, proteins are disassembled into individual amino acids, and fats break down into fatty acids. The nutrient building blocks are absorbed from the intestine into the bloodstream and are then are used to build and repair our tissues. The circulatory system makes sure that the nutrients are properly distributed throughout the body.

Chapter 3 mentions that wholesome carbohydrate foods are loaded with nutrients, vitamins, and minerals. This chapter explains the special role carb foods play in terms of *fueling* our bodies. Glucose is a critical source of energy.

Filling Your Tank and Fueling Your Cells

Have you ever really thought about what happens to the food once you've eaten it? It's more common to let food occupy our attention when grocery shopping and planning meals. Effort and focus goes into food preparation and serving the meal. We savor the flavors and textures while eating. But after we finish a meal and clear the table, we are usually off to thinking about something else and moving on to the next thing on our agenda.

In this section, I pick up where we typically leave off. I want to focus on what happens after the last bite has been enjoyed. Figure 4-1 sets the stage for this discussion by depicting the journey that glucose takes through the body. Carbohydrate foods are emptied from the stomach, digested in the intestine, and absorbed into the bloodstream. Glucose then travels through the bloodstream to fuel the body's cells and contribute to glycogen stores in the liver and muscles.

Settling in your stomach

The digestive system starts in your mouth. You've likely heard of a delicious meal being described as "mouth-watering." Seeing or smelling foods and sometimes just thinking of food gets the saliva flowing. Saliva contains an enzyme called amylase that begins the process of digestion. Chewing moistens food and breaks it into smaller particles. Swallowing moves food down through the esophagus and into the stomach.

The stomach serves as a temporary holding tank where food is mixed and churned and prepared for digestion. The stomach secretes hydrochloric acid, which helps to break up the food. It also serves as a defense mechanism as acid kills any bacteria that may have hitched a ride in with the food.

TECHNICAL STUFF

The top of the stomach has a sphincter that is supposed to prevent food from coming back up into the esophagus. We call it heartburn when the acidic stomach contents percolate back up into the sensitive esophagus. Fat and caffeine are known to relax the esophageal sphincter and can make heartburn worse.

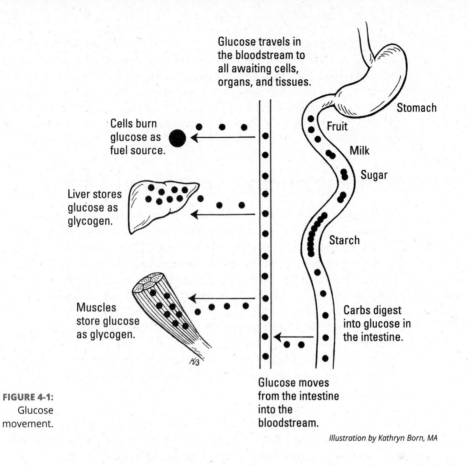

Glucose travels in the bloodstream to all awaiting cells, organs, and tissues.

Stomach

Fruit

Milk

Sugar

Cells burn glucose as fuel source.

Liver stores glucose as glycogen.

Starch

Muscles store glucose as glycogen.

Carbs digest into glucose in the intestine.

Glucose moves from the intestine into the bloodstream.

Illustration by Kathryn Born, MA

FIGURE 4-1: Glucose movement.

The contracting stomach is supposed to move the food downward. The pyloric sphincter at the lower end of the stomach regulates the passage of food from the stomach into the upper intestine. Next stop on the journey is the small intestine where digestion and absorption take place.

Extracting glucose via digestion

Once food has transited the stomach, it enters the *duodenum*, which is the uppermost part of the small intestine. The pancreas secretes bicarbonate into the duodenum to neutralize the stomach acid and enzymes to digest the slurry of foods. Specific enzymes break down each macronutrient: carbs, proteins, and fats. Digestion is complete when macronutrients are broken down into their separate building blocks: glucose (from carbs), amino acids (from proteins), and fatty acids (from fats).

Individual building blocks are small enough to be transported through the intestinal wall into the network of blood vessels surrounding the intestine. Vitamins and minerals are absorbed into the bloodstream via specific channels. Fiber isn't digestible, so it continues downward and transits through the entire intestine. Fiber helps keep the intestine clean and healthy. Once glucose has been absorbed into the bloodstream, it begins its journey throughout the body (refer to Figure 4-1).

Pumping through your bloodstream

The circulatory system is like a complex road map. Take California, for example. The state is made up of countless cities, communities, and people that are connected by freeways, highways, boulevards, rural routes, alleys, and streets. Delivery trucks can bring goods from any location and deliver them directly to your doorstep. Similarly, the circulatory system is made up of blood vessels of varying sizes from main arteries to tiny capillaries. Nutrients are picked up from the digestive tract and transported through every blood vessel to be delivered to each cell in the body. The heart pumps tirelessly to keep the blood moving. (Fun fact: The average adult heart beats 115,200 times each day!) Red blood cells also take advantage of the circulatory system's route to deliver oxygen from the lungs to all tissues. Carbon dioxide waste is carried away and then taken back to the lungs to be exhaled.

Glucose and blood cells share the blood vessels traveling side by side just like cars and trucks share the roadway. Everyone is going about his business. There may have been times when you've been at home waiting for an important package to be delivered to your doorstep; likewise, the cells in your body are awaiting delivery of glucose and other key nutrients.

Fueling your cells

To stay with the analogy in the preceding section, sometimes the delivery truck needs you to be home to sign for an important package. There are delivery stipulations for glucose too. In most cases the cells need insulin to be ready and waiting to accept the glucose. The brain is unique in that it can access glucose without insulin. People with diabetes have an insulin issue. Either they don't make any of their own insulin, as is the case with type 1 diabetes, or they have insulin that doesn't work very well, as is the case with type 2 diabetes. (See Chapter 2 for more details on what causes diabetes.)

After the insulin transports glucose into the cell, the glucose becomes the fuel that provides energy for cellular functions. Cells need a steady supply of glucose. Because we don't nibble around the clock, there has to be a mechanism for storing glucose to be used later. The body solves that issue by storing glucose as *glycogen*, which can then be used later, as discussed next.

Saving Some for Later: Glycogen, the Storage Form of Glucose

It isn't uncommon for families to do a major weekly shopping trip to load up on groceries and the essentials. Perhaps a nice meal is prepared a few hours later, but most of the groceries are unloaded and put away in the pantry, the refrigerator, and the freezer. We stock up, saving some for later. It's good to have reserves. We keep our cupboards stocked because we wouldn't want to run completely out of food. Neither does your body. Carbohydrate foods need to provide enough glucose for immediate use and to have some left over to stash away for later. The storage form of glucose is called *glycogen*. Glycogen is made when glucose molecules form bonds with other glucose molecules to create a long polymer, a chain of glucose molecules. Only specific tissues can store glycogen: the liver and the muscles. The following details elaborate on the process.

Making a layover in the liver

When foods digest and are absorbed into the bloodstream, the first stop is the liver. The liver takes what it wants. Glucose and other nutrients, including minerals and fat-soluble vitamins, can be stored in the liver and accessed later as needed.

A balanced meal that contains a mixture of carbohydrate, protein, and fat takes about four hours to fully digest. As the meal is digesting, the carbs from the meal turn to glucose. Some glucose is distributed for immediate use by the body, and some goes into storage as glycogen (refer to Figure 4-1). After the meal has finished digesting, the liver releases a steady stream of glucose until the next meal is eaten.

REMEMBER

A significant amount of time passes between dinner and breakfast. The liver supplies glucose all night long while you sleep. Sometimes glucose levels rise while you sleep. That glucose is coming from your liver. If your fasting glucose levels are typically above target, that calls for a medication adjustment. Speak to your healthcare provider if you face this situation.

About 20 percent of the body's glycogen reserves are held in the liver. The liver breaks the glycogen back down into individual glucose molecules and releases the glucose into the bloodstream as needed. The liver tries to make sure that blood-glucose levels don't fall too low. When glycogen stores are depleted, the liver can even be called upon to make new glucose. That process is detailed later in this chapter.

Maintaining the muscles' glucose reserves

The muscles can't boast the ability to make new glucose from scratch, but they certainly do their part by storing up glucose to have at the ready for immediate use when muscle power is needed (refer to Figure 4-1). Muscle glycogen accounts for about 80 percent of the body's total glycogen reserves.

The glycogen that is stored in the muscles stays in the muscles and feeds only the muscles. It cannot be mobilized or transported elsewhere in the body. The likely reason is so the muscles will always have immediate fuel for any fight-or-flight situations. Even if blood-glucose levels drop, the glucose stays put inside the muscles to be used by the muscles.

TIP

Regular exercise and fitness help to build and condition the muscles, which increases the glycogen storage capacity. People who exercise and stay fit can store more glycogen than those who are sedentary. Glycogen is not stored in body fat. Flip to Chapter 14 for more information on fitness.

Noting What Happens When Glucose Levels Remain Elevated

Without diabetes, the normal range for blood glucose is about 70–140 milligrams per deciliter (mg/dl) all the time. Type 1 and type 2 diabetes can both lead to blood-glucose levels that rise far above the normal limits. Elevated blood glucose over time can lead to complications associated with poorly controlled diabetes. The kidneys try to do their part to assist, as I describe in the next section.

Spilling glucose into the urine

Each time the heart beats, blood is pushed throughout the body. Blood is continually making a pass through the kidneys along its journey throughout the body. The kidneys are filled with miniature filters called *nephrons* that filter the blood and decide what stays in the blood and what gets taken out. The filtered waste that is removed by the kidneys is sent to the bladder and disposed of in the urine.

When glucose levels rise too high, the kidneys decide to filter out some of the excess glucose. Long before blood-glucose monitors were available, the glucose levels in the urine were checked. The process was woefully inaccurate, and the results were hard to interpret. Urine can accumulate in the bladder over several hours. High glucose in the urine didn't necessary reflect glucose levels *in the blood* at any particular time. It just indicated that blood glucose had been high enough in the preceding hours for the kidneys to filter out some of the glucose. Figure 4-2 shows the kidneys removing excess glucose and dumping it into the bladder.

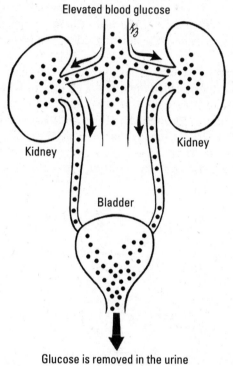

Elevated blood glucose

Kidney

Kidney

Bladder

FIGURE 4-2: Kidneys remove excess glucose.

Glucose is removed in the urine

Illustration by Kathryn Born, MA

WARNING

Keep in mind that glucose is food and has calories. Losing glucose in the urine contributes to the unintended weight loss when diabetes is out of control. When glucose levels are significantly elevated, some of the glucose can attach to tissues in the body as explained in the next section. You sure wouldn't want to gunk up those little filters in the kidneys, because there is no effective way of repairing damaged nephrons.

Sticking glucose where it doesn't belong: Glycosylation

Glucose has a real affinity for protein. Glucose can glom onto proteins in the body and is very reluctant to ever let go. Glucose sticking to tissues is called *glycosylation*. Our bodies are made out of protein, and the bloodstream has the ability to expose all areas of the body to excess glucose when levels are high. Blood vessels are made of protein, so unfortunately, glucose has the opportunity to damage blood vessels. As I mention in the previous section, the tiny filters in the kidneys are vulnerable; so are the retinas of the eyes and the nerves throughout the body. Uncontrolled diabetes even increases the risk of heart attack. The damage isn't easy to see. You can't get a camera into the tiny kidney filters to take a look around.

There is a test that can be used to estimate the risk that glycosylation poses to delicate tissues. It's a lab test called the A1C, which measures the amount of glucose that has attached to hemoglobin A1, a protein on the surface of red blood cells. (See Chapters 2 and 23 for more details on A1C.) Figure 4-3 illustrates glycosylation of red blood cells. Red blood cells travel side by side through the bloodstream along with glucose. They share the road, so to speak. When blood-glucose levels are high, more glucose attaches to the surface of the blood cells.

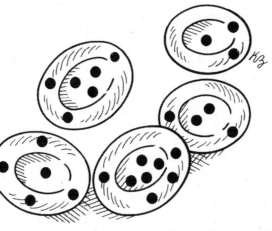

FIGURE 4-3:
Glycosylation of red blood cells.

Illustration by Kathryn Born, MA

Red blood cells live about three months. Every day some new red blood cells are created while some old ones are eliminated. The older cells have more glucose attached to them. It's possible to estimate the *average blood glucose* over the previous three months by knowing the A1C; see Table 4-1. A person without diabetes would have an A1C below 5.7 percent. In general, the target A1C is below 7 percent for adults with diabetes and below 7.5 percent for adolescents with diabetes.

Sometimes, such as during pregnancy, the targets are set lower. Conversely there are medically complex situations that may warrant a less-stringent target, such as below 8 percent.

TABLE 4-1

A1C and Estimated Average Glucose (eAG)

A1C Percent	eAG in mg/dl
5	97
6	126
7	154
8	183
9	212
10	240
11	269
12	298
13	326
14	355

WARNING

Keep in mind that while A1C can provide information about the *average* blood-glucose control in the previous three months, it doesn't show any detail whatsoever in terms of how high or how low the blood glucose has been. The reason the target A1C for an adult is below 7 percent (instead of aiming for an A1C in the normal nondiabetic range of below 5.7 percent) is because the lower you aim, the more significant the risk of causing severe hypoglycemia (for insulin users). See Chapter 15 for more on hypoglycemia.

To clarify further: An A1C of 6 percent indicates an estimated average blood-glucose level of 126 mg/dl. If a person is not on medications, there is no risk of hypoglycemia. The blood-glucose range may be stable and hover just above or below 126 mg/dl. However, another person could have the same A1C of 6 percent but have erratic blood-glucose levels with values as low as 40 mg/dl and as high as 350 mg/dl. In other words, A1C doesn't provide enough information. The home blood-glucose monitoring results are crucial for making regimen adjustments to decrease the variability. That's a good reason to share your blood-glucose records with your healthcare team. If they have only the A1C to work from, they don't have enough information to safely adjust medications.

TIP

Table 4-1 lists A1C in whole numbers, but your result may be a decimal. The American Diabetes Association has an A1C calculator. Just enter your A1C percentage and it converts it to your estimated average glucose. For example, an A1C of 7.4 has an estimated average glucose of 166 mg/dl. Access the calculator at www.diabetes.org and then click the "Living with Diabetes" tab and look under the "Treatment and Care" heading for "A1C."

Recognizing the Risks of Undereating Carbs

You need enough carb to meet the fuel demands of the day and to keep your glycogen reserves stocked so your liver can dole out carbs overnight while you sleep, as described earlier in this chapter. When glucose levels are too low, you can't perform or think at your best. The brain can't store any glucose, so it must have a constant supply. Lack of concentration and trouble completing mental tasks may be a sign of hypoglycemia (glucose deficiency). If you chronically eat fewer carbs than your body needs, you won't have enough carbs available to keep glycogen stores well-stocked. There are possible consequences to undereating carbs, as explored in this section.

TIP

Body size, age, gender, and level of physical activity all determine how much carbohydrate your body requires. It's not an exact science, but Chapter 5 provides some guidance on how much carb you may want to aim for.

Depleting glucose reserves and dealing with hypoglycemia

If you don't consume enough carbs at mealtimes, your body has little choice but to tap into the glycogen reserves. The liver can break down glycogen and send it back into circulation for use by other tissues. The glycogen stored within the muscles can be used by the muscles. Muscle glycogen stores prefer to be fully stocked, so when glycogen supplies are low, the muscles pull glucose from the bloodstream to replenish the glycogen reserves. As muscle glycogen is being refilled, blood-glucose levels may drop too low in individuals who inject insulin or take medications that stimulate insulin production. The muscles don't really care if sucking glucose out of the bloodstream to fill glycogen stores ends up causing hypoglycemia. People without diabetes don't share the same risks because when the pancreas is working properly, it turns insulin production on and off as necessary to prevent hypoglycemia.

Hypoglycemia is only a risk if you take insulin or certain pills that stimulate your pancreas to produce extra insulin. But if you're on a medicine that can cause hypoglycemia, then consider this: Depleted glycogen stores draw glucose steadily from the bloodstream until glycogen storage sites are full. That could lead to unexpected hypoglycemia anytime and especially during the night. Hypoglycemia requires carbs to treat the low blood-glucose level, and sometimes you end up with a high blood-glucose level after treating a low-glucose level. It can be quite a roller coaster. It is easier to simply eat the right amount of carb in the first place. (See Chapter 15 for details on handling hypoglycemia.)

If hypoglycemia isn't a risk for you, it still makes sense to eat a balanced diet with the proper amount of carbohydrate. Many people are cutting the carbs to try to lose weight. It's better to cut the overall calories and still keep the proper balance between carbs, proteins, and fats. Most people who strive to lose weight want to lose body fat, not muscle. Poorly planned diets can lead to the loss of muscle and ketone production, which I cover at the end of this chapter.

Making glucose but losing lean body mass

The liver is at the hub of metabolic activity. As previously mentioned in this chapter, the liver is able to store glycogen and release it as glucose later when needed. Although the muscles can store glycogen, the glycogen in the muscles can't be shared or released. Glycogen in the muscles stays in the muscles to be used solely for the muscles. The liver glycogen stores can be depleted, especially if there are long periods of time between meals. The glycogen is broken back down into glucose and released to fuel hungry cells when no glucose is forthcoming from digestion. The liver glycogen stores are tapped into during exercise too.

The bottom line is that the liver stores a finite amount of glucose, and when it's gone, the liver switches gears and produces brand-new glucose. The process is called *gluconeogenesis*; gluco (glucose) plus neo (new) plus genesis (beginning) translates to making new glucose. We all know you can't make something from nothing. You have to have an ingredient to start with that can be converted to glucose.

When there is no food digesting and no more glycogen in the liver, the liver can convert amino acids into glucose. Muscles are made of protein, and protein is made out of amino acids. Amino acids are made out of carbon, hydrogen, oxygen, and nitrogen. If you remove the nitrogen and rearrange the other elements, you can create glucose. The scientific abbreviation for carbohydrate is CHO, which represents carbon, hydrogen, and oxygen. See Figure 4-4 for a look at the starvation mode of metabolism.

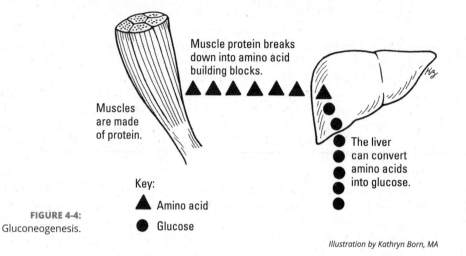

FIGURE 4-4:
Gluconeogenesis.

Muscle protein breaks down into amino acid building blocks.

Muscles are made of protein.

Key:

▲ Amino acid

● Glucose

The liver can convert amino acids into glucose.

Illustration by Kathryn Born, MA

People are able to survive under extreme food shortages by breaking down their own muscles to produce glucose. It comes at a cost though. You lose healthy muscle tissue. (Unfortunately, fat cannot turn into glucose. During the starvation mode of metabolism, fat turns into ketones, as explained in the next section.)

Producing ketones

Burning fuels always creates some sort of byproduct. Cars have exhaust fumes, for example. Dietary fats can be burned (*metabolized*) to form very safe byproducts, including carbon dioxide (which you exhale) and water (which turns to sweat or urine).

Cells need insulin to transport glucose. Cells also require the proper fuel mix of fat and glucose in order to produce safe byproducts. When the cells lack insulin or have an extreme shortage of glucose, the fat is incompletely metabolized, and the byproducts are ketones.

In Figure 4-5, notice what happens when there is no insulin available, which can happen in the case of type 1 diabetes and missed insulin delivery. Without insulin, the glucose can't enter the cell. The fat can still get in, but it is only partially utilized. Unfortunately, without insulin the fat turns into a different byproduct called ketones. Ketones have a low pH, which means they are acidic like vinegar. They produce a distinctive fruity smell to the breath. The lungs remove some ketones in the exhaled breath. Someone with high levels of ketones may have labored breathing and sweet-smelling breath.

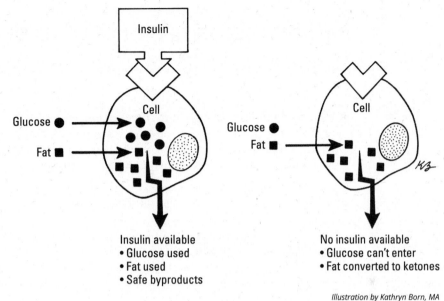

FIGURE 4-5:
Making ketones.

	Cell
Glucose ●	
Fat ■	

Insulin

Insulin available
• Glucose used
• Fat used
• Safe byproducts

	Cell
Glucose ●	
Fat ■	

No insulin available
• Glucose can't enter
• Fat converted to ketones

Illustration by Kathryn Born, MA

TIP

The kidneys filter some of the ketones out of the blood and dispose of them in the urine. Ketone dipsticks are available from the pharmacy and can be dipped into a urine sample to detect ketone levels. In addition, several meters on the market can measure blood-ketone levels. A drop of blood is applied to a special strip in a manner that mimics blood-glucose monitoring. Blood-ketone testing is more accurate because urine-ketone results may show a delayed picture. Keep in mind that urine can continue to show ketones even when blood-ketone levels have resolved. That's because urine accumulates in the bladder over time, and it takes time to completely wash out of the bladder.

Someone without diabetes may produce ketones when following a very-low-carb diet or fasting for extended periods of time. Ketone levels won't be high enough to cause diabetic ketoacidosis (DKA) because nondiabetic people produce insulin. On a low-carb diet, a person's liver can still crank out glucose by turning amino acids from protein into glucose (gluconeogenesis). Body fat can be turned into ketones. Without diabetes, there will still be insulin and enough glucose to burn alongside the fat such that DKA is not a concern. However, if the body has to resort to digesting itself due to drastic dieting, metabolism may slow down and the body will become more efficient at burning calories; the net effect can make losing weight even harder. (See the nearby sidebar for more about DKA.)

DANGER! KETONES CAN LEAD TO DKA

If you have type 1 diabetes and you have ketones, it means you need insulin. Check your blood-glucose levels.

- If you are on an insulin pump and you have ketones, you shouldn't use your pump to give a correction dose. You should assume that there may be an issue with the pump. Instead, use an insulin syringe or insulin pen to give your dose of insulin. Next you can problem-solve what may be wrong with the pump.

- If you are on injections and have ketones, you may have forgotten a dose, or maybe something is wrong with your insulin and it isn't working properly. Insulin that is past its expiration date loses potency. Your insulin pen or vial can be left at room temperature, but insulin is destroyed by exposure to high heat, so don't leave your insulin in sunlight, near the heater, or in a hot car. Once you start using a pen or vial, you usually have to discard it in 28 days even if it isn't gone. Some types of insulin have a shorter shelf life, so ask your pharmacist about your insulin storage.

If large amounts of ketones accumulate, the pH of the blood can drop. If uncorrected, this can lead to a very dangerous metabolic disturbance called diabetic ketoacidosis (DKA). DKA can lead to complications including electrolyte abnormalities, coma, and death, which is why type 1 diabetes was a fatal disease prior to the discovery and use of insulin. DKA is corrected by administering insulin and fluids for rehydration. DKA requires medical management; speak to your healthcare provide if you have questions about DKA.

Chapter 5

Finding Your Sweet Spot: The Right Amount of Carbs for You

When it comes to diabetes, the age-old question is whether an ideal fuel mix exists: Is there a best ratio of carb, protein, and fat to eat? Studies fail to identify a specific diet pattern that should be prescribed to everyone with diabetes. Diet recommendations should be individualized. However, everyone should strive to consume wholesome foods in reasonable portions because a nutritionally complete diet and weight control improve health outcomes. Favor foods that are less processed and have more fiber. Limit refined grains and cut down on saturated fats, added sugars, and salt. The body definitely needs carbs, but not everybody needs the same amount.

This chapter provides charts and tables to help you estimate your caloric needs and to personalize your carbohydrate intake goals. First, though, I briefly review general nutrition guidelines from several reputable sources.

Checking Out the Official Diet Guidelines

Popular diets come and go. Well-respected health experts share the opinion that the best diets are balanced, nutritionally complete, and sustainable for the long run. The following institutions have been studying outcomes, setting standards, and forming nutrition policy for many decades. People with diabetes can look to the experts for dietary guidance.

Advice from the American Diabetes Association

The American Diabetes Association (ADA) says that diet plans should be individualized while keeping in mind calorie goals and other health conditions. They encourage choosing carbohydrates from whole grains, vegetables, fruits, legumes, and dairy sources. They suggest limiting sugary foods and completely avoiding sugar-sweetened beverages.

The ADA doesn't make a specific recommendation about how much carb should be consumed, but by observation they note that people with diabetes tend to eat about 45 percent of their calories as carbs. They report that there is no clear evidence that supplementation with vitamins, minerals, herbs, or spices can improve diabetes. The ADA encourages people with diabetes to adhere to the dietary guidelines for the general population when it comes to fat intake, and it does not set rigid standards for dietary protein intake. For more info, log on to www.diabetes.org and click on the Food & Fitness tab.

The 2015–2020 Dietary Guidelines for Americans

Every five years the U.S. Departments of Health and Human Services (HHS) and of Agriculture (USDA) publish a report containing nutrition guidelines for the general public. These guidelines encourage a variety of nutrient-dense foods including whole grains, fruits, vegetables, nonfat and low-fat dairy products, lean meats, poultry, seafood, eggs, oils, legumes, nuts, and seeds. They suggest limiting solid fats, added sugars, refined starches, and sodium.

The portioning guidelines are embodied in the "Choose MyPlate" image. Half of the plate is divided between vegetables and fruits; just over one-fourth of the plate is for grains, just under one-fourth of the plate is for lean proteins, and a serving of low-fat or nonfat dairy can accompany the meal. They suggest that at least half of the grain servings should be whole grains. You can access more information at www.choosemyplate.gov.

Intakes and allowances from the National Academy of Sciences

Dietary Reference Intakes (DRI): Recommended Dietary Allowances (RDA) are set by the Food and Nutrition Board of the Institute of Medicine, National Academy of Sciences. They determine gender-specific nutrient-intake targets for vitamins and minerals across the various age ranges. They suggest a carbohydrate intake of between 45 and 65 percent of total daily calories. This range is considered the Acceptable Macronutrient Distribution Range (AMDR). The Recommended Dietary Allowance sets a *minimum intake target of 130 grams of carb per day* for ages one year old and above. The AMDR is 10–35 percent of daily calories for protein and 20–35 percent for fat.

Figuring Out Calorie and Carbohydrate Intake Targets

Body size, gender, age, weight goals, health status, and physical activity determine how many calories and how much carb you need. This section provides tools for setting carb intake targets based on your caloric need.

Estimating your caloric needs

Tables 5-1 and 5-2 can be used to determine caloric needs. There are two separate tables: for women (Table 5-1) and men (Table 5-2). Find your age range in the left column and then choose your activity level to locate your estimated caloric needs. Sedentary means only the light activity typical of day-to-day life and no additional exercise. Moderately active includes walking about 1.5 to 3 miles per day, and active means walking more than 3 miles per day. Other forms of exercise can be considered instead of walking.

TABLE 5-1   ## Estimated Caloric Needs for Women by Age and Activity

Age	Sedentary	Moderately Active	Active
18	1,800	2,000	2,400
19–25	2,000	2,200	2,400
26–30	1,800	2,000	2,400
31–50	1,800	2,000	2,200
51–60	1,600	1,800	2,200
61 and up	1,600	1,800	2,000

Source: Office of Disease Prevention and Health Promotion, www.health.gov

TABLE 5-2   ## Estimated Caloric Needs for Men by Age and Activity

Age	Sedentary	Moderately Active	Active
18	2,400	2,800	3,200
19–20	2,600	2,800	3,000
21–25	2,400	2,800	3,000
26–35	2,400	2,600	3,000
36–40	2,400	2,600	2,800
41–45	2,200	2,600	2,800
46–55	2,200	2,400	2,800
56–60	2,200	2,400	2,600
61–65	2,000	2,400	2,600
66–75	2,000	2,200	2,600
76 and up	2,000	2,200	2,400

Source: Office of Disease Prevention and Health Promotion, www.health.gov

TIP

Tables 5-1 and 5-2 consider only three variables: gender, age, and activity level. Therefore, they approximate your caloric needs. Apps and online calculators that also consider your height and weight can provide a more accurate estimate of actual needs:

>> See the United States Department of Agriculture's list of medical calculators available at https://fnic.nal.usda.gov/dietary-guidance/interactive-tools/calculators-and-counters.

>> Calculate exact body mass index (BMI) online at this link or using any other BMI calculator: www.nhlbi.nih.gov/health/educational/lose_wt/BMI/bmi-m.htm. Find out more about BMI in the next section.

Adjusting calories for your weight target

Body mass index (BMI) compares weight to height and is an easy tool for estimating weight status for men and women, as shown in Figure 5-1. Locate your height in the left column and follow the horizontal line to the right to find the weight that is closest to your weight. From that weight, follow the column directly up to find your BMI.

BMI → Height (inches) ↓	19	20	21	22	23	24	25	26	27	28	29	30	35	40
	Weight (pounds)													
58	91	96	100	105	110	115	119	124	129	134	138	143	167	191
59	94	99	104	109	114	119	124	129	133	138	143	148	173	198
60	97	102	107	112	118	123	128	133	138	143	148	153	179	204
61	100	106	111	116	122	127	132	137	143	148	153	158	185	211
62	104	109	115	120	126	131	136	142	147	153	158	164	191	218
63	107	113	118	124	130	135	141	146	152	158	163	169	197	225
64	110	116	122	128	134	140	145	151	157	163	169	174	204	232
65	114	120	126	132	138	144	150	156	162	168	174	180	210	240
66	118	124	130	136	142	148	155	161	167	173	179	186	216	247
67	121	127	134	140	146	153	159	166	172	178	185	191	223	255
68	125	131	138	144	151	158	164	171	177	184	190	197	230	262
69	128	135	142	149	155	162	169	176	182	189	196	203	236	270
70	132	139	146	153	160	167	174	181	188	195	202	209	243	278
71	136	143	150	157	165	172	179	186	193	200	208	215	250	286
72	140	147	154	162	169	177	184	191	199	206	213	221	258	294
73	144	151	159	166	174	182	189	197	204	212	219	227	265	302
74	148	155	163	171	179	186	194	202	210	218	225	233	272	311
75	152	160	168	176	184	192	200	208	216	224	232	240	279	319
76	156	164	172	180	189	197	205	213	221	230	238	246	287	328

FIGURE 5-1: Body mass index table.

© John Wiley & Sons, Inc.

The key to interpreting BMI is as follows:

BMI	Weight Status
Below 18.5	Underweight
18.5–24.9	Healthy or normal weight
25–29.9	Overweight
30 and above	Obese

REMEMBER

Keep in mind that BMI doesn't differentiate between lean muscle and body fat. A muscular athlete might have a high BMI but be totally fit. The calorie target in Table 5-1 (for women) or Table 5-2 (for men) is the number of calories needed to *maintain your current weight.* If you desire weight loss based on your BMI result, you should reduce your caloric intake. One pound of body fat stores about 3,500 calories. Weight loss occurs when you consume fewer calories than you burn. To lose one pound per week, you would need to use 500 calories from body fat stores each day. For example, if Table 5-1 indicated you need 2,000 calories per day to stay the same weight, then you could consume 1,500 calories per day to lose weight. Tapping into 500 calories from body fat every day would lead to losing one pound per week. If you only reduce your intake by 250 calories per day, you can be on your way to losing half a pound per week.

Deciding on carb intake targets

I discuss the Dietary Reference Intakes (DRI) for Americans earlier in this chapter. The DRI minimum for carbohydrate is 130 grams per day, and the suggested carb intake range is calculated at 45–65 percent of caloric targets. Some people with diabetes opt to go somewhat lower, such as 40 percent. Targets should be individualized based on preference and health considerations.

After you've estimated your caloric needs using Table 5-1 or Table 5-2 or by using an online calorie calculator, you're ready to use the chart in Figure 5-2 to estimate carbohydrate intake targets. Find your desired calorie level in the left column. Decide what percentage of your daily calories you want to allocate to carbohydrate as indicated along the top row, from 40–65 percent. (Note the suggested minimum carb intake per DRI guidelines is 130 grams per day, so the table doesn't go below that number.)

Calorie Level	Number of Suggested Grams of Carb per Day Based on Percentage of Calories Coming from Carbs)					
	40%	45%	50%	55%	60%	65%
1,200	130	135	150	165	180	195
1,300	130	146	163	179	195	211
1,400	140	158	175	193	210	228
1,500	150	169	188	206	225	244
1,600	160	180	200	220	240	260
1,700	170	191	213	234	255	276
1,800	180	203	225	248	270	293
1,900	190	214	238	261	285	309
2,000	200	225	250	275	300	325
2,100	210	236	263	289	315	341
2,200	220	248	275	303	330	358
2,300	230	259	288	316	345	374
2,400	240	270	300	330	360	390
2,500	250	281	313	344	375	406
2,600	260	293	325	358	390	423
2,700	270	304	338	371	405	439
2,800	280	315	350	385	420	455

FIGURE 5-2:
Daily carb intake targets by calorie levels.

© John Wiley & Sons, Inc.

REMEMBER

If your blood-glucose levels are running above target, it may be wise to choose a lower level of carb until control improves. Gaining control of your diabetes may require diet modifications, exercise, and medications. Once medications are properly adjusted, I usually suggest starting with 45–50 percent of daily calories as carbs. If you prefer a lower carb intake, 40–50 percent is fine. The lowest carb intake in the table is 130 grams per day to comply with the minimum dietary intake recommended by the National Institutes of Health. If you're active and can control blood-glucose levels while eating more carbs, then you may aim for carb intakes of 50–55 percent of calories. It may be difficult to control blood-glucose levels with 60–65 percent of your calories from carb unless you are an athlete who is getting a lot of exercise.

Here's an example using Figure 5-2: Consider a moderately active person who wants to eat 1,600 calories each day and opts for 40–50 percent of calories to come from carbs. Locate the 1,600-calorie level in the far left column. Find the column headings for 40–50 percent. Line up the horizontal 1,600 calorie line with the vertical 40–50 percent columns. The daily carb intake goal would be 160–200 grams. Blood-glucose levels will be best controlled if the carbs are budgeted between meals and snacks. (See the next section for more information.)

Distributing carb intake

Having a daily carb budget in mind is helpful, but even more helpful is to have an idea of how many carbs to eat at each meal and snack. (Snacks are *not required*.) Consider two women who each have chosen to aim for 150 grams of carb per day. They both have type 2 diabetes and take the same type of oral medication.

>> Natalie skips breakfast, has 30 grams of carb for lunch, and then she eats the remaining 120 grams of carb for dinner. Not surprisingly, she has significant blood-glucose elevations in the evening.

>> Cassie, on the other hand, divides her carbs more evenly and has 40 grams of carb at breakfast, 50 grams at lunch, and 60 grams at dinner. She finds it much easier to control her blood-glucose levels because she spreads her carb intake into manageable amounts.

See Chapter 6 for guidelines on establishing carb intake targets at meals.

Leaving room on your plate for protein and fat

Although this chapter focuses on establishing a reasonable carbohydrate intake, a balanced diet also requires appropriate intakes of protein and fat. It pays to limit saturated fats, so opt for lean protein sources. The type of fat found in fatty cuts of meat is linked to heart disease. A reasonable portion of meat is roughly the same size as the palm of your hand. Another heart-healthy tip is to choose liquid oils in place of solid fats.

Chapter 8 provides portioning tips, and Chapter 13 elaborates on choosing healthy foods. See Appendix A for a list of lean proteins and heart-healthy fats. See Part 5 for menu ideas.

WHY DEALING WITH HIGH-CARB MEALS CAN BE HARD

Type 2 diabetes means your insulin doesn't work as well as it should. The more carb you eat at one time, the higher the blood glucose is likely to go because glucose levels build up in the blood while waiting for their turn to get transported into the cells. It can take many hours for the elevated glucose levels to resolve. (See Chapter 4 for more details.)

Even if you take pills to treat your diabetes, you still need to limit how much carb you consume at one time. You can out-eat any medication, including insulin. Even insulin has its limitations. The action times of the insulin and the digestion timing of the meal must match so that the insulin is working while the foods are digesting. (See Chapter 6 for more on the importance of timing.)

Carbohydrates are a very important part of a balanced diet, but they are best tolerated when distributed between three main meals. Small snacks may be included if you're hungry between meals or as needed to support exercise or prevent hypoglycemia.

Tweaking Your Carb Intake Target When Conditions Change

Carbohydrate requirements can change throughout life. Your carb demands may even change seasonally if your activity levels vary according to the time of year. The following sections explore situations that may call for making adjustments to your carb intakes.

Changing needs throughout the life cycle

Childhood and adolescence are times when dietary needs are constantly changing. It is important that children with diabetes get the same amount of nutrition and carbs as recommended for all children. Hormones and changing activity patterns call for more frequent visits with the diabetes team to make sure insulin and other medications are adjusted as needed to support a balanced and adequate diet.

Pregnancy and breastfeeding increase the demand for carbohydrates and other nutrients, so close monitoring is required with a team of experts who specialize in high-risk pregnancies.

Elderly individuals typically see a decrease in their calorie and carbohydrate needs as metabolism changes. Their vitamin and mineral needs don't shift much, however, so they need to focus on nutrient-dense food choices.

Flip to Chapter 17 for details on managing diabetes during different life stages.

Altering intake to account for activity

Varying activity is a typical reason for adjusting carb intake. Exercise uses up more calories in the forms of carb and fat, so needs change on active days. If you aren't at risk for hypoglycemia, you may not need or want a snack, especially if you're trying to lose weight. If you're at risk for low blood glucose due to insulin use or other medications, you can monitor blood-glucose levels to decide whether you need to add a snack to prevent hypoglycemia. You should always carry carbs to eat as needed and quick forms of sugar or juice for treating lows. Insulin doses can be adjusted on active days to reduce the risk of hypoglycemia. Speak to your health-care provider for tips on medication. For more info on exercise, see Chapter 14.

Adjusting portions when blood glucose is out of control

The American Diabetes Association sets pre-meal blood-glucose targets at 70–130 milligrams per deciliter (mg/dl) and post-meal blood-glucose targets at under 180 mg/dl. What should you do if your blood glucose level is significantly elevated, perhaps even above 180 mg/dl *before* eating?

REMEMBER

Your own insulin, as well as any insulin that is injected, doesn't work as effectively when you're hyperglycemic. Follow your doctor's advice about how to adjust insulin to correct glucose elevations. Limit carbs and fill up more on salad, non-starchy vegetables, and protein foods to give your blood glucose a chance to return to target levels. If you're frequently above target before meals, you likely need a medication tune-up and should see your doctor for advice. You can't be expected to skip carbs on a regular basis.

Managing sick days

REMEMBER

Being sick can make diabetes management a real challenge. Talk to your health-care providers in advance to make a plan about how to manage illness. Your body responds to illness with stress hormones, which can cause blood-glucose levels to rise. Monitor your blood-glucose levels more frequently when you're sick. People with type 1 diabetes should be monitoring their glucose levels *at least every four hours,* and people with type 2 should check at least four times daily when sick.

Illness increases the risk of producing ketones, so people with type 1 diabetes should have supplies for checking ketones. You're less likely to have ketones if you have type 2 diabetes, but it is possible if you're very ill.

Stick to your usual meal plan if possible. Staying hydrated is important, but that can be difficult to do if you have vomiting or diarrhea. Keep sipping fluids. Choose noncarb fluids, including water, diet drinks, broth, and tea. If you can't eat normal foods, try substituting bland foods such as crackers, toast, cooked cereals, boiled potatoes, soups, yogurt, pudding, applesauce, and canned fruits.

If you can't handle solids, get your carbs from liquids, such as diluted fruit juices, sports drinks, gelatin, popsicles, sherbet, and soft drinks (regular — not diet — in this case).

WARNING

Vomiting, diarrhea, persistently elevated blood-glucose levels, difficulty breathing, dehydration, or having ketones are all reasons to seek medical attention.

REMEMBER

Discuss sick-day management with your doctor. Make a plan in advance. Ask your doctor for the appropriate phone numbers for whom to contact after hours and on weekends. Don't stop taking your diabetes medications when you're sick. Illness can cause blood-glucose levels to rise even if you aren't able to keep any food down. People with type 1 diabetes may require even higher than usual doses of insulin during illness.

Chapter **6**

Timing Your Carb Consumption

C hapter 5 provides assessment tools to help determine *daily* carbohydrate intake targets. But knowing how much carb to eat in a day is only part of the picture. It's equally important to distribute the carb budget between meals, and possibly snacks, throughout the day. Blood glucose can be difficult to control if too much carb is consumed at one time. This chapter helps you establish a reasonable carb intake target for individual meals.

This chapter also explains the relationship between food and some of the medications used to treat diabetes. Whether you are controlling your diabetes with diet alone, pills, insulin, or a combination of medications, there is a lot to be said for timing. *How much* you eat is one factor, but *when* you eat is another. In order to optimize blood-glucose control, the timing of meals and meds is critical. If you use insulin, it's especially important to grasp insulin action profiles for the specific types of insulin you use. Carb intake and insulin must be strategically balanced to assure safety and effectiveness. Discuss managing your meals and meds with your healthcare provider to get personalized advice.

Distributing Your Daily Carb Intake

Achieving blood-glucose control is easier if you eat reasonable portions and distribute your carbohydrate intake throughout the day instead of overeating at one time. This section explains the importance of carbohydrate distribution and meal timing.

WARNING

Skipping meals is not advised. Missing breakfast or lunch often leads to overeating later in the day. Excessive carb intakes at dinner can drive blood-glucose levels way up. Hyperglycemia in the evening can be slower to resolve because many people are less active at that time of day.

Striving to eat three meals per day

A balanced meal that contains carbohydrate, protein, and fat typically takes about four hours to fully digest, with the highest blood-glucose level around one to two hours after eating. Some foods, such as yogurt and fruit, digest quicker than that, while other foods digest slower. Deep-fried and fatty meals can take longer to digest because fat delays digestion. In Chapter 4 I explain that as a meal digests, some of the glucose becomes available for immediate use but that glucose is also delivered to the liver and muscles to be stored as glycogen. Glycogen stored in the muscles can be used later, but only by the muscles. Glycogen stored in the liver can be released as needed and shared with the other cells and organs throughout the body.

REMEMBER

Eating three meals and spacing them roughly four to six hours apart keeps a steady supply of glucose and nutrients available to the body. An example of well-spaced meals would be breakfast at 8 a.m., lunch at 1 p.m., and dinner at 6 p.m. There is certainly room for personal preference, and you don't have to start your day at 8 a.m. The main idea is that once you have breakfast, whatever time that happens to be, aim to have lunch four to six hours later, and then dinner four to six hours after lunch. Meals are typically finished digesting in about four hours, so your liver will tide you over between meals by releasing glucose from glycogen storage as needed until the next carbs are consumed.

Chapter 5 provides guidelines for establishing daily carbohydrate intake targets. Once you have a sense of how many carbs your body needs in a day, you can then decide how to divvy up the carbs into separate meals. Table 6-1 is designed to help you establish a reasonable mealtime carb target. The recommended carb ranges are based on gender and variables such as age, caloric needs, and activity. Consider the criteria in the left column when picking your carb intake target.

TABLE 6-1   **Establishing Mealtime Carb Targets**

Women	Grams of Carb Each Meal
Calorie controlled; for middle- to older-age, less-active women	30–60 grams
Maintenance calories; for younger to middle-age, moderately active women	45–75 grams
Higher calorie; for young women and active exercisers	60–90 grams (possibly more)
Men	**Grams of Carb Each Meal**
Calorie controlled; for middle- to older- age, less-active men	45–75 grams
Maintenance calories; for younger to middle-age, moderately active men	60–90 grams
Higher calorie; for young men and active exercisers	75–105 grams (possibly more)

Carb targets are expressed in ranges. A range allows for flexibility and variation in appetite, activity, and blood-glucose trends. For example, if you choose a range that calls for 45 to 75 grams of carb *per meal*, the assumption is that you will have three meals per day and each meal will have between 45 and 75 grams of carb. For example, breakfast could have 45 grams of carb, lunch might contain 60 grams of carb, and you could have another 55 grams of carb at dinner. All three meals are within the carb-range budget.

REMEMBER

Saving up the carbs from one meal to have a bigger amount at a different meal doesn't really work. You shouldn't skip lunch and have twice as much at dinner. The point is to distribute carbs in manageable amounts throughout the day. The range sets an upper and lower limit of how many carbs to eat at each meal. Having diabetes inherently makes it difficult to tolerate very large carb intakes in one sitting. You're bound to benefit from spacing out your meals and controlling your portions, whether you take diabetes medications or not. Having a mealtime carb budget that you stick with most of the time helps stabilize blood-glucose levels. If the higher end of the range isn't well-tolerated, aim for the lower end of the range.

Opting for smaller meals with controlled snacks

Some people find it easier to control post-meal blood-glucose spikes by eating four to five smaller meals per day rather than three main meals. You may choose to distribute your daily carb intake into three smaller meals and one or two between-meal snacks. Plan to wait at least two hours after a meal before adding a carb-containing snack. If you face a long period of time between lunch and dinner, having a snack midway between the meals may be beneficial. An afternoon snack may curb hunger and help with portion control at dinner. Going into dinner ravenously hungry can lead to overeating.

For example, if you're aiming for 160–200 grams of carb per day, you can have three meals with 45 grams of carb each and two snacks with 20 grams of carb each. Such a pattern equals 175 grams of carb total. You have room for some flexibility while staying within the daily carb target range. (See Chapter 5 to choose your daily carb intake range.)

TIP

It's fine to fit in a noncarb snack whenever you desire (as long as excess calories aren't leading to unwanted weight gain). String cheese, for example, doesn't raise blood glucose, so it can be an "anytime" snack.

By definition, snacks are supposed to be small. It can be easy to get carried away. A snack with up to 15–20 grams of carb is reasonable. You may tolerate a snack with 30 grams of carb, especially if you are fitting in a walk or some form of activity.

REMEMBER

Be mindful of your snacking. It all adds up. Read labels. Don't eat directly out of a multi-serve container or you may end up eating multiple servings. If you do consume too many carbs while snacking, your blood-glucose level at the next mealtime may be higher than desired. If your blood glucose is already elevated when you eat your meal, your glucose levels will likely climb even further. Plenty of snacks have few or no carbs. Raw veggies are low in carbs and calories. Dipping veggies in Ranch dressing or scooping up guacamole won't increase the carb count much at all (just the calories). Cottage cheese, a hard-boiled egg, or a few nuts can curb hunger without driving up blood-glucose levels. For more carb-controlled snack ideas, see Chapter 22.

Stabilizing Blood-Glucose Levels at Breakfast and Dinner

The following practical pointers regarding the first meal of the day and the last meal of the day may help you stabilize blood-glucose levels.

Breaking your fast: The importance of breakfast

TECHNICAL
STUFF

Some people say breakfast is the most important meal of the day. There are lots of reasons to eat breakfast:

>> Research has shown that people who eat breakfast have a mental edge with enhanced memory, attention, reasoning, creativity, and problem-solving skills.

>> Children who eat breakfast consistently perform better at mental tasks.

>> Many studies show that eating breakfast is actually correlated with a reduced incidence of obesity.

There is usually a long period of time without food in the hours between dinner and breakfast. The last meal of the previous day is done digesting in a few short hours. When the final meal has digested, you survive on the glucose that was previously stored as glycogen in your liver. Once glycogen reserves are gone, your body resorts to the starvation mode of metabolism, which means you turn your muscles and body fat into fuel. Going 8 to 10 hours without food isn't unusual, but skipping breakfast can easily increase the period of fasting to 12 or more hours, which is too long. Breakfast breaks that cycle. (See Chapter 4 to find out more about how the liver is able to create glucose out of muscle and ketones out of fat.)

The hormones that direct the liver to release glucose from glycogen stores are called *counter-regulatory hormones.* These hormones surge at or before dawn and cause transient insulin resistance, which may contribute to elevations in fasting blood-glucose levels. Your healthcare provider can assess the need for medication adjustments to resolve this problem. If you find your blood-glucose levels are more difficult to control at the morning meal, then choose breakfast foods that contain complex carbohydrates, such as oatmeal or whole-grain toast, and pair them with protein such as eggs or peanut butter. Breakfast foods and fluids that digest rapidly can lead to steeper rises in blood glucose. (See Chapter 10 for more about the variables affecting digestion rates and glucose control.)

Considering the merits of an earlier dinner

Type 2 diabetes is characteristic of insulin resistance. Insulin sensitivity is enhanced with physical activity. A moving and contracting muscle is a muscle that is burning glucose. If you go to bed shortly after eating, your muscles will be relaxed and therefore less able to help your insulin transport glucose. Any activity after a meal helps muscles use glucose. Exercise, an after-dinner walk, or even light housekeeping improves the way insulin works.

A meal takes about four hours to fully digest, with blood-glucose levels peaking about one to two hours after eating. If your blood-glucose peaks are above target when you go to bed, you may find that blood glucose stays higher all night and potentially contributes to elevated fasting-glucose levels the next day. If that is an issue for you, try to eat dinner about three to four hours before going to sleep. For example, if you go to bed at 10 p.m., eat dinner by 6 or 7 p.m.

Understanding Insulin Action

When the pancreas is working properly, it produces just the right amount of insulin to keep blood glucose controlled within a fairly narrow range. People who do not have diabetes have blood-glucose levels between 70 and 140 milligrams per deciliter (mg/dl) all the time, regardless of what they eat. "Normal" fasting blood glucose is 70–99 mg/dl. Post-meal blood-glucose levels remain below 140 mg/dl if you don't have diabetes.

REMEMBER

The American Diabetes Association (ADA) recommends fasting and pre-meal blood-glucose levels of 80–130 mg/dl. The ADA suggests peak post-meal blood-glucose levels below 180 mg/dl. Notice the ADA is not suggesting that everyone with diabetes should achieve normal nondiabetic blood-glucose levels. Blood-glucose targets are lower during pregnancy and may be less stringent in other situations. Discuss your personal blood-glucose targets with your healthcare providers.

As you find out in Chapter 4, carbohydrate-containing foods digest and turn into glucose, which then enters the bloodstream. A functioning pancreas produces a surge of insulin to match the amount of carbohydrate in the meal. Some glucose is stored in the liver and the muscles as glycogen. During extended periods of time without food, such as while you sleep, the liver releases glucose from glycogen storage because the body needs a steady supply of glucose. A working pancreas releases just enough insulin to match the glucose that is being slowly released from the liver.

Insulin replacement therapy for someone with type 1 diabetes should mimic physiologic insulin as closely as possible. Rapid-acting or short-acting insulins are used to cover the carbs at mealtime. Intermediate-acting or long-acting insulins are used to cover the glucose that is released from the liver between meals. Insulin types and action times are covered in this section.

Comparing insulin options

Everyone with type 1 diabetes and many people with type 2 diabetes use insulin. Insulin is typically administered with insulin syringes, insulin pens, or an insulin pump. Type 1 diabetes treatment requires the use of two types of insulin unless an insulin pump is used (I discuss pumping insulin later in this chapter). There must always be baseline insulin, typically one of the long-acting insulin options. In addition, insulin is needed to handle the carbohydrate in meals. Rapid-acting insulin options are the best match for the digestion timing of meals.

See Table 6-2 for a list of the insulins currently on the market. To better grasp the way insulin works, use Table 6-2 to locate the type of insulin you use in the left column and then note the action times to the right. The key differences have to do with the onset, peak, and duration times. To clarify further:

» **Onset:** The time before the insulin reaches the bloodstream to begin working

» **Peak:** The time that the insulin is working at maximum strength

» **Duration:** How long the insulin continues to lower blood glucose

TABLE 6-2 **Insulin Action Profiles**

Insulin	Onset	Peak	Duration
Rapid-Acting: Lispro (Humalog); Aspart (NovoLog); Glulisine (Apidra)	15 minutes	1 hour	Under 5 hours
Regular or Short-Acting: Humulin R; Novolin R	30 minutes	2–3 hours	5–8 hours
Intermediate-Acting (NPH): Humulin N; Novolin N	2–4 hours	4–10 hours	10–16 hours
Long-Acting: Detemir (Levemir); Glargine (Lantus, Basaglar, Toujeo)	2 or more hours	Minimal	Up to 24 hours
Degludec (Tresiba)	1 hour	Minimal	At least 42 hours

Checking out concentrated insulins

The standard concentration for insulin in the United States is U100, which means 100 units of insulin per milliliter. The following insulin products offer more-concentrated versions so you use a smaller volume of insulin to get the same number of units:

» **Humulin Regular** offers U500, which is a version that is five times the concentration of Regular insulin. There are 500 units per milliliter.

» **Lispro (Humalog)** offers a U200 version with 200 units of insulin per milliliter.

» **Toujeo U300** is a more concentrated form of glargine. It has 300 units of insulin per milliliter.

» **Degludec (Tresiba)** offers two concentrations: U100 with 100 units per milliliter and U200 with 200 units per milliliter.

Looking at blended insulin preparations

In addition to the concentrated insulins in the preceding section, there are also combination insulins. Rapid- or short-acting insulin is blended with intermediate- or long-acting insulin in one solution. The mixture is a set percentage. For example, 70/30 is 70 percent intermediate-acting insulin mixed with 30 percent rapid- or short-acting insulin. In this instance, 10 units of 70/30 would provide 7 units of intermediate-acting insulin, and 3 units of rapid- or short-acting insulin. When you increase or decrease the dose, you change the amounts of both types of insulin in the blend. If you want, or need, to independently adjust the components, you need separate bottles of the two types of insulin.

The blended insulin options include

» 70/30 with NPH and Regular

» 50/50 with NPH and Regular

» 70/30 with insulin aspart protamine and Aspart

» 75/25 or 50/50 with insulin lispro protamine and Lispro

» 70/30 with Degludec and Aspart

Combination insulins are typically administered twice daily: one injection before breakfast and one before dinner.

» **The morning injection** provides insulin coverage for breakfast (the rapid- or short-acting part kicks in first), and the intermediate-acting insulin provides the second peak effect, which covers the carbs in lunch. The pros: One shot covers two meals and you don't have to draw up and mix two types of insulin in the same syringe. The cons: You are locked into a specific lunch meal in both *timing and amount of carb*. The insulin that is injected in the morning is set to peak at lunch, and there is no stopping it.

» **The pre-dinner injection** covers the carbs in the dinner and the glucose that is released from the liver overnight.

I provide more info on managing meals with blended insulin later in this chapter.

REMEMBER

You cannot fine-tune doses, because increasing or decreasing the dose affects both types of insulin in the blend. For that reason, blended insulin preparations are not ideal for managing type 1 diabetes; however, they may be appropriate for certain people with type 2 diabetes. Your medical professionals can help personalize an insulin plan that is best for you.

Pumping and inhaling insulin

An insulin pump, which is worn externally, is a programmable device that delivers insulin continually via an *infusion set* (small catheter), which is inserted under the skin into fatty tissue. The infusion set is typically replaced every two to three days. Some pumps are waterproof and submersible, while others have a quick-release to remove the pump for bathing. Numerous pumps are on the market, and their features vary.

An insulin pump holds only one type of insulin (rapid-acting), but it has two main modes of insulin delivery:

>> The *basal rate* is a programmable rate of insulin that is delivered continuously. It replaces the need for intermediate- and long-acting insulins. Insulin delivery patterns can be customized to an individual's needs considering things such as exercise and hormonal fluctuations.

>> The *bolus mode* of delivery refers to the amount of insulin that is needed for a meal as determined by carbohydrate counting, or for correcting blood-glucose elevations. The pump user presses a button to deliver the desired amount of bolus insulin.

REMEMBER

Individualized carbohydrate ratios and correction ratios are programmed into the pump. You just need to let the pump know what your blood-glucose level is and how many carbs you plan to eat, and the pump does the math. The pump has a memory that tracks total daily insulin administration, and data is downloadable for computer printout. Pump initiation requires a prescription and a team of experts to train and monitor the pump user.

Afrezza is an inhaled version of rapid-acting insulin. It is used in combination with long-acting insulin. It begins working within 5 minutes (onset), reaches maximum strength in 12 to 15 minutes (peak), and is done working in about three hours (duration).

THE APPROVAL OF THE FIRST HYBRID CLOSED-LOOP SYSTEM

September of 2016 marked a historic advancement in the management of type 1 diabetes. The FDA approved the MiniMed 670G — the first hybrid closed-loop system in the world. The device combines two current technologies: an insulin pump and a continuous glucose monitor. What has changed is that the two technologies are now being allowed to "talk to each other."

- The pump can adjust basal insulin delivery according to the blood-glucose fluctuations detected by the sensor. Insulin delivery will automatically suspend if blood-glucose levels fall too low. Automated insulin adjustments minimize high- and low-glucose levels. The user still needs to count carbs and enter the amount of carbs into the pump. The pump then calculates the correct insulin dose for the food and displays the recommended dose. The user just needs to "accept" the dose.

- Finger-stick blood-glucose monitoring is still indicated for calibrating the sensor and making insulin bolusing decisions.

The system is approved for nonpregnant adults and youth 14 years and older who have type 1 diabetes. The approval of the device, which is slated to be available in the spring of 2017, marks a significant milestone.

Coordinating Insulin Action with Meals

Rapid-acting and short-acting insulins are used to cover the blood-glucose rise after a meal. Insulin doses and action times need to match the amount of carb and the timing of digestion. This section explains two common approaches to determining how much insulin to take at mealtimes: insulin-to-carb ratios (ICR) and sliding-scale insulin (SSI). Blended insulins, such as 70/30 insulin, impose the need to be regimented with mealtimes and carbohydrate intake amounts, as I explain in detail.

WARNING

This section provides *examples* of insulin dosing. Actual insulin requirements vary greatly from one person to the next. Do *not* change your insulin regimen based on the theoretical discussion in this book. Speak to your diabetes specialist about your insulin plan.

Enjoying the flexibility of insulin-to-carb ratios

Insulin-to-carb ratios allow for flexibility in carb intake. The general concept is that 1 unit of rapid- or short-acting insulin will "cover" a set amount of carb. For example, a ratio of 1:10 means 1 unit covers 10 grams of carb, and a ratio of 1:15 means 1 unit covers 15 grams of carb. The mealtime or snack dose is determined by the amount of carbohydrate planned as well as the ratio. For example, consider a meal with 60 grams of carb. The recommended dose could vary for three different people. A person with a ratio of 1:10 would take 6 units for 60 grams of carb. Someone else might be on a 1:12 ratio and need 5 units, and yet another person might be on a 1:15 ratio and need 4 units.

Ratios can also change within the day for the same person. Morning hormonal surges can cause insulin resistance at that time of day, so a stronger ratio may be required at breakfast than is needed for lunch or dinner. For example, a person might need a ratio of 1:10 at breakfast but 1:15 at lunch and dinner. Ratios can also vary on active versus sedentary days.

The insulin-to-carb ratio only covers the carbs in the meal. It doesn't address the current blood-glucose level. If blood glucose is above target range at mealtime, a correction ratio is also needed. This ratio can vary from one person to the next. For the sake of providing an example, say someone needs 1 unit of rapid-acting insulin for every 50 mg/dl their blood glucose is elevated above a target pre-meal number. If the blood-glucose target is set at 120 mg/dl but the pre-meal blood glucose is 220 mg/dl, then a person with a correction ratio of 1 to 50 would take 2 units for the correction (here's the math: 220 minus 120 is 100; 100 divided by 50 is 2).

REMEMBER

When using insulin-to-carb ratios, the mealtime insulin dose is *the sum* of the two separate calculations: the amount of insulin needed for the food (insulin-to-carb ratio) *plus* the amount of insulin needed to bring blood-glucose levels back into target range (known as the correction ratio or the insulin sensitivity factor).

The benefit of using ratios is that you can adjust your own dose according to how much you want to eat. You aren't locked into eating the exact same amount of carb at every meal of every day. Ratios also allow you to make corrections to blood-glucose levels. Use a calculator if needed; most phones have one. It's a new skill, and it takes some practice.

REMEMBER

Get your doctor's advice on how to initiate ratios. After you start using ratios, you'll want to assess how well the ratios are working. Figuring out what your ratios should be takes a little trial and error. Gather data. Record the pre-meal blood glucose, the carb count, and the dose of insulin. Be sure to count carbs as accurately as possible. Check blood-glucose levels again about four hours after the meal to see whether your level is near target. Gather and review at least one to two weeks' worth of data in order to fine-tune the ratios. Keep in mind other variables can affect blood-glucose results. Blood-glucose levels may be lower after exercise and higher if you're sick or stressed. There will always be some variability in blood-glucose results simply because injected insulin isn't quite the same as a pancreas that does it all for you automatically.

Keeping carbs consistent when using sliding-scale insulin dosing

Sliding-scale insulin dosing isn't as precise as using ratios (see the preceding section), but it may be simpler. Sliding-scale insulin is when your insulin dose is based solely on your current blood-glucose level. Your medical provider designs a dosing scale, and the number of units of insulin recommended increases incrementally as blood-glucose levels rise.

Table 6-3 shows a glimpse of what the layout of a sliding-scale insulin regimen may look like. This sort of insulin dosing plan relies on having the same amount of carb at each meal. The need for a pre-set and consistent carb budget is often overlooked. The dose of insulin injected can't possibly cover the carbs in every meal consumed if carb intakes are variable. For example, a dose of 6 units may be too much insulin for a low-carb meal but may not be enough insulin for a high-carb meal.

TABLE 6-3 **Example of Sliding-Scale Insulin**

Blood Glucose	Units of Insulin
70–100	The doctor would fill in for your needs.
101–150	. . .
151–200	. . .
And so on . . .	. . .

TIP

While sliding-scale dosing is simpler, it doesn't erase the need to understand how to quantify carbohydrate portions. See Chapter 7 to brush up on label reading and Chapter 8 to find out how to count carbs.

Basing injection timing on pre-meal blood-glucose levels

Rapid-acting insulin is designed to be injected five to ten minutes before eating a meal. If pre-meal blood-glucose levels are running higher than desired, injecting a few minutes earlier may help by giving the insulin a head start at lowering glucose levels. If you check your blood glucose 20–30 minutes before the meal, you'll have the opportunity to inject early if desired. The insulin then has a chance to lower the blood glucose somewhat before the pending meal digests and adds even more glucose to an already elevated level. On the flip side, if pre-meal blood-glucose levels are lower than desired, you may opt to eat half of the meal before injecting the rapid-acting insulin to give the food a head start. (For pre-meal hypoglycemia, treat the low blood glucose as described in Chapter 15.) Regular insulin is slow to get started and is always supposed to be injected 30 minutes before the meal. However, if blood-glucose levels are elevated, it can be injected 45 minutes before the meal. Most people aren't in the habit of stopping to check blood glucose a full 45–60 minutes prior to eating, which makes using regular insulin less convenient than rapid-acting insulin.

Being regimented if you use 70/30 insulin

I discuss blended insulin options in the earlier section "Looking at blended insulin preparations." There are several different blends, but all contain a mixture of two different insulins: a longer-acting type and a shorter-acting type.

Figure 6-1 illustrates the action profile of 70/30 insulin. The horizontal axis is a 24-hour timeline that shows the onset, peak, and duration times of the insulin. This figure illustrates the insulin action timing of two injections of 70/30 insulin — specifically, the blend with rapid-acting and intermediate-acting insulins.

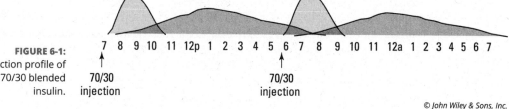

FIGURE 6-1: Action profile of 70/30 blended insulin.

© John Wiley & Sons, Inc.

The first injection is at 7 a.m. The blended insulin has two phases of action:

>> The rapid-acting portion covers the breakfast meal and wears off by 11 a.m.

>> The intermediate-acting portion doesn't even begin to work for almost two hours. It then works over a sweeping length of time. You can see by the darker shading that it ramps up and works before, during, and after lunch.

REMEMBER

One critical thing to remember is that it's necessary to eat lunch about four to six hours after the morning injection because the intermediate-acting insulin is set to peak. You need to provide carbs to go with it. The second point to keep in mind is that the dose of insulin doesn't vary, so the amount of carb needs to be consistent every day. You can't eat a low-carb salad one day and a carb-heavy pasta meal with garlic toast the next day.

The second injection of the day in this example is at 6 p.m. The rapid-acting part (indicated by the light shading) covers dinner and the intermediate-acting portion of the blend (indicated by the darker shading) works while you're sleeping. As described in Chapter 4, the liver releases glucose all night long. The glucose coming out of the liver is covered by the intermediate-acting portion of the blended insulin. If the dose is appropriately set, you shouldn't get hypoglycemic overnight.

WARNING

Some people with type 2 diabetes do fine with this regimen because the blended insulin adds a layer of help to the insulin already being made in the body. Twice-daily injections of blended insulin are less than ideal for someone with type 1 diabetes, however, because the insulin can't be fine-tuned adequately. Notice also that the insulin wears off fairly early in the morning (by 7–8 a.m. in this example), which means someone with type 1 diabetes would "run out" of insulin and start making ketones if she didn't get up and take another injection — so no sleeping in.

Another issue is that most people release a surge of hormones in the pre-dawn hours, and those hormones can cause blood-glucose levels to rise. It's known as the *dawn phenomenon.* Hormones cause blood glucose to rise in two ways: Hormones can stimulate the liver to release extra glucose, and hormones can increase insulin resistance, so insulin doesn't work as well. The net result can lead to elevated fasting blood-glucose levels. Instead of using blended insulin, some people inject the rapid-acting and intermediate- or long-acting insulins separately, enabling doses to be independently adjusted. Given the option, it is usually more effective to inject NPH insulin at bedtime rather than at dinnertime. That way the NPH peaks later and lasts longer into the morning hours, which can improve fasting blood-glucose levels.

There are pros and cons when using blended insulins. Insulin dosing plans need to be carefully crafted with the help of a medical provider well-versed in managing diabetes.

Managing Carbs on Oral Diabetes Meds

Some people with type 2 diabetes are treated with a combination of insulin and oral agents (pills), while others take only insulin, only pills, or nothing at all. Numerous oral medications are currently available for treating diabetes, with more yet to come. There are injectable medications other than insulin. This section reviews the importance of dietary diligence when using diabetes pills.

Review your medications with your healthcare provider. Ask *when* you should take your doses and what to do if you miss a dose. Some pills should be taken *before* the meal, while others are best tolerated *with* the meal. Find out whether the meds you take have the potential to cause hypoglycemia.

Keeping the carbs appropriate

If blood-glucose levels aren't being controlled by lifestyle modifications, medications may be needed to manage type 2 diabetes. Many medications are available, which may be used alone or in combination. Long-standing type 2 diabetes often requires several medications to successfully reach blood-glucose targets. Eat a healthy, balanced diet with adequate carbs. Don't overdo carb intake because excessive carb loads make the pancreas have to work too hard. But don't undereat carbs either. Use Chapter 5 to find the right amount of carbs for you.

Blood-glucose levels that are persistently elevated (when eating an appropriate amount of carb) indicate the need for initiating or adjusting medications. Some of the medications used for diabetes management require attention to carb intake, as discussed next.

Any medication that stimulates the pancreas to produce extra insulin may cause hypoglycemia if not enough carbs are consumed:

>> A class of medications known as *sulfonylureas* stimulates sustained insulin release over a period of many hours. The typical dosing schedule is once or twice daily. If you take one of these medications, it is important to stick with your meal plan and eat an appropriate amount of carbohydrate. Don't skip meals or skimp on carbs, or you could end up hypoglycemic. Aim for three

meals spaced four to six hours apart. See Chapters 19, 20, and 21 for menu plans with consistent carb amounts.

>> *Meglitinides* are medications that also stimulate insulin release; however, the effect is shorter lived. The dose taken before a meal stimulates insulin release for just that meal, not all day. Due to the short duration of action, there is less risk of hypoglycemia, but you should still be cognizant of eating carbs.

Biguanides (Metformin) decrease the amount of glucose that is released from the liver. Hypoglycemia is unlikely because insulin secretion isn't affected. It is best to take this medication with food to reduce the risk of upset stomach.

Knowing your limits

REMEMBER

Medications can help you achieve control of your diabetes, but dietary management will always be at the foundation of treatment. There is no medication that erases the need to pay attention to what you eat. *Simply put, you can out-eat any medication.* Part 2 of this book gets to the nitty-gritty of carb counting. Use the information in this book to establish a reasonable carbohydrate plan with healthy diet principles. Monitor blood glucose and share the results with your doctor. Work with your healthcare providers to determine and monitor your medication needs.

2

Carb Counting: From Basic to Advanced

Get the most out of the Nutrition Facts food label.

Find out how to count carbs in fresh, bulk, and unpackaged foods.

Gather carb-counting resources in print, online, and through apps.

Make carb counting the cornerstone to controlling blood glucose when you have type 1 diabetes.

Employ simpler portioning protocols with type 2 diabetes.

Increase carb-counting accuracy with weights and measures.

Chapter **7**

First Things First: Reading and Deciphering Food Labels

When learning to count carbohydrates, it makes sense to start with the basics, and the place to start is food labels. Food labels are mandatory for packaged foods in the United States. The U.S. Food and Drug Administration (FDA) is the agency that regulates and oversees label laws. Other countries may or may not offer labeling, and they may give their information in a different format. For example, some countries provide nutrition information per 100 grams of the weight of the food product. In the United States, the serving sizes are more tangible and vary depending on the food.

Periodically the Nutrition Facts food labels get a face lift — and change is soon upon us! In May 2016, the FDA approved final updates on the new Nutrition Facts food labels. The updated design is due to go live in July 2018. A grace period will allow time for all manufacturers to get onboard and comply. That means that for a while, both types of labels — old and new — may end up in your cupboard at the same time, so I explain the similarities and differences of both versions in this chapter.

Here I also walk you through all the information you find on a food label and prep you for reading labels at the grocery store.

Rest assured, manufacturers are held accountable for providing accurate information on their Nutrition Facts labels. Strict rules also govern what wording is allowable on the front of the package in terms of label claims. For example, you may find a label on a product containing oats that claims that soluble fiber may reduce the risk of heart disease. In order to make that particular claim, the food must be low in fat, saturated fat, and cholesterol, and specify the source and amount of the soluble fiber. Sufficient evidence proves that those properties may indeed reduce your risk of heart disease, so the claim is allowed. On the other hand, you won't find a food label that promises to reverse the aging process or guarantees that you will shed ten pounds in a week, because those claims are simply not possible and are not backed by scientific evidence.

Finding Your Way around Food Labels

All consumers should be cognizant of the overall composition and nutritional quality of the foods they choose. Often when people with diabetes read a food label, they zero right in on the grams of total carbohydrates or the sugars and may end up ignoring other important information. While the carbohydrate information is certainly important when it comes to regulating blood-glucose levels, it doesn't mean that you should ignore the info on calories, fats, and sodium. The information on the Nutrition Facts labels can be very useful when trying to achieve weight targets, heart health, and blood-pressure control. Labeling can also help you assure adequacy in protein, fiber, and certain key vitamins and minerals. Keep the big picture in mind and use the whole label when thinking about your overall health. (I go into detail on all the information you find on food labels in the later section "Scrutinizing the Nutrition Facts.")

In the following sections, I point out the importance of paying attention to grams rather than percentages on all food labels, and I introduce the setup of both traditional food labels and newly designed food labels, which are set to debut in 2018.

Paying particular attention to amounts

The total fat, saturated fat, trans fat, total carbohydrate, fiber, sugar, and protein amounts on a food label are listed in grams (g), while cholesterol and sodium amounts are listed in milligrams (mg). Off to the right side of the label you find the %Daily Value in bold. The %Daily Value is sometimes abbreviated %DV. The tricky thing is that the food labels are comparing each nutrient to the %Daily Value for a person who needs 2,000 calories per day to reach weight and health targets.

Looking at the Total Carbohydrate amount is important because carbohydrates digest and eventually turn into glucose, which ends up in the bloodstream. Having diabetes means you should be paying attention to how much carbohydrate you're eating. Food labels help you do just that, but you need to look for the *grams* of carbohydrate, not the %Daily Value. You want to focus on the grams of carb, not the %Daily Value, because insulin dosing is based on the actual grams of carb, not the percent. Carbohydrate grams and %Daily Value are listed on the same line on Nutrition Facts labels, as you can see in Figure 7-1.

Nutrition Facts

Serving Size 1/2 cup (115g)
Servings Per Container About 4

Amount Per Serving

Calories 250	**Calories from Fat** 130

	% Daily Value*
Total Fat 14g	**22%**
Saturated Fat 9g	**45%**
Cholesterol 55mg	**18%**
Sodium 75mg	**3%**
Total Carbohydrate 26g	**9%**
Dietary Fiber 0g	**0%**
Sugars 26g	
Protein 4g	

Vitamin A 10%	Vitamin C 0%
Calcium 10%	Iron 0%

* Percent Daily Values are based on a 2,000 calorie diet.

© *John Wiley & Sons, Inc.*

FIGURE 7-1:
Total Carbohydrate is listed in grams.

Because %Daily Value is written in bold and off to the right side of the label, and lined up neatly with the actual amount, it is easy to allow your eye to zero in on the %Daily Value rather than the actual amount in grams. However, knowing that you're getting 26 g of carbohydrate is far more important than knowing that you're getting 9% of the Daily Value for a person who should be eating 2,000 calories per day. (That is, unless you're in the subset of people who happen to need exactly that many calories and therefore fall into the "reference range.")

The %Daily Value on the Nutrition Facts label is useful when you're trying to determine whether a product is high or low in a given substance. Note that 5%DV or less is considered *low* in that nutrient, and 20%DV or more is considered *high* in the nutrient. When looking at total fat, saturated fat, cholesterol, and sodium, it pays to choose foods that are low (5%DV or less). When looking at fiber, vitamin A, vitamin C, calcium, and iron, it is a good idea to aim for choices that are high (20%DV or more).

Viewing versions of traditional labels

Several versions of the Nutrition Facts labels are currently in use. The most extensive label includes additional information at the bottom of the label. This footnote section is often a source of confusion. Figure 7-2 points out the lower segment of the label, which provides the reference information in a footnote.

Notice that target intakes are provided for two calorie levels. One column heading is for a 2,000-calorie intake target, and another column heading is for a 2,500-calorie intake target. Total fat, saturated fat, cholesterol, sodium, total carbohydrate, and fiber daily targets are set for the two reference calorie levels.

Nutrition Facts

Serving Size 2/3 cup (55g)
Servings Per Container About 8

Amount Per Serving

Calories 230	Calories from Fat 72

	% Daily Value*
Total Fat 8g	12%
Saturated Fat 1g	5%
Trans Fat 0g	
Cholesterol 0mg	0%
Sodium 160mg	7%
Total Carbohydrate 37g	12%
Dietary Fiber 4g	16%
Sugars 1g	
Protein 3g	

Vitamin A	10%
Vitamin C	8%
Calcium	20%
Iron	45%

* Percent Daily Values are based on a 2,000 calorie diet. Your daily value may be higher or lower depending on your calorie needs.

	Calories:	2,000	2,500
Total Fat	Less than	65g	80g
Sat Fat	Less than	20g	25g
Cholesterol	Less than	300mg	300mg
Sodium	Less than	2,400mg	2,400mg
Total Carbohydrate		300g	375g
Dietary Fiber		25g	30g

© *John Wiley & Sons, Inc.*

FIGURE 7-2: Label reference information.

The upside of this information is that it allows consumers to have a rough idea of what intake targets to aim for in a day. The downside is that lots of people simply don't fall into those calorie target ranges. Many women, especially those who are older or trying to lose weight, should be aiming for a much lower calorie goal. Clearly, if you're limiting your intake to 1,200 to 1,500 calories per day, then the nutrition information related to 2,000 and 2,500 calories is simply irrelevant and could lead to overconsumption.

An abbreviated version of the food label is also acceptable for manufacturers to use. Some food packages use a version that omits the footnote details from the bottom of the label and simply provides the key nutrition facts, such as the label in Figure 7-1.

Taking a sneak peek at newfangled food labels

The current food label imagery (as shown in Figures 7-1 and 7-2) has been in use for over 20 years. The Nutrition Facts label has recently been redesigned, revamped, and improved. Changes reflect the latest scientific, nutrition, and public-health research. Health experts and the general public provided feedback, which helped shape the label transformation. The new design should make it easier for the public to make informed decisions about what they are consuming. Manufacturers have some time to gear up and get the new image rolling, but they are mandated to go live by July 2018. Smaller companies have an additional year to make the changes.

Figure 7-3 shows the old and the new, in a side-by-side view. The label on the left is the design currently in print. The label on the right is the sneak peek of the upcoming new and improved label.

Here's the scoop on what you can expect to see:

>> **More realistic serving sizes:** The first line on the new label specifies the number of servings in the container. Suggested serving sizes have been reconsidered on various foods. Changes have been made so that suggested serving sizes will be more likely to reflect actual intake. For example, the serving size on the new label will reflect the reality that a 20-ounce beverage is likely to be sucked down by one person, not 2.5 people. However, a 12-ounce beverage will also indicate that the container holds one serving. Let's be honest; most of us don't tend to share our beverages, and once the beverage is opened, it's usually finished off in one sitting.

Nutrition Facts

Serving Size 2/3 cup (55g)
Servings Per Container About 8

Amount Per Serving

Calories 230   Calories from Fat 72

	% Daily Value*
Total Fat 8g	**12%**
Saturated Fat 1g	**5%**
Trans Fat 0g	
Cholesterol 0mg	**0%**
Sodium 160mg	**7%**
Total Carbohydrate 37g	**12%**
Dietary Fiber 4g	**16%**
Sugars 1g	
Protein 3g	
Vitamin A	10%
Vitamin C	8%
Calcium	20%
Iron	45%

* Percent Daily Values are based on a 2,000 calorie diet.
Your daily value may be higher or lower depending on
your calorie needs.

		Calories:	2,000	2,500
Total Fat	Less than		65g	80g
Sat Fat	Less than		20g	25g
Cholesterol	Less than		300mg	300mg
Sodium	Less than		2,400mg	2,400mg
Total Carbohydrate			300g	375g
Dietary Fiber			25g	30g

Nutrition Facts

8 servings per container
Serving size   **2/3 cup (55g)**

Amount per serving

Calories   **230**

	% Daily Value*
Total Fat 8g	**10%**
Saturated Fat 1g	**5%**
Trans Fat 0g	
Cholesterol 0mg	**0%**
Sodium 160mg	**7%**
Total Carbohydrate 37g	**13%**
Dietary Fiber 4g	**14%**
Total Sugars 12g	
Includes 10g Added Sugars	**20%**
Protein 3g	
Vitamin D 2mcg	10%
Calcium 260mg	20%
Iron 8mg	45%
Potassium 235mg	6%

* The % Daily Value (DV) tells you how much a nutrient in
a serving of food contributes to a daily diet. 2,000 calories
a day is used for general nutrition advice.

© *John Wiley & Sons, Inc.*

FIGURE 7-3:
Current label and
updated label
comparison.

>> **Per serving versus per package notation:** Some labels will provide dual columns to show nutrition information for *per serving* as well as *per package*. For example, if you eat the whole pint of ice cream, you'll be able to easily identify calories and nutrition facts for not only one portion but also the full container. Being more aware may help people to limit their intake to the suggested "one serving."

>> **Bigger, bolder serving-size and calorie fonts:** Looking further at the new label design, on the right, you may notice how the serving size will be noted in large, bold font. The calorie level will be in even larger and bolder font. They want to make sure everyone knows that one large bag of potato chips isn't a single-serving container.

>> **No inclusion of calories from fat:** The calories from fat will no longer be listed. There will still be a requirement to identify the Total Fat grams and the amount of unhealthy Saturated and *Trans* Fats.

>> **Specification of "added" sugar:** One significant change coming to the new label relates to sugar. Current labels already list the amount of sugar in the product, but the new food label will add more clarity. It will not only list the total amount of sugar per serving, but it will also tell you how much of the sugar is "added" versus naturally present in the food. In the example of the updated label shown in Figure 7-3, there are 12 total grams of sugar, but of the 12 grams, 10 grams have been *added* during manufacturing and process- ing. You can deduce that 2 grams of sugar were naturally occurring, such as the sugars found in milk or fruit.

WARNING

Added sugars are going to be identified on the new labels to help consumers be more aware. Added sugars, honey, syrup, and other processed sweeteners tend to add too many "empty calories." Those calories, if not kept in check, can lead to unwanted weight gain and a rash of other health concerns, not to mention the impact on blood-glucose control if you have diabetes.

>> **Updated %Daily Value targets:** Daily values for nutrients like sodium, fiber, and vitamin D are being updated based on newer scientific evidence from the Institute of Medicine and other reports such as that from the 2015 Dietary Guidelines Advisory Committee. In Figure 7-3, for example, 8 grams of Total Fat is listed as 12% of Daily Value on the label on the left (the original label), but the same amount of fat is listed as 10% of Daily Value on the label on the right (the revised label). The difference is due to the newly established targets.

>> **Inclusion of micrograms and milligrams for vitamins and minerals:** Old labels fall short, as they currently list only the %Daily Value for vitamins A and C and for the minerals calcium and iron. Current labels don't indicate exactly how many milligrams of calcium, for example, are provided. The new labels will continue to list information on calcium and iron, and will start to list the specific amounts in milligrams in addition to the %Daily Value.

>> **Addition of vitamin D and potassium info:** Another notable change will be the addition of vitamin D and potassium information:

- Many folks fall short in the vitamin D department. Vitamin D is critical for bone health, and lab results are showing that many of the people who are being screened have low blood levels of this crucial vitamin. Vitamin D content will be listed in micrograms and in %Daily Value.

- Listing potassium on the new label will bring more attention to this important mineral, which, among other things, helps with blood-pressure regulation. Potassium content will be listed in milligrams, which will be useful for individuals with kidney failure who need to limit or track their intake of potassium. The %Daily Value will also be listed.

>> **Omission of vitamins A and C:** New labels will no longer be mandated to include details on vitamin C and vitamin A. You may wonder why those two nutrients are being booted off the new label. It's simply because deficiencies are far less frequent these days as most individuals have adequate intakes for both vitamins A and C.

Scrutinizing the Nutrition Facts

When it comes to scrutinizing the Nutrition Facts food label, I start at the top of the label and work my way down. I'll be focusing on the current labels as they exist now, since the new label design won't be out until the summer of 2018. Refer to Figure 7-4 as you read through this section. Key content is identified in bold font throughout the label and includes Calories, Total Fat, Cholesterol, Sodium, Total Carbohydrate, and Protein.

Nutrition Facts

Serving Size 1 cup (55g)
Servings Per Container 4

Amount Per Serving

Calories 216	Calories from Fat 72

	% Daily Value*
Total Fat 8g	12%
Saturated Fat 1g	5%
Trans Fat 0g	
Cholesterol 5mg	2%
Sodium 490mg	20%
Total Carbohydrate 30g	10%
Dietary Fiber 4g	16%
Sugars 2g	
Protein 6g	

Vitamin A	4%	·	Vitamin C	8%
Calcium	0%	·	Iron	10%

* Percent Daily Values are based on a 2,000 calorie diet.

Serving Size is 1 cup.

The number in parentheses is weight. One serving weighs 55 grams.

There are 4 servings in the package.

One serving, which is 1 cup, provides 30 g of total carbohydrate.

Fiber does not digest so you can subtract the grams of fiber from the total carbohydrate grams.

30 g carb minus 4 g fiber = 26 grams of digestible carb.

The grams of sugar are already included in the total carbohydrate count.

© John Wiley & Sons, Inc.

FIGURE 7-4: Sample Nutrition Facts label.

Sorting out serving sizes and servings per container

The very first line tells you what is considered to be one serving. Next to the serving size, in parentheses, you find the weight of the product. For example, if the label says Serving Size 1 cup (55 g), it means that one serving, or 1 cup, weighs 55 grams on a food scale.

The next line down tells you how many servings are in the container. In Figure 7-4, the serving size is 1 cup and there are 4 servings in the container, so the full container has 4 cups.

TIP

Sometimes it's easier to measure a serving using the Servings Per Container information. For example, a frozen lasagna may say the Serving Size is 1 cup, and Servings Per Container 6. Using a measuring cup to serve lasagna would end up being a sloppy mess. Instead, take the lasagna out of the oven and cut it into six even pieces. It will look a lot nicer served with a spatula. Each piece is about a cup.

REMEMBER

All the nutrition information provided on the label is correct only for exactly one serving. Be sure to note what's identified as the serving size. If you eat more or less than the specified serving size, do the math. If you eat two portions, you should double all the information on the label as you manage your carbs.

Calling out calories

REMEMBER

Calories matter. If you eat more calories than you need, no matter what the source, you will gain weight. If you eat fewer calories than your body requires for its day-to-day functioning, then you will lose weight. Be sure to take the time to look at calories and compare products. Use this information as part of your decision-making process when shopping.

The product in Figure 7-4 has 216 calories per serving. If you eat two servings, you end up with 432 calories. Eating the whole container would be four servings with a total intake of 864 calories. Next to the calories, on the same line, the current food label lets you know how many of the calories come from fat. The new food labels will do away with that notation and will just focus on the total number of calories.

Finding the fat

The total amount of fat per serving is given in both grams and %Daily Value. Providing information on the *unhealthy* types of fat is required. Labels must tell you the amount of saturated fat and trans fat per serving. Labels are not required to list the details on the heart-healthy types of fats, known as unsaturated fats. Some manufacturers proudly choose to do so, so you may end up with a label that does show you how many grams of monounsaturated fat and polyunsaturated fat are provided per serving. That info is optional.

Toting up the total fat

The sample label in Figure 7-4 shows 8 grams of Total Fat, 12% of Daily Value. Indented below the Total Fat you always find the information on the Saturated Fat and the Trans Fat. The goal is to eat as little saturated fat and trans fat as possible. Both types are linked to raising LDL cholesterol, which is the bad kind of cholesterol in your blood.

REMEMBER

While some fats are good for your heart and others are not so good, all fats have the same effect on your hips because they have the same number of calories. Flip to Chapter 16 for tips on eating smart for both weight and heart.

Breaking out the saturated fat

Saturated fats are *not* heart healthy. Look for this number to be as low as possible when reviewing labels; the example in Figure 7-4 shows 1 gram of saturated fat (5% of Daily Value). Saturated fats occur naturally in many different foods, predominantly animal products such as fatty meats and full-fat dairy products. It pays to compare labels and aim to lower your intake of saturated fats. One thing to be aware of is that a label can say 0 g of saturated fat as long as a serving provides under 0.5 grams per serving.

Tallying trans fats

Trans fats are especially bad for your health. Trans fats are a double whammy. They not only raise the LDL, which is the bad kind of cholesterol in your blood, but they also lower the HDL, which is the good kind of cholesterol in your blood. There has been a big push to reduce the amount of trans fat in our food sources. Manufacturers have responded by reformulating many products to reduce trans fat.

You should definitely compare labels and look for items with zero grams of trans fat (like the one in Figure 7-4). The label can say 0 g trans fat as long as a serving provides less than 0.5 grams per serving.

Noting the cholesterol content

Cholesterol content is listed in milligrams (mg). Expert opinion has shifted somewhat in terms of the recommendations on intake of dietary cholesterol. The focus has shifted away from the cholesterol in the foods we eat, and the attention is zeroing in on the *type* of fat. New recommendations are allowing for more cholesterol than previously allowed. The attention is focused on limiting saturated and trans fats. Prior guidelines set an upper limit at 300 milligrams of dietary cholesterol per day. The current guidelines say, "While adequate evidence is not available for a *quantitative* limit for dietary cholesterol in the 2015–2020 Dietary Guidelines, cholesterol is still important to consider when building a healthy eating style." It's a good idea not to go overboard. The product in Figure 7-4 provides 5 mg of cholesterol per serving, which isn't much.

Surveying the sodium

Salt is a significant source of sodium. Common table salt is made from sodium and chloride. Sodium intake is linked to high blood pressure, so if you have hypertension, you should take note of the amount of sodium you eat. Packaged foods make it easy by listing the milligrams per serving.

Guidelines for Americans encourage keeping sodium intake to under 2,300 mg/day. Depending on your overall health, doctors may suggest that you keep your intake below 1,500 mg/day. The product in Figure 7-4 has 490 mg of sodium, which is considered high. Anytime the %Daily Value is 20 percent or more, it's considered high.

For more information on making heart-healthy choices and further details on sodium, dietary fats, and cholesterol, see Chapter 16.

Focusing on total carbohydrate

The Total Carbohydrate grams represent the lump-sum total from all carbohydrate sources, including the starch, the fiber, the sugars, and any and all other types of carb, such as sugar alcohol.

The subsets indented below the Total Carbohydrate identify the specific amount of carbohydrate coming from fiber and from sugar. The sample label in Figure 7-4 has 30 grams of Total Carbohydrate, of which 4 grams come from fiber and 2 grams come from sugar. Nutrition Facts labels don't list how much of the Total Carbohydrate comes from starch, but it's pretty easy to figure out. Because fiber and sugar are providing 4 g and 2 g respectively, the remainder must be from other carbohydrates, which is *generally* the starch. In this case, add 4 grams of fiber and 2 grams of sugar to get 6 grams, and then subtract 6 from 30 grams of total carb; your answer is 24 grams of starch.

Carbohydrates from starch and sugars are digested and eventually turn into the individual sugar molecules that are absorbed into the bloodstream. The sugar in the bloodstream is called blood glucose, abbreviated BG. Carbohydrate foods provide the glucose that the body needs to function normally. Having diabetes doesn't mean that you should over-restrict, or avoid, carbohydrates. Managing diabetes does mean that you should learn to identify which foods have carbs and how much of those foods you should eat. Portion size matters. Take note, though, that not all carbohydrates affect the blood-glucose levels in the same way.

The following sections delve deeper into the two types of carbs called out on food labels: fiber and sugar.

TIP

Find out which foods have carbohydrates in Chapter 3. For more details on how carbs fuel the body, see Chapter 4. Get an idea of how much carb you need by delving into Chapter 5. For more about digestion rates and how food composition can impact your blood-glucose readings, see Chapter 10.

Accounting for fiber

Fiber is unique because it is a form of carbohydrate that doesn't digest. Fiber comes from plant foods such as whole grains, legumes, fruits, and vegetables. (Meats, dairy products, fats, and oils don't have any dietary fiber.) Dietary fiber is what remains after digestion; it's the indigestible part of the plant. Fiber makes its way all the way through the intestine, pushing things along as it goes, which helps promote regularity in bowel movements. Fiber is important for intestinal health. Fiber is made out of glucose molecules all linked tightly together. It doesn't break down into individual glucose molecules in the same way that starch does.

REMEMBER

Bottom line: When counting carbs, you don't need to count fiber since it doesn't end up raising your blood-glucose levels. You can subtract the grams of fiber from the grams of Total Carbohydrate. In Figure 7-4, 30 grams of Total Carbohydrate minus 4 grams of fiber leaves you with 26 grams of digestible carbs.

TIP

If you inject insulin, you should definitely subtract the fiber *if it is going to make a difference to your insulin dose.* However, if you have diet-controlled Type 2 diabetes, you really don't need to worry about subtracting the fiber.

When adjusting insulin doses to the amount of carbohydrate eaten, precision is important. Calculating your own doses of insulin allows for flexibility in what you eat, but getting the proper dose of insulin relies on you counting the carbohydrates accurately. Consider the two tortilla labels shown in Figure 7-5.

Nutrition Facts	
Serving Size 1 Tortilla (41g)	
Servings Per Container 14	
Amount per serving	
Calories 60	Calories from Fat 5
	% Daily Value*
Total Fat 0.5g	1%
Saturated Fat 0g	0%
Trans Fat 0g	
Cholesterol 0mg	0%
Sodium 95mg	4%
Total Carbohydrate 13g	4%
Dietary Fiber 1g	4%
Sugars 0g	
Protein 1g	

Nutrition Facts	
Serving Size 1 Tortilla (36g)	
Servings Per Container 10	
Amount Per Serving	
Calories 50	Calories from Fat 15
	% Daily Value*
Total Fat 2g	3%
Saturated Fat 0g	0%
Trans Fat 0g	
Polyunsaturated Fat 0.5g	
Monounsaturated Fat 1g	
Cholesterol 0mg	0%
Sodium 210mg	9%
Total Carbohydrate 10g	3%
Dietary Fiber 7g	28%
Sugars 0g	
Protein 5g	

FIGURE 7-5:
Fiber comparison.

© *John Wiley & Sons, Inc.*

The label on the left shows that the total carbohydrate count is 13 grams and the fiber is a mere 1 gram. If you subtracted the gram of fiber and counted the carbs as 12 grams, you would be very unlikely to change your dose of insulin on that basis. For example, if your doctor recommended that you take 1 unit of rapid-acting insulin for every 12 grams of carb you eat, you would end up taking just 1 unit of insulin regardless of whether you counted this tortilla as 13 grams of carb or as 12 grams of carb.

WARNING

The insulin-dosing examples used in this book are only to make a point. Individual insulin requirements vary significantly. Do not make changes to your insulin plan without conferring with your doctor.

Next, look at the label on the right. That's a different story. There are 10 grams of carb per tortilla, but 7 of those grams come from fiber. Keep in mind that fiber doesn't digest. Subtract the fiber: 10 grams of carb minus 7 grams of fiber leaves you with just 3 grams of digestible carb. That means only 3 grams will turn into glucose and enter your bloodstream. Anyone calculating insulin-to-carb ratios would want to subtract the fiber in order to calculate the right dose of insulin. If a person took insulin to cover 10 grams but digested only 3 grams, then that person might end up with low blood glucose as a result of taking too much insulin. Eating two high-fiber tortillas amplifies the discrepancy.

TIP

A food label can say it's a "good" source of fiber if it provides 10 percent of the Daily Value for fiber, or at least 2.5 grams per serving. An excellent source of fiber provides at least 5 grams of fiber per serving, or 20 percent of the Daily Value.

Sizing up the sugar content

REMEMBER

The grams of sugar are already included in the Total Carbohydrate count. First and foremost, look at the labels for the Total Carbohydrate count. The number of grams of sugar noted on the Nutrition Facts label is a number that includes *all forms* of sugar in the product. That means the grams of *naturally occurring* sugars in milk and fruit are counted together with the grams of *added sugars* (for example, from honey, syrups, white sugar, or any other sugar). Don't panic when you notice your milk carton shows 13 grams of sugar. That is from the naturally occurring sugar in milk, lactose. If fruit is packaged, you see the same thing: The carbs that are found in fruit are technically sugars.

There are no arbitrary rules on how many grams of sugar to choose or avoid. When you count carbs, look at the total grams of carb and consider the fiber as mentioned in the previous section. Consider the health properties of food rather than the grams of sugar on the label. In the case of breakfast cereals, it won't hurt to compare labels and choose cereals with less sugar. Choose wholesome whole-grain cereals rather than sugary refined breakfast cereals.

Pinpointing the protein

Labels indicate the amount of protein per serving. Figure 7-4 shows that one serving of this product (1 cup) provides 6 grams of protein. Protein needs vary significantly based on age, gender, and other factors, so the food labels don't provide information regarding the %Daily Value for protein. Most Americans have no problems meeting their protein needs; in fact, most people get a lot more than what the body requires. Chapter 8 provides tips on portioning and planning balanced meals.

Taking note of other valuable nutrients

Currently, food labels provide information on vitamin A, vitamin C, calcium, and iron. (This will change with the labels debuting in 2018, as I note in the earlier section "Taking a sneak peek at newfangled food labels.") However, only the %Daily Value is provided. Labels do not specifically tell you how many micrograms or milligrams are provided.

Figure 7-4 shows that one serving provides 4 percent of the Daily Value for vitamin A, 8 percent for vitamin C, and 10 percent for iron, but it does not provide any calcium at all. As I note in the earlier section "Paying particular attention to amounts," 5%DV or less is considered low in the nutrient, and 20%DV or more is high in the nutrient.

Investigating the ingredients

Food labels must include an ingredients list. Ingredients are listed in descending order by weight. That means that the ingredient that weighs the most is listed first, and the ingredient that weighs the least is listed last. Everyone benefits from eating wholesome foods, so look for whole grains, as I describe later in this chapter. For heart health, steer clear of hydrogenated oils, as I discuss further in Chapter 16.

Identifying allergens

The Food Allergen Labeling and Consumer Protection Act requires that packaged foods clearly identify the eight most common food allergens. While many foods can elicit an allergic response in a sensitive individual, just eight main foods account for 90 percent of all food allergies. If a packaged food contains milk, eggs, fish, crustacean shellfish (such as shrimp, crab, or lobster), tree nuts, peanuts, soybeans, or wheat, it must be clearly noted on the label.

Allergens may be noted in the actual ingredient list, but if the ingredient isn't a commonly known source of the allergen, then the source must be listed in parentheses. The allergen may or may not be written in bold font, so look closely at each label. For example:

> **Ingredients:** wheat flour, corn oil, eggs, honey, whey (**milk**), vanilla, lecithin (**soy**), salt.

It is obvious that the product contains wheat and eggs. It is less obvious that whey indicates a milk product or that lecithin is made from soy. To clarify, the common words "milk" and "soy" must be noted in parentheses to clarify the less-common ingredient names.

An alternate way to note the allergens is to do so below the ingredient list, by saying "contains" and then listing the allergens. For example:

Ingredients: wheat flour, corn oil, eggs, honey, whey, vanilla, lecithin, salt.

Contains: wheat, eggs, milk, soy

Heading to the Grocery Store

Make use of the information on the Nutrition Facts food labels when you go to the grocery store. Take some time to compare products. Go shopping in off-peak hours so you can feel relaxed about browsing the aisles. It's easy to become a creature of habit and always grab the same items as you dash in and out of the store. New products are frequently introduced, and many great choices are available. Some not-so-great items are also available (if not abundant), so take yourself on a grocery store tour and be your own tour guide. For tips on choosing foods wisely, see Chapter 13.

The following sections cover label claims to watch for, help you prepare a shopping cheat sheet, and encourage you to read labels faithfully.

Being skeptical about label claims

Manufacturers want to catch your attention as you browse the grocery aisles. This section clarifies some of the terminology you may see on packaging.

Net carbs

Manufacturers try to get your attention by using terms like net carbs, impact carbs, or active carbs. Manufacturers may subtract the grams of carb that come from fiber, sugar alcohol, and glycerin, claiming that those things don't impact blood-glucose levels that much, if at all.

REMEMBER

The problem is that most sugar alcohols *do digest*, at least in part, and do contribute some glucose to the bloodstream. If you're using insulin-to-carb ratios, trying to figure out just how much insulin you should take gets tricky. Fiber doesn't digest, so subtracting fiber grams from the Total Carbohydrate is fine (see the earlier section "Accounting for fiber" for details). However, it's estimated that roughly half of the sugar alcohol in a product will likely be digested. If a product contains sugar alcohol, it will be listed under the Total Carbohydrates below the grams of fiber and sugar. For example, if there are 10 grams of sugar alcohol per serving, about 5 grams of that will probably be digested, enter the bloodstream, and require insulin. Adjust your dose accordingly. Keep in mind that the remaining sugar alcohol that is not digested may cause gas and bloating. Complicating matters further, there are quite a few different forms of sugar alcohol, and some are more digestible than others.

Zero trans fat

A package is allowed to say the product contains zero trans fat if it has less than 0.5 grams of trans fat per serving. If you're having multiple servings, or if you're having several items throughout the day, they could add up to a significant amount of trans fat. In other words, a product just has to have slightly less than *a half of a gram* of trans fat per serving to say "0"; this doesn't guarantee that there is none whatsoever.

Whole grain

The term "whole grain" means the product contains all three portions of the wheat — the germ, bran, and endosperm — and has at least 51 percent whole-grain ingredients by weight per serving. Look for products that claim to contain 100 percent whole grain. Items are listed in descending order by weight on ingredients lists. An item may contain more than one kind of grain, so choose items that have "whole grain" listed at, or near, the top of the ingredient list.

WARNING

Keep an eye out for the following products and terms:

>> Cereals may have three or four different kinds of sugar added. If manufacturers keep the weight of each *individual* type of sugar lower than the weight of the whole grain, then they can still list whole grain first on the ingredient list — even if combining all the sugars together may actually outweigh the grain! Yikes! Check those cereal boxes carefully.

>> Beware, the following terms do not necessarily mean that you are getting whole grain: wheat flour, 100 percent wheat, bran, seven grain, multigrain, enriched, or stoneground. None of those terms indicate 100 percent whole grain. Saying that the product is made *with whole grains* doesn't cut it either.

REMEMBER

When reading label claims and ingredients lists, look for the word "whole" in front of the word indicating the grain. Examples include "whole wheat" and "whole grain."

The Whole Grains Council is helping to clear up confusion in the supermarket. They've developed a stamp of approval for whole-grain products. See Figure 7-6. If a product has the "100% whole grain" stamp, it means all the grain ingredients in the product are whole grain and that a serving provides a minimum of 16 grams of whole grain. The basic stamp indicates the product has at least 8 grams of whole grain but may also contain refined grains.

TIP

Have you seen *white whole-wheat* bread and wondered whether it really was whole grain? Well, the answer is that white whole-wheat flour does contain all three components of the wheat — the bran, germ, and endosperm — so yes, it really counts as a whole grain. This light-colored whole wheat has a milder flavor, so fans of white bread should find it very palatable.

No sugar added

This term simply means that no sugars have been added in manufacturing or processing. The product may contain naturally occurring sugars, however. Yogurt is made from milk, and milk contains lactose, which is technically a form of sugar. You can't find a yogurt that says "sugar-free," but you can find one that says "no sugar added." The same holds true if you look at no-sugar-added applesauce. It is still going to look like it is 100 percent sugar when you check the grams of sugar on the Nutrition Facts food label. Milk sugar and fruit sugar both show up on the label as grams of *sugar*. (Check out the earlier section "Sizing up the sugar content" for more information.)

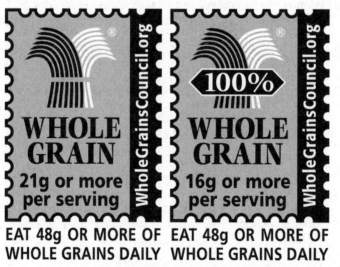

FIGURE 7-6:
The whole grain stamp.

Courtesy Oldways and the Whole Grains Council, wholegrainscouncil.org

Sugar-free

A product can make the claim "sugar-free" if it has fewer than 0.5 grams of sugar per serving. Be aware that products that are sweetened with sugar alcohol are allowed to say sugar-free on the front of the package but may have a surprising amount of carbohydrate. When you look at the Nutrition Facts label on sugar-free products, the *sugar* grams are indeed zero. Total Carbohydrates are not necessarily zero, because sugar alcohol is a form of carbohydrate. Some candies have a regular version and a sugar-free version. Both usually end up having the same number of calories, fats, and carbs. The only difference is that the carbs are being counted as sugar alcohol instead of sugar. Always look at the total carbohydrates. (Find out more about sugars and various sweeteners in Chapter 12.)

Preparing your carbohydrate cheat sheet

TIP

The Exchange Lists in Appendix A provide information on single foods but not mixed dishes. You can create a cheat sheet by doing a little investigative work at your local market. Take a note pad or index card (or keep notes on your phone) and head to the supermarket when you have some spare time. You can discover a thing or two about the carb counts in mixed dishes and ethnic foods. Think about some of the foods that you eat but are unsure about how to count. Do you count tamales, pizza, calzones, or ravioli? How about egg rolls, pot stickers, or Indian foods? Head to the frozen foods section in the store and look for foods similar to those that you eat in restaurants or make at home. Glance at the food label and make note of the portion size and the carb count. You can at least get an idea of how much carb is in quiche or lasagna if you look at a label on a similar item. Keep a running list of carb counts on mixed dishes and ethnic foods that you can refer to in the future when you next eat those foods.

Developing supermarket savvy

Next time you're shopping, take a look at labels. Choose with health in mind. Try new foods. Look at the upper and lower shelves. Keep in mind that just because an item is at eye level on the supermarket shelf, it doesn't mean it's the best choice. Check out your options and read labels carefully; the more you practice, the easier it'll be. Eating healthfully pays off.

REMEMBER

While it is fairly easy to count carbs using food labels on packaged foods, don't be afraid to buy fresh foods or produce just because they lack a label. Some of your best choices will be in the perimeter of the store. Produce, reduced-fat dairy products, lean meats, poultry, fish, and whole-grain breads are usually in the outer perimeter. See Chapter 8 for details on how to count carbs in foods that don't have a food label, such as bulk foods and produce.

Chapter **8**

Mastering Carb Counting and Portioning Fundamentals

Reading labels on packaged foods makes it fairly easy to count carbs. Many foods, however, don't come with labels. It would be a shame to limit yourself to packaged foods just because the carbs are easier to count. If you would like a detailed review on deciphering food labels, see Chapter 7.

This chapter moves beyond label reading and explains several other methods for controlling and quantifying carbs. It's important to make healthy food choices and eat appropriate portion sizes. That means eating the right amount of carb; it doesn't mean entirely avoiding or over-restricting healthy foods to the point of compromising nutrition.

Controlling carb intake is at the foundation of diabetes management. Carb counting is an especially important tool to learn if you have type 1 diabetes, because blood-glucose control hinges on balancing insulin with carbohydrate intake. Carb counting is also an effective method of portion control if you have type 2 diabetes. Whether carb counting is a new concept or you're a seasoned carb counter who's ready to take it to the next level, this chapter offers tips that will build on your skills.

Simple visual methods for carb portioning work well enough for many people with type 2 diabetes. The plate model and the hand method are two easy-to-use strategies that I explore in this chapter. The chapter begins by introducing the Exchange Lists and showing how these food composition tables can be used for counting carbs. Other topics explored in this chapter include measuring and weighing food as well as handling special carb-counting cases.

Estimating Carb Counts for Foods without Labels

A wide variety of foods, including fresh produce, breads, legumes, and grains, don't come with a food label. Foods are also often combined into mixed dishes rather than consumed separately, which can make carb counting trickier. Whether you're preparing meals at home or being served in restaurants, it's important to be able to accurately estimate carb counts, and the following sections can help. *Note:* You'll need a standard set of measuring cups to count carbs effectively; I discuss the use of measures and weights later in this chapter.

Relying on food composition lists

For many years food composition lists have been referred to as the Exchange Lists. The main concept is that foods are separated into groups according to their macronutrient composition: carbohydrate, protein, and fat. These lists have historically been referred to as "exchange" lists because you can pick any item within a given list and have roughly the same amount of carbohydrate, protein, fat, and calories as any other item on that list. This section identifies some of the more common foods found within each list, but be sure to review all the Exchange Lists in Appendix A.

The six separate Exchange Lists are

>> Starches

>> Fruits

>> Milk

>> Nonstarchy vegetables

>> Meats and proteins

>> Fats

The groups that have the most carbohydrate are the starch, fruit, and milk groups. Nonstarchy vegetables contain carbs, but in lower amounts. The protein and fat groups don't contain carbs, or at least not much.

REMEMBER

Foods within each Exchange List food group are adjusted in portion size to provide roughly the same amount of carb, protein, fat, and calories per serving. Choose wisely within the groups. Whole grains are healthier choices than white refined grains. For blood-glucose control, limit your intake to one serving of fruit at a time. For improved health, choose plenty of nonstarchy vegetables and opt for lean proteins and unsaturated fats.

The starch list

The starch list contains staple foods that are relatively high in carbs. This group includes breads, bagels, tortillas, biscuits, crackers, oats, cereals, noodles, rice, quinoa, millet, and barley. High-carb vegetables are also included in the starch group. Examples of the starchy vegetables included are potatoes; corn; peas; yams; winter squash; and legumes, also known as the dried bean family.

Table 8-1 shows a few examples from the starch list. Each item on the list has 15 grams of carbohydrate in the portion size listed (measured *after* cooking). Each starch exchange also provides about 3 grams of protein, little or no fat, and 80 calories. For example, a half-cup of cooked oatmeal provides 15 grams of carb. It doesn't mean that you have to limit yourself to a half-cup of cooked oatmeal. The portion sizes are simply a tool to help you count carbs in foods that don't come packaged with a label. A whole cup of oatmeal would be 30 grams of carb. A cup of cooked rice has 45 grams of carb; the entire bagel adds up to 60 grams of carb, and so on.

TABLE 8-1

Starch List: Examples = 15 Grams Carb

Food	Portion Size
Bagel, large	¼
Bread, wheat or white	1 slice
Legumes (dried bean family)	½ cup cooked
Oatmeal	½ cup cooked
Pasta, spaghetti, noodles	⅓ cup cooked
Potato	½ cup cooked
Rice, white or brown	⅓ cup cooked
Tortilla, 6-inch flour or corn	1

The fruit list

The fruit list includes fresh fruits, dried fruits, frozen fruits, canned fruits, and fruit juices. Each item on the list has 15 grams of carbohydrate in the portion size listed, 0 grams of protein, 0 grams of fat, and 60 calories. See Table 8-2 for portion sizes.

TABLE 8-2

Fruit List: Examples = 15 Grams Carb

Food	Portion Size
Apple, small	1
Banana, average	½
Blackberries, blueberries	¾ cup
Cantaloupe, honeydew melon	1 cup cubed
Grapefruit, large	½
Grapes, small	17
Orange, small	1
Peach, medium	1

WARNING

Fruits are concentrated sources of natural sugar. Too much fruit at one time can bump up blood-sugar levels sharply, so you may want to stick to one portion at a time. A "small" apple or orange has 15 grams of carb. Small means the size of a tennis ball. A medium peach is about the size of a baseball.

TIP

If you want to take your carb counting to the next level, you can increase precision by using a food scale. I address food scale use later in this chapter.

Note: Although avocados and tomatoes are technically fruits (if you ask a botanist), they aren't grouped with the fruits on the Exchange Lists. Tomatoes are grouped with the nonstarchy vegetables because tomatoes are relatively low in carbs. Avocados are even lower in carbs and they are very high in fat, so they have been adopted into the fats group.

The milk list

The milk list includes milk and yogurt. See Table 8-3 for a partial list. Fat and calories vary depending on the selection, but each portion listed provides about 8 grams of protein. Appendix A has a more complete list, which separates milk and yogurt into three categories: non- and low-fat, reduced fat, and whole milk.

TABLE 8-3

Milk List: Examples = 12–15 Grams Carb

Food	Portion Size
Milk: Nonfat, 1%, 2%, whole	1 cup
Evaporated milk	½ cup
Yogurt, plain	⅔ cup

The carb in milk comes from a natural sugar called lactose. You may wonder why cheese, butter, sour cream, and cream cheese are missing from the milk list. Although they are made from milk, they have very little lactose. Milk contains three macronutrients: carbohydrate, protein, and fat. Fat, the cream, separates and rises to the top. If churned, it turns into butter (no carbs there). If the fat is cultured, it turns into sour cream (that's fat too). Cream cheese is mostly fat. To make cheese, enzymes are added to whole milk causing fat and protein to form a curd. Cheese has only a trace of carb. The low-carb dairy foods are found in the protein and fat Exchange Lists (which I introduce later in this chapter). I discuss nondairy milk substitutes like soy milk in Chapters 11 and 13.

The nonstarchy vegetables list

The nonstarchy vegetables list includes veggies that are low in carb. Each item on the list has about 5 grams of carbohydrate in the portion size listed, 2 grams of protein, 0 grams of fat, and 25 calories. There are advantages to eating lots of low-carb vegetables: They're low in calories yet packed with vitamins, minerals, and fiber. They don't raise blood-glucose levels very much, and they help you feel fuller. Salad greens have such a small amount of carb that most people consider them free foods. I'm convinced you burn as many carbs chewing lettuce as you get out of digesting it, so it sort of balances out.

There's no need to count the carbs in mixed greens, arugula, lettuce, or endive. Whether you should bother to count the carbs in other nonstarchy veggies depends on whether you take insulin to manage your diabetes. (For a more detailed discussion, see the nearby sidebar "To count or not to count, that is the question.")

>> People with type 1 diabetes should consider all carbs when calculating insulin doses. Yet many people with type 1 have been told not to count vegetables. When children are diagnosed with type 1 diabetes at a young age, their families are regularly told not to count the carbs in vegetables. Why? Because young kids simply don't eat large enough portions of broccoli and carrots to make a difference in their blood-glucose readings. (Frankly, some of the vegetables given to kids don't actually get consumed. Kids slip unwanted foods to the family dog. I even had one mom tell me that she found the green beans under the couch cushions.)

Eventually these kids grow up and so do their palates. As adults they learn to love vegetables and may eat substantial amounts. When the portion size begins to make a difference to insulin needs, then it's time to start counting the vegetables.

>> People with type 2 diabetes who aren't on medications or who are only taking diabetes pills such as Glucophage likely don't need to count the carbs in nonstarchy vegetables. In my many years of being a diabetes educator reviewing food and blood-glucose logs, I've never once seen a high blood-glucose result that could be blamed on overeating green vegetables.

Table 8-4 introduces some nonstarchy vegetables.

TABLE 8-4   **Nonstarchy Vegetable List: Examples = 5 Grams Carb**

½ cup cooked or 1 cup raw = about 5 grams carb	
Asparagus	Greens (collard, kale)
Bamboo shoots	Mushrooms
Beets	Okra
Broccoli	Onions
Brussels sprouts	Pea pods
Cabbage	Peppers (all)
Carrots	Spinach
Cauliflower	Sprouts
Celery	Tomatoes
Eggplant	Zucchini

The meat and protein list

The meat and protein list includes all animal protein sources: beef, chicken, fish, lamb, pork, seafood, and turkey. Cheese has no carbs but is high in protein and fat, so it's included on this list and not on the milk list covered earlier in this chapter. Eggs and tofu are likewise protein foods included here. Fat and calories vary depending on selections, but each ounce of meat or cheese provides about 7 grams of protein. Table 8-5 shows a few examples of lean, medium-fat, and high-fat proteins. Appendix A has a more complete list, including the calorie and fat counts.

TABLE 8-5   **Meat and Protein List (No Carbs)**

Lean	Medium Fat	High Fat
Fish and shellfish	Fried fish	Bacon, sausage
Skinless poultry	Eggs	Hot dogs, ribs
Pork tenderloin	Mozzarella cheese	Bologna, salami
Sirloin steak	Corned beef	Cheese

TO COUNT OR NOT TO COUNT, THAT IS THE QUESTION

Many people use insulin-to-carb ratios to calculate mealtime doses (see Chapter 6 for details on these ratios). All of the carbs in the meal need to be accounted for in order to get the proper dose of insulin. A slice of tomato and lettuce on a sandwich aren't significant, but a cup of vegetables may be. It depends on the portion size of the vegetables and the insulin-to-carb ratio. The following two scenarios illustrate the point:

Example 1: Meaghan has type 1 diabetes, and her insulin-to-carb ratio is 1:5. That means she takes 1 unit of rapid-acting insulin for every 5 grams of carb.

For dinner she plans to eat 2 cups of cooked vegetables from the nonstarchy list. Each ½ cup of cooked vegetables has approximately 5 grams of carb. Therefore, 2 cups of cooked vegetables provides 20 grams of carb.

She is supposed to take 1 unit for every 5 grams of carb consumed, so she needs 4 units of insulin for the veggies in the meal. If she doesn't count the carbs in the veggies, she will be under-dosing by 4 units of insulin and may end up with blood-glucose levels higher than expected.

Example 2: Carter has type 1 diabetes, and his insulin-to-carb ratio is 1:20. That means he takes 1 unit of rapid-acting insulin for every 20 grams of carb.

For dinner he plans to eat ½ cup of cooked vegetables from the nonstarchy list. Each ½ cup of cooked vegetables has approximately 5 grams of carb.

With a 1:20 ratio, Carter needs only ¼ unit of insulin for the veggies, which is insignificant. An insulin pump can deliver insulin to the hundredth of a unit, but insulin syringes and insulin pens can only accurately deliver in 1-unit or ½-unit increments.

TIP

Do your heart a favor and use the lean protein list found in Appendix A as a shopping list to pick your proteins. You may be surprised to find out that the options aren't limited to fish and poultry.

The fat list

The fat list has both animal-based and plant-based fats:

>> Animal fats tend to be solid at room temperature and are saturated fats (less heart healthy); butter is one example. Too much saturated fat in the diet can lead to blocked arteries.

>> The plant-based fats that are liquid at room temperature, such as olive oil, are better for blood vessels.

All fats have the same number of calories and affect weight similarly. Each selection on the fat list in Appendix A provides 5 grams of fat and 45 calories. Other than nuts and seeds, the fat group doesn't provide protein or an appreciable amount of carb. Nuts, seeds, and avocados are foods that are high in fat, so much so that they are listed in the fat exchange list. Table 8-6 separates fats into three categories: monounsaturated, polyunsaturated, and saturated. For more information on eating for heart health, see Chapter 16.

TABLE 8-6   ### Fats List (No Carbs)

Monounsaturated	Polyunsaturated	Saturated
Avocado	Margarine	Butter
Nuts	Mayonnaise	Cream cheese
Oils: olive, canola	Oils: corn, soy	Cream, sour cream
Olives	Seeds	Lard

Solving carb-counting conundrums in mixed dishes and ethnic foods

Food composition lists work great when you're cooking single-ingredient foods such as rice, beans, spaghetti, or oatmeal. Just use your measuring cups and look up the carb count on the reference list.

A BRIEF HISTORY OF THE EXCHANGE LISTS

In years past, people with diabetes didn't have as many management tools. The recommended diet was called a "diabetic diet" and was often handed out as a pre-printed diet sheet based on a calorie goal. The meal plans rigidly directed patients to eat a certain number of servings from the various Exchange Lists at mealtimes and snack times. For example, the lunch plan may have allotted 2 exchanges from the starch group, 1 fruit exchange, 1 milk exchange, 3 protein exchanges, and 2 fat exchanges. The snack assignment might have been 1 starch exchange plus 1 protein exchange. On the plus side, these plans encouraged eating from a variety of food groups. Also, if strictly followed, the plans controlled overall caloric intake and could be used for weight management.

However, these diet prescriptions left very little room for personal preferences or flexibility. Many people found them confusing and cumbersome, and simply gave up on them. The one-size-fits-all approach isn't ideal. Not everyone needs or wants to eat the same thing day in and day out.

Having said that, I think the lists are still useful in many ways. The Exchange Lists can be used for carb counting and portion control. Quite a few people still use the lists to track numbers of "carb servings" instead of counting grams of carbohydrate. The math is easier. For example, you may aim for 3 or 4 carb exchanges per meal, yet mix and match as desired between the three main carb groups: starch, fruit, and milk.

Other foods aren't so straightforward. Consider tamales, enchiladas, pot stickers, spring rolls, dim sum, ravioli, pizza, lasagna, and other mixed dishes, appetizers, and ethnic foods. One strategy for estimating carb counts in foods such as these involves going to a well-stocked grocery store and being a label detective. When you have some spare time, do a little research utilizing labels on packaged foods. If you're trying to figure out the carb count on tamales, for example, look through the frozen food aisles until you find a similar packaged item. Check the food label for the serving size and the carb amount and write it down. Keep a running list of your carb-count estimations on an index card or on your phone. Some people snap a picture of the label and organize the information later.

Visit the canned goods, dry goods, and condiment aisles, too. You may be surprised to see the amount of carbohydrate in some of the Asian stir-fry sauces. Make note of the carbs in condiments, such as ketchup or barbeque sauce, and be sure to include the portion size in your notation. A swipe of ketchup on a bun is negligible, but ¼ of a cup of ketchup is a significant 15 grams of carb. (See the later section "Preparing your carbohydrate cheat sheet" for more information on putting together your research.)

TIP

Nutrition information is also available online for many combination foods, mixed dishes, and ethnic foods. Chapter 9 provides guidance on how to harness the information on the Internet.

Calculating carbs in your favorite recipes

You can figure out how many grams of carb are in your recipes by adding up the carbs in the individual ingredients. Once you know the total grams of carb in the recipe, simply divide by the number of servings to get the carb count in one serving. Take cornbread, for example. If the list of ingredients totals 270 grams of carb and you cut the finished product into nine even pieces, then each piece of cornbread equals 30 grams of carb. 270 grams of carb divided by 9 servings equals 30 grams of carb per serving. Once you've calculated the carbs in your recipe, be sure to mark it on the recipe card. *Note:* Carb counts can be found on the Nutrition Facts labels for ingredients such as flour and sugar (see Chapter 7 for more about reading labels).

Here's another example. The first step in counting carbs in recipes is to identify which ingredients contain carb. In this chili recipe, the carbs are found in the kidney beans; canned chopped tomatoes; canned tomato sauce; and sautéed onions, bell peppers, and celery. The ingredients that don't have carbs are garlic, spices, oil, and vegetable broth. Adding ground beef or turkey, neither of which have any carbs, is optional. If you choose to use vegetarian soy crumbles (which are designed to replace the burger), the package will have a food label that you can review. Beans are especially high in fiber, and because fiber doesn't digest, I subtract the fiber from the total carbs. Now let's count carbs:

>> 15-ounce can of kidney beans: 66 grams total carb minus 27 grams fiber = 39 grams carb

>> 12-ounce can of chopped tomatoes: 14 grams carb

>> 8-ounce can of tomato sauce: 12 grams carb

>> ½ cup each of chopped raw onions and celery, and 1 cup diced raw bell pepper = 10 grams carb

The total amount of carb in the recipe is 75 grams. Divide into three bowls and each bowl has 25 grams of carb.

Preparing your carbohydrate cheat sheet

Each time you make a recipe at home, take the time to calculate the carbs in the recipe. Read labels in grocery stores on combination foods, such as lasagna, and ethnic foods, such as pot stickers (as I explain in the earlier section "Solving carb-counting conundrums in mixed dishes and ethnic foods"). Keep a running list so you can refer to it again in the future when eating those foods. Review a few new labels each time you shop. Create a cheat sheet of sorts that contains carb counts for the foods that you tend to choose. An index card is a good place to start, as the cards are easy to tuck into a purse, a backpack, or the car's glove compartment.

Chain restaurants are required to provide nutrition information for everything they serve. Some restaurants post the info on the wall; others mark it on the menu or may leave a chart in the menu holder on the table. If you find yourself in a restaurant where the information is posted, be a carb detective and write down the details on foods that you may be eating in the future. For example, if a fast-food restaurant says a large order of fries has 500 calories and 60 grams of carb, take note because that may be shocking enough to prevent you from ordering them! Or maybe you'll be more likely to choose the small order, which has 230 calories and 30 grams of carb. The carb counts on fries are comparable from one place to the next. It's the portion size that matters. (I talk more about counting carbs when dining out later in this chapter.)

TIP

All chain restaurants are required to post their nutrition information online, so you can look it up on their website. See Chapter 9 for more on that topic. If the restaurants you eat at aren't chain restaurants, then they aren't required to provide the nutrition information.

Sizing Up Servings with Measures and Weights

The best way to hone your ability to "guesstimate" is to train your eye by measuring precisely. Increase your carb-counting accuracy by using standardized measuring cups, and consider purchasing an inexpensive food scale for the kitchen. I discuss tips in this section.

Measuring with standardized cups and spoons

When you're counting carbs, it's important to use standardized measuring cups and measuring spoons. They are readily available in the kitchen supplies section of many stores. When the Exchange List says "one cup" of cantaloupe has 15 grams of carb, it doesn't mean you can use any mug in the cupboard to measure it. It means an 8-ounce measuring cup. Glass measuring cups have lines that mark the fractions of a cup, whereas stackable cups have individual cups marked as ¼ cup,

⅓ cup, ½ cup, and 1 cup. Some sets throw in additional sizes such as ⅔ cup and ¾ cup. Liquids are most easily measured using the glass cups. The stackable cups are great for measuring dry ingredients, fruits, or cooked grains. (Increase precision on measuring certain fruits by using a food scale, as I explain in the next section.)

TIP

If you plan to eat 45 grams of carb from starches at dinner, for example, you can use a measuring cup to serve the cooked starch directly from the pan to your plate. It saves a step because you're serving and measuring all at once. Use a knife to level off the top.

TIP

Get some practice with measuring cups so that you can eventually eyeball foods more accurately. Train yourself to be able to accurately estimate portion sizes. A glass measuring cup works well for the following exercise:

1. **Measure various starches and fruits in ½-cup and 1-cup portions.**

   Study how those portion sizes look on a plate or in a bowl. Compare the servings to your fist or palm for reference.

2. **Next test yourself by putting a serving of food on your plate without using a measuring cup and guess the amount.**

3. **After guessing, put the food into a measuring cup to see how well you guessed.**

   Practicing helps.

TIP

Another strategy is to find out how much your bowls, cups, and glasses hold. Pour measured amounts of water into the various dishes and take notice of where the water line reaches. When you use that dish in the future, you can serve directly into the dish and be better able to estimate portions and carb counts. For example, if you have a rice bowl that holds exactly one cup, you can use that bowl every time you eat rice and you'll know how much carb you're eating. Pick appropriate-sized dishes to help manage your portions.

TECHNICAL STUFF

Studies show that people perceive being satisfied when their plate looks full, even though they may be eating less because of a reduced-size plate. Using salad-sized plates or smaller bowls typically felt acceptable as long as the dish looked full. People in the study ended up eating less just by using smaller dishes.

Weighing in on whether to weigh foods

Food scales provide an option for increased precision when measuring foods. For example, the Exchange List says that a "small" apple has 15 grams of carb. What *you* consider small may not be what *they* consider small. That's why in parentheses the Exchange List specifies that a small apple weighs 4 ounces. It means 4 ounces on a food scale, not 4 ounces in a measuring cup. Ounces of liquid and ounces of weight are entirely different things:

>> **Measuring cups measure liquid ounces.** There are 16 tablespoons to 1 cup, 2 cups to 1 pint, 2 pints to 1 quart, and 4 quarts to 1 gallon.

>> **A food scale measures weight in grams or ounces.** There are 28 grams to 1 ounce, 16 ounces to 1 pound, and 2.2 pounds to 1 kilogram.

Precision carb counting matters most when using insulin-to-carb ratios (see Chapter 6 for more about these ratios). You can use food scales to weigh fruits (if they're not easy to measure in a cup, as I explain in the preceding section), snack foods, or a slice of bread that you cut off of an unsliced loaf. Have you ever opened a bag of pita chips that says the serving size is eight pita chips, but the chips are all broken into smaller pieces? Food labels tell you the weight of one serving. In the case of the pita chips, the serving size says eight pieces, but in parentheses to the right of the serving size, it notes that the weight of a serving is 28 grams. You can use the food scale to weigh out 28 grams, which is one ounce, to get an accurate portion of the pita chips for a precise carb count.

The following sections go into more detail on using a food scale and counting carbs with a food's weight.

Using a food scale

If you purchase a food scale, make sure that it measures in increments of grams and ounces. Some food scales are designed for heavier items and weigh in increments of pounds. Food scales are available for less than ten dollars, but you can choose to spend more. Some versions have a dial that lines up with markings indicating the weight in grams or ounces, while others are digital. Scales have either a flat weighing surface or a bowl to contain the food. Compact travel scales are also available.

TIP

If you buy snack foods in multi-serve containers, weigh out individual portions and put the measured portions into zip-lock baggies or reusable containers. Mark the carb count on the bag with a permanent marker or write it on a label if using reusable containers.

The Exchange Lists in Appendix A note the weight next to some of the fruits. Use your food scale to compare your fruit to the reference size. For example, the list says that a small (4-ounce) apple has 15 grams of carb. It's unlikely your apple weighs exactly 4 ounces. Most don't. If your fruit weighs 6, 7, 8, or 9 ounces, then you're looking at doing some math, which can get tedious. To simplify, I've created a list of common foods that shows the carb count "per ounce" of the food. See the next section for more on that.

Counting carbs with a food's weight

Table 8-7 is useful because it's designed for you to weigh the fruit with the peel on. Weigh the entire fruit. Don't cut, core, or peel it until after it has been weighed. The inedible waste has been factored in, and the math has been adjusted to account for the part of the fruit that isn't consumed. Fiber grams have already been subtracted from the total carbs.

TABLE 8-7   **Grams of Carb per Ounce of Food**

Fruits	Grams of Carb per Ounce of Fruit (Skin On)	Starchy Foods	Grams of Carb per Ounce of Food
Apple	2.9	Dinner roll	14.0
Apricots	2.5	Kaiser roll	14.2
Banana	3.7	French baguette	14.5
Cantaloupe	1.3	Croissant	12.1
Cherries	3.6	Whole-wheat bread	13.0
Figs, fresh	4.6	Cornbread	12.3
Grapefruit	1.0	Challah bread	14.0
Grapes	4.8	Baked sweet potato	5.0
Honeydew melon	1.2	Baked russet potato	5.4
Kiwi	2.5	French fries	7.0
Mango	2.8	Sweet potato fries	7.3
Nectarine	2.3	Corn on the cob	5.6
Orange	2.0	Potato chips	15.0
Papaya	1.5	Oyster crackers	20.3
Peach	2.3	Tortilla chips	18.0
Pear	3.2	Pita chips	19.0
Plum	2.6	Pretzels	22.0
Tangerines	2.4	Angel food cake	16.0
Watermelon	2.0	Biscotti, almond	17.0

The benefit of using this particular list is that you can weigh all of the bananas in the bunch, one at a time, and get the carb counts figured out in advance. Use a pen to write the carb count in small numbers directly on the peel. Then, a day or two later when you have another banana, the carb counting has already been done. Write on the peel of the orange too. For apples or other fruits that have a sticker, write on the sticker. Office supply stores sell stickers that can be used to mark carb counts.

To use Table 8-7, locate the fruit or starchy food that you want to weigh. The number listed directly to the right of the food indicates the amount of carbohydrate contained in 1 ounce of that food.

Note: Carb content of foods may vary. Data in Table 8-7 was obtained cross-referencing and averaging information from the following two websites:

>> Calorie King: www.calorieking.com

>> USDA National Nutrient Database: https://ndb.nal.usda.gov/ndb/foods

So what kind of calculations do you need to make with this table? Using a food scale, weigh the food (for an entire fruit, include the peel, core, pit, and rind). Be sure to measure in ounces, and multiply the ounces by the number in the next column of the table. For example:

>> For an orange that weighs 10 ounces, multiply 10 by 2 for a total of 20 grams of carb.

>> For an apple that weighs 8 ounces, multiply 8 by 2.9 for a total of 23.2 grams of carb (you can round down to 23).

>> For a baked sweet potato that weighs 3 ounces, multiply 3 by 5 for a total of 15 grams of carb.

Fruits come in a wide range of sizes. Weighing fruit allows for a more accurate carb count. You don't have to weigh every fruit from here on out, but by going through the motions and weighing periodically, you refine your ability to guess correctly. After weighing a few oranges, you'll get pretty good at guessing the carb counts in the future.

Weighing food is something that a family member, friend, or roommate can do for the person with diabetes. Pre-weighing and marking carb counts saves time in the long run, and everyone learns to estimate carbs more accurately. When kids with diabetes repeatedly see the carb counts on foods, they learn to estimate better themselves.

Dealing with Special Cases

This section provides guidance on managing carbs when you're dining away from home. Some restaurants, primarily chain establishments, provide nutrition information and carb counts either in the restaurant or on a website. Chapter 9 provides details on how to zero in on resources that assist with quantifying carbs. Use your carb-counting cheat sheet too, as I discuss earlier in this chapter.

Controlling carb intake when eating out

Getting down to the nitty-gritty of carb counting in a restaurant may be a bit tougher because most of us aren't going to whip out our handy-dandy measuring cups. Using measuring cups at home improves your ability to recognize serving sizes when you're out, as I explain in the earlier section "Measuring with standardized cups and spoons." The hand method of portioning is also useful and discussed in more detail later in this chapter. An average woman's tightly clenched fist is about 1 cup.

Here are some additional pointers for watching your carbs when you eat out:

» Some restaurants serve big portions, which makes it easy to overeat. Ask for a to-go container as soon as the food is served. The best time to pack your leftovers is before you even take your first bite. Leave an appropriate amount on your plate to savor, but pack the rest and take it home to enjoy for tomorrow's lunch.

» Start your meal with a green salad and order an extra side of vegetables to accompany your entrée if you want a larger volume of food. Salad and vegetables are usually lower in calories and carbs than most other selections; just go light on the salad dressing.

» Another strategy for controlling intake in restaurants is to share an entrée. You can also create your own meal from a combination of smaller appetizers and side dishes.

WARNING

» Desserts in restaurants can be deceptively high in carbs and best to avoid. A couple forkfuls of a shared dessert may be the second-best approach.

One key to controlling carbs and calories is to choose the small-sized offerings. Over the years portions have grown, and so have our collective waistlines. Does anyone remember when a soda was in a 6.5-ounce bottle? That same soda is now sold in a 20-ounce bottle. Movie theaters and convenience stores sell buckets of soda with refills. Portion distortion is plaguing the United States. Years ago an order of fries was 210 calories. Today's large order is more than 600 calories.

A small hamburger is close to 300 calories, but deluxe versions range from 600 to more than 1,000 calories.

If you typically inject insulin at mealtime, be sure to bring your insulin with you when going out to a restaurant to eat. Rapid-acting insulins such as Humalog, NovoLog, and Apidra are commonly used to cover the carbs at mealtime, and they are designed to be injected within a few minutes of the meal. Follow your doctor's advice on when to inject. If you have been told to take your insulin 5 to 15 minutes before the meal, then you need to do that with restaurant meals as well. If you take "regular" insulin, then the typical timing is to inject it 30 minutes before the meal. Do not take your injection at home and then drive to the restaurant. If you take your insulin earlier than you should, you stand the risk of having your blood glucose drop too low. What if there is traffic, or you get to the restaurant and there is a waiting list to be seated, or someone bumps the plate out of the waiter's hand as he is delivering your meal? There are no guarantees, so wait to inject your rapid-acting insulin until the food is in front of you. Regular insulin is supposed to be injected 30 minutes prior to eating, which means making your best guess on injection timing when it comes to restaurant meals. Be sure to have carbohydrate foods handy in case the meal you ordered is delayed. Flip to Chapter 6 for more information on timing insulin.

Keeping track of the carbs you drink

For the most part, eating your carbs is better than drinking them. There are a few exceptions. For example, milk is a nutritious beverage and can be consumed without derailing your blood-glucose control.

Just keep in mind that liquids are rapidly digested and absorbed, so liquid carbs get into the bloodstream quickly. Sugar-sweetened beverages should be avoided. Keep a cautious eye on juice too. Juice isn't necessarily the best way to start your day if you have diabetes.

For more information on best-bet beverages, see Chapter 11.

Guesstimating: When Carb Counts Aren't Critical

For many people with type 2 diabetes, blood-glucose levels can be controlled with simpler portioning guidelines. Certainly carb counting is an option, but it may not be necessary. If you want to keep things simple or if you don't like math, charts, and measuring, then the two options covered in the following sections are great alternatives to carb counting. Manage portions and plan a balanced meal with the plate model. You can also learn to use your own hand as a measuring device with the hand method.

REMEMBER

Type 2 diabetes means your insulin is having a hard time helping you to properly use the glucose from the foods you eat. The more you eat at one time, the harder it is to control blood-glucose levels. The first step is to distribute food among three main meals, with optional snacks if needed. Keep the snack portions controlled. See Chapters 19, 20, and 21 for main meal menu ideas and Chapter 22 for tips on reasonable snacks.

Balancing your plate with the plate model

Policy makers and health experts try to guide Americans to eat healthier. For many years the Food Pyramid was used to guide nutrition, but now the pyramid has been replaced with the Choose MyPlate image. The plate image is visually simple to understand. The idea is to choose from a variety of food groups and to control portion sizes. Simply fill your plate in the manner shown in Figure 8-1. Imagine a line down the middle of your plate. Half the plate goes to grains and proteins with a little over one-fourth of the plate going to starch and the remainder allotted to protein. The other half of the plate is for fruits and vegetables, with the vegetable portion a little bit bigger than the fruit portion. A serving of milk is included if desired. (If you aren't a milk drinker, see Chapter 11 for tips on best-bet beverages.)

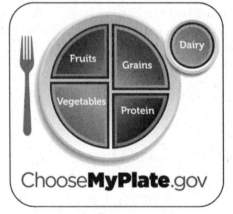

FIGURE 8-1:
The Choose MyPlate image created by the U.S. Department of Agriculture.

Source: U.S. Department of Agriculture

TIP

ChooseMyPlate.gov is a great place to find information on how to choose healthy options within each food group. You can find tips geared specifically to preschoolers, school-aged children, teens, college-aged students, adults, and for pregnancy. The educational materials and online tools are well worth exploring.

When using the MyPlate method to manage portions with diabetes, use vegetables from the nonstarchy vegetable list to fill the "vegetable" section. The starchy vegetables and legumes should be counted in the grains group because they are similar in carb composition.

It is fine to modify your plate to include even more vegetables than the Choose MyPlate model encourages. See Figure 8-2 for a meal-planning alternative that allows for more vegetables. Feel free to fill half of your plate with nonstarchy vegetables and add a leafy green salad if desired. When learning to cut back on other foods, salads and vegetables are the perfect foods to fill the void. Fruit can be consumed with the meal or as a between-meal snack. Use the Exchange Lists in Appendix A to identify fruit portions that are equal to 15 grams of carb. Fruit served at the end of the meal may satisfy your sweet tooth and make it easier to skip dessert. A little whipped topping over berries feels decadent but doesn't add that many extra calories, carbs, or fat.

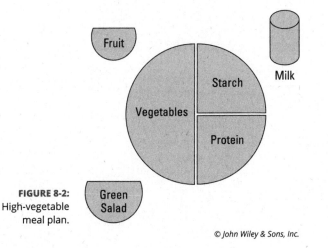

FIGURE 8-2: High-vegetable meal plan.

© John Wiley & Sons, Inc.

Handling portions with the hand model

TIP

Portion control is literally at your fingertips. If you want to keep things simple, you can use your own hands to visually guide serving sizes. Hands are certainly convenient, as you never leave home without them!

>> **Cooked starches:** Serve the size of your tightly clenched fist.

>> **Protein:** Serve the size and thickness of the palm of your hand.

>> **Vegetables:** Serve enough to fill your two cupped hands.

>> **Fruit:** Serve the size of your tightly clenched fist.

>> **Fat:** Limit serving to the size of your thumb.

Chapter **9**

Adding Tools for Carb-Counting Ease and Accuracy

L abel-reading and carb-counting concepts are detailed in Chapters 7 and 8. Don't stop there. You can include additional tools in your "diabetes tool chest." This chapter touches on some of the many resources available, both printed and digital, that can further sharpen your skills and simplify carb counting and diabetes management.

Reviewing the Printed Resources

It's always good to get things in writing. Keep printed carb-counting lists and food-composition reference books handy and refer to them as needed. You'll likely start to memorize some of the foods you frequently consume. Take advantage of the useful printed resources outlined ahead.

Reading the fine print for carb counts

Try some of the following printed materials for carb counts:

>> Compose a carb-counting cheat sheet detailing the foods you eat frequently (see Chapter 8 for details). Tape the list to the inside of your kitchen cupboard door where it's neatly out of sight yet readily accessible.

>> Keep your eyes on the Nutrition Facts food labels. Packaged foods provide the details needed to count carbs accurately and choose foods wisely. Stay tuned for the newly revamped food labels, which will be even easier to use and should be in widespread use by the summer of 2018. You can take a sneak peek at the label's new look in Chapter 7.

>> Keep Exchange Lists, such as those in Appendix A, handy for estimating carb counts in foods that don't have labels.

Additional literature to add to your carb-counting collection may include books, brochures, and menus that identify carb counts and food composition.

TIP

Bookstores are a great place to browse. Look for cookbooks with healthy recipes that list the nutrition details. If you use cookbooks that don't have the carb counts listed, you can look up the carb value of each ingredient. Add up the totals for all the ingredients and divide by the number of servings to estimate how many grams of carb the dish contains per portion. To help with this task, purchase carb-counting reference books, look up nutrition information online, or utilize apps as discussed later in this chapter.

Some chain restaurants have brochures that provide detailed nutrition information for each menu item. Collect them, compare them, and use the brochures to choose foods wisely. More and more restaurants will be providing nutrition details in the future. That's good news since Americans consume about one-third of their calories away from home. (The next section explains new regulations that mandate certain eateries to post nutrition details for the items they serve.)

Looking at labeling regulations for chain restaurants

The U.S. Food and Drug Administration (FDA) passed food labeling regulations that will require calorie information to be clearly displayed on menus and menu boards in chain restaurants as well as foods sold in certain vending machines. Here's the scoop:

>> **Who must comply?** Calorie labeling will be required for all chain restaurants that have 20 or more locations and all vending machines from companies that

have 20 or more vending machines. The labeling rules will apply to ice cream shops, coffee shops, bakeries, movie popcorn, convenience stores, and the cafés in warehouse stores as long as they fit the criteria of "chain establishments."

» **What nutrition info do they have to provide?** Only the number of *calories* needs to be prominently displayed. However, other nutrition details must be "available upon request." You may request information on total carbohydrates, fiber, sugar, protein, cholesterol, sodium, and fats. Restaurants can opt to display the additional nutrition information on posters, tray liners, signs, counter cards, handouts, booklets, computers, or onsite kiosks. If you don't see it, be sure to ask for it!

» **When do the regulations take effect?** The compliance deadline was set for December 1, 2016. Calorie labeling for the restaurant menus must be available by May of 2017 to avoid penalties. In some instances vending machines will have until July of 2018 to abide by the new regulations.

Tapping into Online Resources

Some people like to scroll through their printed materials digitally. That works. The landscape of diabetes management is ever changing and evolving. Technology is at our fingertips, linking us to a digital world full of useful information. If you've been hesitant to hop onto the tech train, it isn't too late. Whether you're using a computer or a mobile device, you can access important nutrition information, carb-counting tools, diabetes management software, blood-glucose tracking programs, and more. The following sections can point you in the right direction.

Digging up chain restaurant food facts

As I mention earlier in this chapter, the FDA is requiring chain restaurants with 20 or more locations to make nutrition information available. However, many chains already list the nutrition details online through their websites. From the restaurant's homepage, look for the "nutrition information" or "menu" tab.

TIP

Oftentimes you can download and print a page that lists all menu items along with the standard nutrition facts, including calories and total carbohydrate counts. Print off the nutrition details for the restaurants that you frequent and keep a copy in the glove compartment of your car. Compare menu options so you can make healthier choices and keep track of carbs, calories, fats, and sodium.

Foraging through Internet food databases

There are numerous nutrition databases online. For example, the USDA Food Composition Database is very detailed. It may provide more information than you really need, and it can be cumbersome to use. But, it's accurate and very thorough. It can be found at https://ndb.nal.usda.gov/ndb/.

Other food databases are more user-friendly. Calorie King is one example. Nutrition information is displayed in the Nutrition Facts food label format that consumers are already familiar with.

Log on to www.calorieking.com to find several useful tools. Under the "tools" tab, locate the BMI calculator to assess your weight status. Next, find out how much you should be eating by using the calorie estimator (click on "How many calories should you eat?"). The interactive calculator considers gender, age, height, weight, and activity level. Toggle between calorie targets based on whether you want to lose weight, maintain current weight, or gain weight.

Calorie King has an extensive food database. Use the search window to look up nutrition information on any food. The results are displayed in their "default" serving size. However, you can change the serving size to get the nutrition details on any particular portion size as discussed in further detail at the end of this chapter.

Using your search engine to count carbs

Whether you use Google, Yahoo!, Firefox, Bing, or any other search engine, you can do a quick search for nutrition information for just about any food. Simply use the search bar and type in your query. For example, if you type "nutrition facts butternut squash," you will end up with numerous search results that display calories, carbs, and key nutrients.

Enlisting the Assistance of Apps: One More Reason to Love Your Smartphone

Applications, or apps as they are more commonly referred to, are self-contained software programs designed to fulfill a particular purpose. Web apps are used online with your desktop or laptop computer. Mobile apps run on mobile devices such as your smartphone or tablet. Some apps are free, some have a one-time purchase fee, and others have a monthly subscription charge.

To search for apps on your smartphone or mobile device, simply locate the app store icon and click on it. Apple devices have an App Store icon; for Android devices, look for the Google Play icon. The search feature, which looks like a magnifying glass, allows you type in keywords to search for desired apps. This section illustrates how apps can help you manage your diabetes and diet.

Finding useful diabetes apps

Browse apps for carb counting, diabetes tracking, blood-glucose logbooks, diabetes management, and so on. The options are overwhelming. My app store search for "carb counting" produced a list of 93 apps to choose from. My search for "diabetes" apps resulted in 1,641 options. Ask and you shall receive! Hone your search results by being very specific about what functions you're looking for.

With so many apps available, choosing can be overwhelming. As you scroll through the available apps, you can investigate the details about each one. First, click on the app. You'll then have the option to review "details" about the app, read "reviews," and find "related" apps. Apps are rated by users and can score from 1 to 5 stars. In parentheses is a number that indicates how many users rated the app. An app that received 5 stars and has been rated by 1,853 users is an app that has loads of positive user feedback. The rating isn't as useful if the app has been rated by only two people. Read several of the user reviews to find out what people liked or didn't like about the app.

TIP

Give free apps a try. If they don't suit your needs, you can simply erase them. Before purchasing an app, spend a little extra time going through the review process to make sure the app offers the utility you desire.

Diabetes management apps can help you track food, activity, medication doses, blood-glucose data, health screenings, lab values, and more. They allow you to generate food records, blood-glucose charts, and reports that can be reviewed with your healthcare providers. Some diabetes management apps link to journals, message boards, blogs, educational videos, articles, nutrient databases, and recipes.

There are many diabetes apps to choose from. For example, there is a free app provided by Sanofi-Aventis called Go Meals. It has tools for healthy eating and a nutrient database powered by Calorie King (which I describe in the earlier section "Foraging through Internet food databases"). An activity tracker syncs with a Fitbit account to merge technologies. The blood-glucose tracker organizes blood-glucose data. Other free apps that get the nod of approval from users include "Diabetes in Check" and "Glucose Buddy."

Educational apps can help you build your diabetes knowledge base. Reputable information is literally in your back pocket if you download the right apps. Here are two examples:

>> The American Association of Diabetes Educators (AADE) offers a free app called AADE Diabetes Goal Tracker. It allows you to set and track self-care goals and empowers you to make positive changes to behaviors in order to enhance health.

>> The American Diabetes Association (ADA) has a free app for its online journal "Diabetes Forecast." The journal features articles on living with diabetes and offers tips for exercise, fitness, and nutrition (including recipes).

Integrating apps and a food scale

Apps can be helpful in deciphering carb counts. The Calorie King nutrient database, discussed earlier in this chapter, offers a free app for iOS so you can download the database to your Apple device. For Android systems, simply access the web version. Calorie King is interactive and can display nutrition details for weighed foods. Use a food scale to weigh your item (for example, a piece of fruit or a bread roll) and then enter the weight into your search results. If you're using Calorie King, first look up the food. Next, use the drop-down menu so results will be provided by weight in ounces or grams. Then enter the actual weight of your food item and the app will calculate and display the results.

For example, you can look up a baked potato on either the online or app version of Calorie King. The results page will list several different options for baked potato: russet potato, sweet potato, red potatoes, and so on. If you click on baked "russet" potato, the default size is small, 2 inch, (4.9 oz). You don't have to settle for the default size. You can change it by using the drop-down menu. Options include using a measuring cup or a food scale weight. To use a food scale, switch the serving size to oz (1 ounce). Weigh your own baked potato and enter the number of ounces in the space provided on the Calorie King program. Once you indicate the weight of your potato, Calorie King will calculate and display a nutrition facts food label for a baked russet potato of the size you entered.

Another popular app is MyFitnessPal, which helps you track your foods and physical activity. It also has a massive food database. The benefit of pairing a food database with a food scale is added accuracy in carb counting.

3

Going Beyond Counting Carbs

Find out why some foods raise blood-glucose levels more than others, even when they have the same carb counts.

Optimize blood-glucose control by aligning insulin action to digestion timing.

Imbibe best-bet beverages and think twice before drinking sodas and juices.

Know the risks when it comes to alcohol and diabetes.

Sort through sugars, sugar alcohol, and sugar substitutes.

Chapter **10**

Accounting for Variations in Digestion and Absorption Rates

M anaging carbohydrate intake is an important part of managing diabetes. While basic portion-control methods work well for some people, others rely on detailed carb counting to calculate mealtime insulin doses. Carb portioning and counting are key concepts, but the next layer is to understand how digestion rates differ among foods and how that influences blood-glucose levels.

This chapter moves beyond the basics in Parts 1 and 2 and explores other dietary variables that affect blood-glucose outcomes. Not all carbs are created equal. As carbs are digested, glucose becomes available. Whether the glucose races into the bloodstream or enters gradually depends on how long it takes for the food to digest. It may take ten minutes or it may take five hours, which makes a big difference. Fast digestion can result in a sharp rise in blood glucose. Very slow digestion may cause blood-glucose levels to rise hours after the meal.

The concepts in this chapter apply to everyone with diabetes, whether or not medications are used. Blood-glucose levels are simply easier to control if you understand the variables that influence digestion and absorption of food and then use that information to your advantage. Carbs and meds are two big pieces of the diabetes puzzle, and it's crucial that those two pieces fit together.

If you take insulin, you need a firm grasp of how that insulin works. See Chapter 6 to review the specifics on insulin action times. You'll want to make sure your insulin action matches the digestion timing of your meals. Discuss your insulin regimen questions with your healthcare provider.

Comparing Digestion Speeds for Fluids and Foods

This section identifies key factors that alter the rate of digestion and ultimately the absorption of the carbs in a meal. Blood-glucose levels reflect not only the *amount* of carb you eat but also the *type* of carb you choose.

Looking at liquid carbs

Liquids move through the stomach and into the intestine quickly. Therefore, sugary beverages can raise blood-glucose levels sharply. Sodas, juices, smoothies, milkshakes, specialty coffee drinks, and other sugar-sweetened beverages can derail blood-glucose management efforts. This is especially true if you have insulin resistance, as is the case with type 2 diabetes. See Chapter 11 for tips on choosing best-bet beverages.

High-carb beverages are rapidly digested and absorbed, so blood-glucose levels rise within minutes. If you polish off a bottle of soda or juice, the carbs from the drink will likely reach the bloodstream before the peak effect of injected insulin. The rapid-acting insulins peak in about one hour, and the duration of action is about four hours. That means the insulin works far longer than the digestion timing of the liquid carbs consumed. Beverages that are concentrated in carbs tend to cause a blood-glucose spike initially, but hypoglycemia may occur later. It can be hard to predict.

For the most part, it's best to avoid sugary liquids. An exception to the rule is if you're experiencing hypoglycemia. A blood-glucose level that falls below 70 milligrams per deciliter (mg/dl) is considered too low. Hypoglycemia indicates an imbalance in medication, activity, and carb intake. Drinking 4–6 ounces of fruit juice or regular soda is an appropriate choice for treating hypoglycemia. Exercise is another time when controlled amounts of liquid carbs can be used to fuel muscles during prolonged or strenuous exercise. For more on exercise, turn to Chapter 14.

Singling out sugars

One tablespoon of sugar, honey, or syrup contains almost 15 grams of carbohydrate. For perspective, that's the same amount of sugar as a whole cup of cantaloupe. Sugars and syrups have nearly 60 grams of carb in ¼ cup. The carbs in sugars add up quickly. Desserts and treats typically contain a lot of sugar, so controlling portion sizes is important.

As described in Chapter 3, sugar is a simple carbohydrate. Its effect on blood glucose depends on the amount of sugar consumed and what the sugar is mixed with:

>> Candies that are pure sugar digest quickly so they can raise blood-glucose levels swiftly. Examples of pure-sugar candies are jelly beans, gummy bears, and hard candies. These types of candy can be used to recover from hypoglycemia because they are digested and absorbed within 10–15 minutes.

>> Candy that contains fat or nuts, such as a candy bar, is digested and absorbed more slowly. Chocolate and nuts are both high in fat. Fatty foods are retained in the stomach longer, as described later in this chapter. Slower digestion and absorption means blood-glucose levels tend to rise less sharply. Chocolate candies can take well over an hour to be digested completely. For this reason, chocolate isn't the best choice for treating hypoglycemia.

See Chapter 15 to find out more about the causes, symptoms, and effective treatment of hypoglycemia.

Figuring out fruit

Fruit offers health benefits and should be consumed as part of a balanced diet. However, the natural sugars in fruit tend to raise blood-glucose levels sharply if eaten in excess. There's no starch, protein, or fat in fruit, just natural sugars along with fiber and important vitamins and minerals. Fruit digests more quickly than most other foods. When it's eaten alone, it may be fully digested in under 30 minutes. When it's eaten as part of a meal that contains protein and fat, however, then the entire meal is digested together and the rate of digestion depends on the amount of protein and fat in the meal.

TIP

Aim to keep fruit portions similar to the sizes listed in Appendix A. Generally that means a piece of fruit about the size of a tennis ball. For melons, berries, and mixed fruits, have up to one cup at a time. It's okay to have fruit several times per day, but blood glucose is easier to control if you spread out the servings of fruit and eat just one portion at a time. It takes several servings of fruit to make a glass of juice, so skip the juice and eat the fruit instead. You don't always need to pair fruit with fat, but it's worth considering if you do want to slow digestion, which blunts the blood-glucose peak. If you have a little cheese or peanut butter with your apple, for example, then the apple is digested more slowly because fat delays digestion.

Focusing on complex carbs and fiber

Complex carbs and simple carbs are made out of the same building blocks, as you find out in Chapter 3. Simple carbs such as fruit and sugar have only one or two sugar molecules, whereas complex carbs have many sugar molecules bound together. Starch and fiber are considered complex carbs:

>> **Starches:** Starches can be broken down into individual sugar molecules during digestion. Those sugars are absorbed into the bloodstream.

>> **Fiber:** Fiber is different. It can't be digested. Dietary fiber continues through the intestine and is excreted in the stool.

TIP

It's well known that fiber promotes intestinal health and reduces constipation, but did you know that fiber can lower blood-cholesterol levels? See Chapter 16 for details on soluble fiber and heart health.

Higher-fiber foods, such as whole grains, brown rice, oatmeal, and legumes, take longer to digest than refined white breads and white rice. Quick-digesting carb foods result in a steeper blood-glucose rise. White rice and brown rice, for example, both have the same amount of starch, but the brown rice has fiber, which slows digestion. Enzymes have to maneuver around the fiber to digest the starch. Consequently, glucose enters the bloodstream more slowly, and the blood-glucose rise is slightly blunted. Take note of your blood-glucose levels after eating refined versus whole grains to see how much of a difference fiber makes for you.

Take a look at Figure 10-1. The two curves illustrate the rise and fall of blood-glucose levels after eating refined grains, as shown in curve A, versus whole grains, as shown in curve B. Notice the refined grains have a steeper blood-glucose rise and are finished digesting sooner than the whole grains. Choosing whole grains instead of refined grains may be one tool for reducing blood-glucose spikes after eating. Slower-digesting foods may also help you feel satisfied for longer and reduce the urge for snacking, which can help with weight-control efforts.

FIGURE 10-1:
Blood-glucose response of refined versus whole grains.

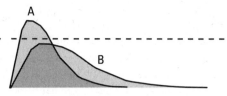

© John Wiley & Sons, Inc.

Recognizing the fat factor

A balanced meal, which includes carbohydrate, protein, and fat, takes roughly four hours to digest. If the meal is especially high in fat, it may take longer. Simply stated, fat delays gastric emptying. Fatty foods are processed in the stomach for a sustained period of time before entering the intestine for digestion. Protein foods can slow digestion too, but that may be from the fat naturally present in the protein food. For example, all meats contain fat — some much more than others. Cheese and nuts have protein but are especially high in fat. Significantly delayed digestion can contribute to blood-glucose issues, especially if you take insulin before your meals.

REMEMBER

If you take pre-meal insulin, it's important that your insulin and your meals are well-timed, as discussed in Chapter 6. A high-fat meal digests slower, so the rise in blood glucose tends to be delayed. The insulin taken prior to the meal can actively lower blood-glucose levels before the fatty meal digests — a mismatch in timing that can lead to hypoglycemia during or shortly after eating. Later, if the insulin wears off before the food has finished digesting, the blood-glucose levels can end up too high and stay high for hours after you eat the meal. Digestion timing and insulin timing need to line up. I discuss strategies for dealing with this situation later in this chapter.

TIP

The focus of this chapter is to highlight variables that affect digestion and absorption rates. Besides delaying digestion, fat content also correlates with calories consumed, which in turn influences body weight. For guidance on fitting in favorite foods yet eating for overall health, see Chapter 13.

Considering other variables

A few other things can influence digestion rates and alter blood-glucose results, at least somewhat:

>> **Particle size:** Grains that are pulverized into a powder digest quicker than larger grain particles.

>> **Degree of processing and addition of sugars:** I frequently hear complaints about blood-glucose spikes from people who have dry cereal and milk for breakfast. The issue is that many breakfast cereals are made from highly processed grains, so digestion is quick. Additionally, cereals often have added sugars. If you aren't accustomed to checking your blood glucose after breakfast, you may not have noticed how you respond to different meals. To observe the effect, check your blood-glucose levels an hour or two after breakfast and see whether meal composition makes a difference.

>> **Level of cooking:** How long a food is cooked may have some effect. Pasta cooked al dente takes longer to digest than pasta that is soft-cooked or overcooked.

>> **Degree of ripeness:** Riper fruits may digest more quickly or have more readily available sugars than unripe fruits; for example, your blood-glucose response may not be the same for a greener banana versus a riper banana.

>> **Length and type of grain:** When it comes to rice, blood-glucose results may differ depending on whether it's short-, medium-, or long-grain. Not everyone responds the same way to the same foods. Pay attention and see whether you note any differences between basmati, jasmine, red, black, or any other kind of rice that you eat. Certainly the portion size eaten is one of the most significant factors.

REMEMBER

Before you start splitting hairs over the potential differences among the many varieties of apples, or what part of the country the food was grown in, or the soil conditions . . . reel those thoughts back in and focus on the most influential factors. They may boil down to the portion size of carbohydrates consumed, the fiber content, the level of processing, whether the carb is solid or liquid, and the composition of the foods eaten at the same time as the carbs. The American Diabetes Association (ADA) has a commonsense suggestion: Replace refined carbohydrates and added sugars with whole grains, legumes, fruits, and vegetables.

Gauging the Glycemic Index and Glycemic Load

The *glycemic index* (GI) is a tool to measure how individual foods are expected to impact blood-glucose levels. A food is scored on a scale of 0 to 100 according to how much it raises blood-glucose levels as compared with blood-glucose levels after the consumption of 100 grams of glucose. GI tables separate foods into three categories: low (0–55), medium (56–69), and high (70–100). High GI foods tend to be digested and absorbed quickly and cause a steeper rise in blood glucose. Low GI foods are expected to digest slowly and produce a more gradual rise in glucose levels.

Foods are evaluated one at a time. To determine the GI of a food, 50 grams of digestible carbohydrate (total carbohydrate minus grams of fiber) are consumed on an empty stomach after an overnight fast. Blood glucose is checked every 15 to 30 minutes for the next two hours. Finger-stick blood samples are monitored. The blood-glucose responses of ten people are averaged to determine the GI of each food.

According to GI tables, apple juice has a low GI, yet it is commonly used to treat hypoglycemia. Carrots have a high GI, but most people can munch them without a significant rise in blood glucose. According to GI scoring, white rice can fall in the low, medium, or high GI range. It depends on the type of rice, how it's cooked, and even whether it's reheated after being previously cooked. Numerous GI tables and calculators can be found in print and online, yet there are many inconsistencies in the GI scores when you compare sources. It can get pretty confusing.

Here are a few more things to consider:

>> Most people do not eat one single food at a time on an empty stomach. When foods are eaten in a mixed meal that contains carbohydrate, protein, and fat, the glycemic effect differs. Meals are blended and churned in the stomach, and foods are digested together, not as separate components. The glycemic index score doesn't predict how blood glucose will respond when foods are consumed in a mixed meal.

>> The 50 grams of carbohydrate used to derive the GI score don't necessarily coincide with normal portion sizes. A slightly rounded cup of cooked rice provides 50 grams of carb, which is a fairly common portion size. However, it may take close to 6 or 7 cups of cooked carrots to reach 50 grams of digestible carb. Most people simply don't eat that many carrots at one time. When a typical portion of carrots is consumed, such as a half cup, blood-glucose response is quite flat.

>> GI scores are based on a relatively small sample size of people.

Because the portion sizes studied were not always consistent with usual intakes, an alternate system was developed. The *glycemic load* (GL) is based on the typical portion sizes consumed. Glycemic load ranks the blood-glucose effect of foods when eaten in normal portion sizes, not the arbitrary 50 grams of carbohydrate used in constructing the glycemic index tables. Glycemic load has more utility simply because it reflects usual portions. For example, watermelon has a high glycemic index but a low glycemic load as long as portion size is controlled.

The question remains: Should consumers be looking at GI or GL tables before writing out their shopping lists? There's no solid consensus among healthcare professionals. If glycemic tables help you reach your blood-glucose targets, it can be argued that they work for you. Evidence is mixed when you review study results. The ADA's 2016 Standards of Care note the complexity of the glycemic index concept. The ADA cites several studies related to GI, but the results are mixed and inconclusive. Some studies showed that use of lower glycemic load carbs improved A1C values by 0.2–0.5 percentage points. Other studies showed no appreciable effect. It may be that portion control and exercise make a more significant impact on diabetes control than using glycemic tables.

Reducing Blood-Glucose Fluctuations: Tips and Tricks

Have you identified any particular foods that wreak havoc with your blood-glucose control? If those foods happen to be foods that you're very attached to, finding solutions that enable you to include those foods — at least once in a while and in small portions — is important. (There's no magic here — unfortunately, there are some limits to what your body can tolerate when you have diabetes.) The strategies in the following sections may help you fit in a favorite food without significant consequences to blood-glucose control.

REMEMBER

Food choices matter when you have diabetes. Table 10-1 highlights key dietary factors that influence blood-glucose results (see the earlier section "Comparing Digestion Speeds for Fluids and Foods" for more information). If you consider these points when planning meals and snacks, you may find it easier to reach your blood-glucose targets.

TABLE 10-1   Dietary Variables Affecting Glycemia

Variable	Consideration
Portion size	Excess carb intake can sabotage blood-glucose control efforts. The larger the portion, the larger the amount of glucose that enters the bloodstream.
Form	Liquids digest rapidly, so they have the potential to raise blood-glucose levels more sharply than a comparable amount of carb in a solid food.
Processing	White, refined breads and processed grains typically cause a sharper blood-glucose rise than the same amount of the whole-grain version.
Meal composition	Having a balanced meal with carb, protein, and fat is usually better tolerated than just eating carbohydrate by itself.
Concentrated sugars	Sugar, honey, and syrups have concentrated amounts of carb in small servings. It's important to use caution when sweetening foods or having desserts.
Glycemic variance	Individual variation exists. You may notice that certain foods affect your blood glucose more than other foods. It may have to do with particle size, level of cooking, or simply the way your body handles that food.

Controlling portion sizes of foods that pack a blood-glucose punch

Reaching into the box of chocolates and taking one piece of candy isn't a make-or-break situation when it comes to blood-glucose control. One such candy may contain roughly 10 grams of carb and 80 calories. It just boils down to how much willpower you have. If the candy is too tempting, keeping a box of chocolates on your kitchen counter may not be a great idea. If you can muster the self-control to limit your intake, keeping mini treats on hand is feasible.

WARNING

Fruit juice has the potential to raise blood-glucose levels sharply for several reasons: It's liquid, it's concentrated in simple sugars, and it has no protein or fat to slow down digestion. Very small servings may be tolerated, provided your blood-glucose levels are near the lower end of your target range. Large portions of juice are unforgiving even if you eat something with protein and fat at the same time. Tolerance is tough simply because juice is concentrated in carbs. Fruit juice may be used in moderation before or during exercise sessions to prevent hypoglycemia. Blood-glucose results depend on your starting blood-glucose levels, the intensity and duration of the exercise, what type of diabetes you have, and whether or not you use medications such as insulin.

REMEMBER

Use Chapter 5 to set reasonable daily carbohydrate intake targets. Chapter 6 provides guidelines on how to best distribute the carbohydrate into manageable meals and snacks. As long as your diet is balanced and healthy for the most part, you can budget in occasional special treats. Account for the carbs by fitting them into your usual meal plan. That may mean eating a lower-carb meal when you plan to fit in a dessert with carbs. You can also counteract the effects of carbs somewhat by increasing your activity level, which is the focus of the next section.

Adding activity for extra carbs

If you end up slightly overdoing the carb budget, you may be able to offset the effects by adding exercise. A stationary bike or treadmill comes in handy when you need to add a quick exercise session. Weather permitting, a walk outside is another option for burning off the extra carbs and calories. However, you may need to walk or cycle for 20 to 30 minutes just to burn off 100 calories, so think twice before reaching for that pastry with 500 calories. Check out Chapter 14 for more about fitness.

Combining foods to reduce glycemic effect

Digestion rates are affected by how foods are combined. For example, white rice and white bread are refined and low in fiber, so they tend to bump up blood-glucose levels more sharply than whole grains. Putting peanut butter or almond butter on the white bread slows down the digestion and absorption of the bread, which may blunt the blood-glucose rise. Likewise, serving rice with stir-fried vegetables and fish, beef, chicken, pork, or tofu may reduce the glycemic effect of the rice. Of course, you still need to control the portion size of the rice! Plan balanced meals using the simple plate model as discussed in Chapter 8, or view sample meal plans and snack ideas in Part 5.

Altering the order in which you eat the components of your meal

TIP

Sometimes blood-glucose levels are higher than desired when you're about to sit down to have a meal. If you typically take insulin to cover your carbs, it may not hurt to give the insulin a head start when you're hyperglycemic at mealtime. After injecting the insulin, you can opt to start with the low-carb or carb-free foods first. Begin with salad, and then work your way through most of the protein and vegetables. Doing so allows the insulin a chance to chisel down the blood-glucose levels somewhat before you munch on carbs.

REMEMBER

If you're battling to get blood-glucose levels into a reasonable range, don't try to fit in sweets and treats. Don't overdo the carb portions when your blood-glucose levels are up. Sometimes it takes a few lower-carb meals to get blood-glucose levels back into the target zone. If your blood glucose remains elevated despite diet modification efforts, you may need medication dosage adjustments. Ask your healthcare provider for advice on meds.

Aligning Insulin and Digestion Rates

It's important to follow your doctor's recommendations and take insulin as prescribed. However, having a firm understanding of how your insulin works is very helpful. Numerous kinds of insulin are available to treat diabetes, and they differ. Some types of insulin are designed to cover the carbs in the meal, while others have profiles that are meant to match the glucose that is being released from your liver between meals and while you sleep. Chapter 6 describes the onset, peak, and duration times for the various insulins. When, specifically, does the insulin start to work? How long does it take for the insulin to reach its peak (strongest) effect? And how long does the insulin continue to work before it wears off? "Insulin insight" is a powerful tool that you can use to problem-solve and improve diabetes management.

Mealtime insulin must be aligned with digestion timing. If insulin gets into the bloodstream before the carbs digest, blood-glucose levels can drop. If the carbs digest quickly and enter the bloodstream before the insulin is working, blood-glucose levels can spike. I'm tempted to repeat the cliché that "timing is everything," but there are too many important variables to say that, so I'll settle for *timing matters.*

This chapter focuses on factors that affect how long it takes for foods to digest: liquids being faster than solids, refined grains digesting quicker than whole grains, and fat slowing down digestion by delaying gastric emptying. When a meal contains carbohydrates, proteins, and fats in reasonable amounts, the meal takes about four hours to digest. The highest blood-glucose level is about one to two hours after eating the meal. Rapid-acting insulin tends to be a good fit for most meals because it works its hardest an hour after being injected and wears off in about four hours. But some meals take longer to digest, especially meals that are high in fat, are fried, or have significant amounts of meat or cheese. When high-fat meals digest slowly, the timing of rapid-acting insulin may no longer match the digestion timing of the meal.

Understanding insulin action times as well as how long it takes for foods to digest allows you to make decisions about how to best align the two, as described in the upcoming sections.

Optimizing mealtime insulin coverage

Blood glucose is expected to be at its highest level about one to two hours after a meal, as long as it is a fairly balanced meal and not excessively high in fat. The meal should be finished digesting in roughly four hours. Rapid-acting insulin works its hardest (peaks) about an hour after being injected and finishes working in about four hours. See Figure 10-2. The dotted line represents the onset, peak, and duration of rapid-acting insulin. The shaded curve represents the blood-glucose levels rising and resolving after eating. As illustrated, the insulin action and the digestion and absorption of glucose from the meal line up nicely.

FIGURE 10-2:
Rapid-acting
insulin and a
balanced meal.

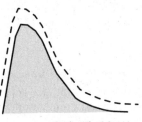

© John Wiley & Sons, Inc.

Recall that fatty meals digest slower. Figure 10-3 illustrates what may happen when rapid-acting insulin is taken before a meal that has a significant amount of fat. Again, the dotted line represents the timing of the insulin and the shaded curve represents the blood-glucose levels resulting from a high-fat meal. It may be a meal composed of fried foods, large portions of fatty meat, a cheesy meal, or a meal with a lot of added fats: butter, mayo, sour cream, salad dressing, or guacamole.

The rapid-acting insulin works at its normal rate, but the fatty meal digests slower than a normal meal. Consequently, the insulin may peak before the meal digests, which could cause hypoglycemia during the meal. Later, when the food finally digests, the insulin has passed its peak and doesn't have enough strength to lower the blood glucose, so glucose levels remain elevated. Such a situation can lead to high blood-glucose levels at bedtime after eating a high-fat dinner.

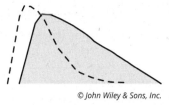

FIGURE 10-3:
Rapid-acting insulin and a fatty meal.

One solution may be to take the insulin midway through the meal or toward the end of the meal. Giving a fatty meal a head start can improve the way the insulin and the blood-glucose timings align.

REMEMBER

Discuss adjustments to injection timing with your healthcare provider prior to making changes to your regimen.

Using your insulin pump's fine features

An insulin pump has a feature that comes in handy when trying to match insulin action to slowly digesting fatty meals. If you aren't familiar with an insulin pump, a quick overview is needed. An insulin pump is a small, battery-driven, computerized device that delivers insulin. The pump contains only one type of insulin: rapid-acting. The pump has two main modes of insulin delivery: basal and bolus.

>> **Basal delivery:** The basal rate delivers tiny doses of insulin continuously. It's like a steady drizzle. Basal insulin delivery replaces the need for long-acting insulin. The basal rate matches the glucose that is being released from the liver.

>> **Bolus delivery:** This type of delivery comes into play when the user directs the pump to release a dose of insulin to cover the carbs in a meal. You can also bolus a correction dose of insulin if blood-glucose levels are above target.

A doctor who specializes in diabetes helps determine appropriate basal rates and bolus ratios.

An insulin pump can release a programmed insulin dose that more closely matches a slow digesting fatty meal. See the dotted line in Figure 10-4, which illustrates insulin action in a "combo bolus," also known as a "dual wave." The user can direct the pump to deliver part of the insulin dose *before* the meal and part of the dose *in small bursts over one or more hours.*

FIGURE 10-4:
Insulin pump
combo-bolus with
a fatty meal.

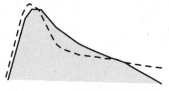

For example, say a person determines her insulin dose for pizza will be 6 units. She can opt to take 3 units up front and 3 units delayed. She can choose to have the delayed portion delivered incrementally over two or three hours, or whatever works for her. She can monitor results by observing her blood-glucose results. If she's not fully satisfied with the results, she can tweak her formula the next time. She might try 2 units up front and 4 units delayed. She can try any number of things. It does take some trial and error to see what works best for pizza versus what works best for a cheeseburger and fries. Diabetes educators and pump trainers can provide tips and guidance.

IN THIS CHAPTER

» Recognizing that sugary drinks can be dehydrating

» Selecting the best beverages

» Understanding that both carbs and calories add up

» Pointing out the risks and effects of alcohol

Chapter 11

Rethink That Drink

E very day you make choices that affect your well-being. What you choose to sip or guzzle can have a big impact on your health, especially your blood-glucose levels. You lose fluid every day through urination, sweat, and simply breathing. It's important to replace lost fluids and to choose your beverages wisely. Staying well-hydrated is essential for proper digestion and nutrient absorption and delivery, as well as for circulation, respiration, and body temperature regulation.

Watch what you reach for, though, because sugary, high-carb beverages can wreak havoc with blood-glucose levels. This chapter calls it like it is when it comes to liquid land mines. Thankfully, many tasty, refreshing beverages work in your favor, whether it's water you reach for or something with flavor.

Noting the Importance of Hydration and Low-Carb Drinks

REMEMBER

Up to 60 percent of an adult's body weight is water, so staying hydrated is critical to good health, especially when you have diabetes. You've probably heard that you should be drinking at least 8 cups of fluid per day. If blood-glucose levels are running above target, you may need more than that. Why? Because when blood-glucose levels are elevated, your kidneys will try to filter out some of the excess glucose, and in doing so they will create more urine. High blood glucose leads to increased urination. Frequent trips to the restroom can lead to dehydration. Dehydration is the result of losing more fluids than you take in. Fatigue, dizziness, muscle cramping, and perhaps rapid heartbeat follow. Dry mouth, dry skin, constipation, and dark-colored urine are also signs that you may be dehydrated. When you are well-hydrated, your urine should appear clear and pale in color. So drink up! But be aware that what you choose to drink can either help or hinder your health.

Consider the carb content of your beverage. If you are drinking sugar-sweetened beverages, regular soft drinks, frappa-yummies, or even fruit juice, you're dumping even more sugar into your system. Your blood-glucose levels will likely rise quickly, your kidneys will work overtime to try to rid your body of the excess glucose, you'll make more trips to the restroom and may end up dehydrated and thirsty . . . and around and around it goes. It's a vicious cycle, as you can see in Figure 11-1.

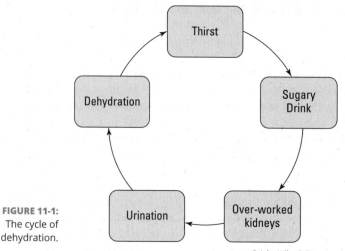

FIGURE 11-1:
The cycle of
dehydration.

© *John Wiley & Sons, Inc.*

The kidneys filter your blood just as the oil filter on your car filters the oil. It's the kidneys' job to decide what stays in the bloodstream and what gets dumped into the urine. The heart pumps blood throughout the body every minute of every day. Each trip around the track takes the blood through the kidneys for filtration. It's a well-known fact that persistently elevated blood-glucose levels can lead to long-term complications, including kidney failure. The oil filter on your car can be changed at regular intervals, the kidneys — not so easily. You're going to want to keep yours healthy, so skip the sugary beverages. (You can opt for some of the beverages in the next section instead.)

NOTICING THE UNQUENCHABLE THIRST

Jesse was in the clinic for his first visit with me. He was recounting the circumstances surrounding his initial diagnosis of diabetes: "In the months before I found out I had diabetes, I was feeling thirsty all the time. I work hard doing landscaping, so I figured that's why I was so thirsty. My morning would start off with a big smoothie, and I would have a large soda at lunch. I might have another soda or a sweetened iced tea in the afternoon. I just couldn't quench my thirst! I was waking up a few times a night to go to the bathroom. Something just didn't seem right, so I went to see my doctor. She checked my blood sugar in her office, and it was 312. Yow! I was drinking plenty of fluids, but all the wrong kinds!"

Jesse started drinking more water. He replaced regular sodas with carbonated water and an occasional diet soda. He switched to unsweetened iced tea with lemon. He's also happy to be sleeping better now that he isn't getting up every few hours to use the bathroom.

Exploring the Pros and Cons of Different Drinks

Sugar-sweetened beverages have come under scrutiny in recent years. Some cities are putting measures on the ballot calling for a soda tax. Health experts are pointing out that sugary sodas are loaded with empty calories. Pediatricians are counseling families to limit the amount of juice they provide to children. Schools are removing soda machines from campuses. What's all the fuss about? The problem is that sweetened drinks are being consumed in mass quantities while the country is reeling from an epidemic of obesity and diabetes.

When you have diabetes, drinking liquid concentrated carbs can cause your blood-glucose levels to rise sharply. The more you drink, the higher your blood-glucose level goes. Sodas, juices, and other sports and specialty drinks need to be carefully considered before you opt to partake; they often send blood glucose sailing above target levels. On the other hand, when treating hypoglycemia, it makes a lot of sense to swig 4–6 ounces of fruit juice to correct the low.

The following sections note the pros and cons of a variety of different drinks. Consider your options carefully!

Giving water a special place in your life

Staying healthy relies, in part, on staying well-hydrated. Every cell in the body requires water to function properly. Although thirst is usually a good indicator that you need more fluid, some people don't feel thirsty until their hydration is already compromised. Plan ahead and prioritize your fluid intake. Aim for at least 8 cups of fluid per day. Water is the obvious choice when promoting hydration, but soup broth, tea, milk, and other fluids count.

Carbonated water, bubbly water, fizzy water, mineral water, bottled water, spring water, tap water, flavored water . . . you can't go wrong with water. Squeeze a lemon or lime into the water for a little added zest. Plan ahead, pack a water bottle, keep a stash in the car, or fill a pitcher with the amount you want to consume each day. Having a pitcher in the refrigerator may get everyone in the house to drink more water.

TIP

You can try infusing the water for added flavor. There are water bottles and pitchers that are designed for infusing. They provide a center cylinder, which is the reservoir to fill with your choice of fresh sliced fruits, vegetables, or herbs. You lower the cylinder into the water bottle or pitcher and allow the flavor to enhance the water. Hikers use these to enjoy refreshing water along the way, and they can always snack on the fruit from the cylinder later. You don't have to be on a hike to enjoy infused water, though. You can infuse water in any pitcher you already own and strain out the fruit later. Favorite recipes include the following:

>> Fill a pitcher with ice water, mint leaves, and lime.

>> Try fresh cucumber slices with lemon slices and cilantro. Citrus peel can taste bitter, so peel the citrus before using.

Lots of recipe ideas are available online for infusing; just do a search for infused water and see what sounds interesting to you.

Sipping and swigging low-carb beverages

If you're looking for flavor, lots of options provide a little pizzazz and still don't drive the blood-glucose levels up. If you want a soda, you're better off with a diet version than a regular sugary soft drink. If you aren't looking for fizz, try drink mixes in powdered or liquid form that can be mixed up in a minute:

>> **Lemonade:** Lemons and limes have very little carbohydrate. Make homemade lemonade by mixing freshly squeezed lemon juice with water and sweeten to taste with your choice of noncaloric sugar substitutes. Start with 2 tablespoons of lemon juice to 8–12 ounces of water, or make it by the pitcher with ½ cup of lemon juice per quart of water, and sweeten according to taste.

Try freezing a more concentrated version of your lemonade in ice-cube trays to add flavor to your water anytime.

» **Tea:** Whether you like herbal, green, or black, caffeinated or caffeine-free, there are countless options. Steep it and drink it hot or chill it for a tall glass of iced tea. Try mixing half a glass of iced tea with half a glass of the lemonade you made in the preceding entry.

» **Diet drinks:** Most sugar-sweetened soda brands offer a diet version. Diet is the way to go when you're watching your blood-glucose levels. (Regular soft drinks wreak havoc.) Nobody benefits from getting hundreds of empty calories from beverages sweetened with sugar or high-fructose corn syrup. Diet sodas shouldn't displace nutrient-rich milk or other calcium-fortified milk replacements, but a diet soda here and there isn't going to hurt. For more information about the sugar substitutes used in diet soft drinks, see Chapter 12.

» **Sugar-free drink mixes:** Check your supermarket shelves for sugar-free drink mixes that you can mix up by the glass or by the pitcher. They come in powdered form or in liquid drops. Look for resealable, multi-serve containers as well as boxes with single-serve packets. Or, buy sugar-free beverages bottled and ready to drink.

When dining out, carry single-serve, sugar-free powdered drink mixes to stir into your glass of water. Stir up a serving of no-sugar-added lemonade or a fruit-flavored beverage. You win in two ways: You get a noncaloric diet drink that doesn't raise your blood sugar, and you save money. You can also carry the brands that come in liquid concentrate and plop a few drops into your ice water.

» **Coffee:** Don't worry. I'm not going to be the one to take away your coffee! Plain, brewed coffee doesn't affect your blood sugar, whether it is caffeinated or not. It boils down to what you put in it. A packet of your choice of sugar substitute doesn't add carbohydrate. A splash of milk or half and half doesn't add up to very much carb (unless you drink cup after cup). So just check the labels on what you're stirring into your coffee. The latte or café con leche carb count depends on the amount of milk you use, whether it's the moo kind or the soy variety. (Check out the next section for more on milk.)

Mentioning the merits of milk and nondairy milk substitutes

Milk has carbs and is liquid, but the carb count is really reasonable. An 8-ounce glass of milk contains somewhere between 12–16 grams of carb. Milk is an excellent source of protein, packing in 8–10 grams per cup. It also boasts some of the highest calcium counts per serving, with a whopping 300 milligrams per cup.

A large percentage of kids don't meet their daily calcium needs. (In truth a majority of adults don't meet their calcium goals either.) That's in part due to the over-consumption of soft drinks. When kids are sucking down soda rather than milk, they rack up the grams of sugar and empty calories, and they lose out on the protein, calcium, and other vitamins and minerals.

The recommended daily allowance for calcium is 1,000 milligrams per day for adults. With aging comes the risk of osteoporosis, so the calcium target bumps up to 1,200 milligrams per day for women aged 51 and older as well as men aged 70 and older. Kids aged 9–18 have the highest calcium needs, so their target is 1,300 milligrams per day. Three 8-ounce glasses of milk per day provide 900 milligrams of calcium, and four 8-ounce servings provide 1,200 milligrams of calcium.

The fat content of milk varies depending on whether you choose nonfat, low-fat, reduced fat, or whole. Your choice affects the calorie count and the saturated fat count, so choose wisely. The butterfat that is in milk is not a heart-healthy type of fat. Calories, carbs, protein, and fat are the same whether the milk is organic or not.

If you love, love, love milk and drink more than 3 or 4 cups per day, you may be driving up your blood-glucose levels and your weight. Calories in milk may range from 90–150 per cup, depending on the version (from fat-free to whole). Milk is a liquid carb, so it makes sense that having too much at a time, or too much in a day, can cause issues if you have diabetes.

If lactose makes you gassy, try lactose-free milk. The carb count is the same; it's just that the "double-sugar" lactose has been broken down into its two single sugar units so it's easier to digest.

If you prefer nondairy milk substitutes, you have many options to choose from: soy milk, almond milk, other nut milks (like cashew), hemp milk, coconut milk, and rice milk. Other options will likely be available in the future. Look at labels to compare carbohydrate, protein, fat, and calories, and don't forget to check for calcium. Many milk substitutes offer calcium-fortified versions that provide as much calcium as milk — or sometimes even more. For more label-reading tips, see Chapter 7.

Food labels give calcium information as a percentage, but you can easily decipher the milligrams of calcium provided. Many milk replacements are fortified to provide the same amount of calcium as milk, 300 milligrams per cup. The %Daily Value for calcium is based on 1,000 milligrams a day. Thirty percent of 1,000 milligrams is 300 milligrams. A label that says a serving provides 20 percent for calcium contains 200 milligrams. If your label boasts 40 percent, then you're getting 400 milligrams. You simply drop the percent sign and add a zero. (Read yogurt labels too.) The Dietary Reference Intake (DRI) for calcium varies by age and gender. DRI tables for a complete list of vitamins and minerals are available online.

Facing the facts about fruit juice

REMEMBER

Fruit digests quickly, which is why it's usually better for blood-glucose control to eat smaller amounts of fruit throughout the day rather than too much at one time. I suggest *if it's small, eat it all.* If it's big, cut the fruit in half. For melons, berries, and mixed fruit, you can ballpark it and aim for a cup of fruit as a suggested serving limit.

Fruit juice digests even faster than whole fruit. You can measure the effect on your blood glucose about 15 minutes after the time you drink it. That's right, from *lips to fingertips* in just a few minutes. The effect occurs so rapidly because liquids digest faster than just about anything else. When you drink juice on an empty stomach, it races through the digestive system like water disappears down the drain (see Figure 11-2). Just as water empties from a sink into the drain, fluids move through the stomach and into the intestine, where the sugars are quickly transferred to the bloodstream.

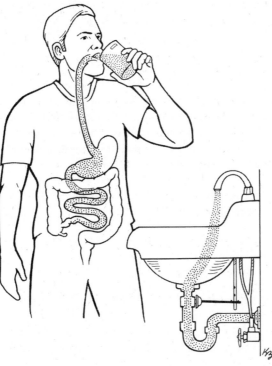

FIGURE 11-2:
Juice goes through your system like water goes down the drain.

Illustration by Kathryn Born, MA

But wait — you may say, "I thought fruit juice was healthy!" Although it's true that fruit is filled with vitamins, minerals, antioxidants, and many nutrients, fruit juice also contains a lot of natural sugar in liquid form. Eating fruit is part of a healthy, balanced diet, but it's better to eat the fruit, not drink the juice. Eating a serving of fruit two or three times each day is recommended, but I don't recommend eating all three portions at one time because large portions of fruit consumed in one sitting can cause a sharp rise in blood-glucose levels. When you drink a glass of fruit juice, you *are* having multiple servings of fruit at one time. The juice of one orange may fill your glass about one inch. A glass of juice is more like several fruits at one time.

TIP

Vegetables have many of the same vitamins and minerals that fruits have but with lower sugar content. You may find that you can enjoy a glass of vegetable juice without the same blood-sugar spike that fruit juice often causes. Portion size matters, so aim for about 4–8 ounces of vegetable juice at a time. An 8-ounce portion may contain close to 10–15 grams of carbohydrate, so you may not want to drink large volumes.

Before you nix juice completely, think about this: Fruit juice can actually come in handy in a couple of key situations. There's no need to keep large bottles of juice in the fridge, though. Single-serving (4–6 ounce) containers can be used for treating and preventing low blood-glucose levels. See details in the following sections.

Treating hypoglycemia

Because juice raises blood-glucose levels quickly, it's an excellent choice for treating hypoglycemia. When blood-glucose levels fall too low, then 4–6 ounces of fruit juice may be just what you need to quickly recover from the low. Remember to recheck your blood glucose again in 15 minutes to make sure you get back into a safe blood-glucose range.

REMEMBER

When blood-glucose levels fall too low, typically defined as less than 70 milligrams per deciliter, then follow the *Rule of 15*:

>> Take *15 grams* of carbohydrate.

>> Wait *15 minutes* and recheck blood-glucose levels.

>> Repeat until blood-glucose levels are back in a safe range.

Four ounces of fruit juice contain approximately 15 grams of quick-digesting carbohydrate. For more tips on treating low blood sugar, see Chapter 15.

REALIZING THAT JUICING WASN'T HELPING

Maria came to a class that I was teaching on diabetes self-management for type 2 diabetes. I was explaining that juice and smoothies can have a big impact on blood-glucose levels, and that for the most part, it's best to simply avoid the concentrated liquid carbohydrate drinks. I noticed her eyes widen as she let out a big sigh. She told the class, "When I was diagnosed with diabetes last month, I decided to take action and eat healthier. I went out and bought a high-powered juicer, and I've been blending orange juice with frozen berries and bananas ever since!"

It's no surprise that Maria's blood-glucose levels were not improving while she was drinking her homemade smoothies. In fact, once she stopped the smoothies and the fruit juices, and added some exercise, her blood-glucose levels improved greatly.

Preventing low blood glucose during exercise

Exercise is another time when juice may come in handy. That doesn't mean that everyone should drink juice before exercising. If you're on insulin or pills that could cause hypoglycemia, check your blood glucose before and during exercise to assess the need for carbs. Small amounts of fruit juice can be used to supply energy to the working muscles so that blood-glucose levels don't fall too low during, or after, exercise. Diluting fruit juice and sipping it during prolonged or strenuous exercise can help prevent exercise-related hypoglycemia. You can choose to use an electrolyte beverage in the same manner, if you need it. Just be sure to check the label for the carb count.

Note: There is much to consider in balancing exercise with carbs and meds. You can find more info in Chapter 14.

It's Not Just the Carbs — It's the Calories Too

WARNING

Liquid carbohydrate sources can have an impact not only on your blood-glucose control but also on your weight. Sugar-sweetened beverages, sodas, juices, smoothies, energy drinks, shakes, and specialty blended coffee drinks all pack in the calories. Too many calories can lead to unwanted weight gain. Excess weight can make it harder for your insulin to do its job of controlling blood-glucose levels. Being overweight worsens insulin resistance and makes blood-glucose management more difficult.

Table 11-1 lists popular beverages with their carb and calorie counts.

TABLE 11-1 ## The Carb and Calorie Counts of Common Beverages

Beverage	Carb Count in Grams	Calorie Count
8.4-oz. energy drink	28	110
20-oz. electrolyte-replacement drink	34	130
12-oz. can of soda	40	150
16-oz. specialty coffee drink	60	250
20-oz. bottle of soda	65	240
16-oz. bottle of juice	70	280
12-oz. fast-food chocolate shake	100	575
32-oz. soda	110	400
28-oz. fruit-juice smoothie	120	509

REMEMBER

The numbers listed in Table 11-1 represent the categories mentioned, but there is certainly variation, so check your Nutrition Facts food labels.

TIP

Did you know that 1 teaspoon of sugar has 4.2 grams of carbohydrate? To calculate the number of teaspoons of sugar in any of the beverages in the table, just take the number of grams of carb and divide it by 4.2.

For example, a 12-ounce can of soda with 40 grams of carbs equals nearly 10 teaspoons of sugar. Even though juice is natural, the standard 16-ounce bottle of juice is equivalent to nearly 17 teaspoons of sugar. Ounce for ounce, juice is similar to soda in sugar content. Whether you're drinking fruit sugar or white sugar, the response in the blood-glucose level is about the same. What about the 12-ounce chocolate shake with 100 grams of carbs? Well, that shakes down to having nearly 24 teaspoons of sugar. A teaspoon of sugar has about 16 calories.

The sugars in sweetened beverages have nearly 4 calories per gram, and with the amount of sugar being swigged in sweetened beverages, the calories can really add up. Some beverages — a milkshake, for example — have additional calories coming from fat.

TIP

The American Diabetes Association (ADA) publishes the annual Standards of Medical Care for Diabetes. Guidelines are updated and released every January in the journal *Diabetes Care*. The ADA emphasizes that "people with diabetes and those at risk should limit or avoid intake of sugar-sweetened beverages to reduce risk for weight gain and worsening of cardiometabolic risk profile." You can view the Standards of Care online by visiting the ADA website at www.diabetes.org. Click on the Professionals section, and then click on Standards of Care.

Last Call for Alcohol: What's the Verdict?

REMEMBER

Having diabetes and having a drink takes a little forethought, besides the usual warnings, such as don't drink and drive and don't drink too much. Managing diabetes safely means you should first discuss alcohol use with your doctor.

The following sections talk about alcohol's risks, effects, carb counts, and calorie counts. You also get information on drinking alcohol safely.

Being informed about the risks

WARNING

Talk to your doctor or nurse practitioner about alcohol use. Review your medication list and your overall health history to find out whether alcohol is safe for you to use in moderation. Alcohol may be unadvisable depending on your health history and the meds you take. If your doctor gives the green light, ask how much and how often you can safely drink.

Some considerations regarding alcohol use that apply to everyone, with or without diabetes, include the following:

>> Alcohol is high in calories and can contribute to weight gain.

>> The more you drink, the more likely you'll suffer from high blood pressure.

>> Drinking too much can raise triglyceride levels (blood fats).

>> Excessive alcohol use can lead to liver disease, pancreatitis, neuropathy (nerve damage), and some forms of cancer.

>> Heavy drinking is linked to depression and dementia.

>> Overconsumption of alcohol increases the risk of heart disease and stroke.

>> Too much alcohol impairs the immune system, making it harder to fight off illness and infection.

WARNING

Alcohol holds an additional risk for a person with diabetes. Alcohol can lower blood-glucose levels and can lead to severe hypoglycemia for insulin users — that means all people with type 1 diabetes, and anyone with type 2 diabetes who is treated with insulin. The risk of hypoglycemia also applies to certain diabetes pills. Specifically, if you take any diabetes medication that stimulates your pancreas to make more insulin, including a class of medications known as sulfonylureas, then you, too, are at risk for hypoglycemia. If you aren't sure, ask your doctor or pharmacist about the medications that you are on to find out whether you're at risk for lows.

Going behind the scenes: How alcohol affects the body

It is important not to drink on an empty stomach. A mini physiology review may shed some light on why it's so important to have carbs digesting when you have a drink.

Blood-glucose levels are at their highest typically one to two hours after eating a mixed meal. (A mixed meal is a meal that contains carbs, protein, and fat.) Protein and fat cause the carbs to digest slower. A mixed meal takes roughly four hours to finish digesting. During digestion, carbs are breaking down into glucose and entering the bloodstream. Normally, some of the glucose from the meal is packed away in the liver and saved, to be used later as needed. When the meal is completely done digesting, the liver is supposed to release the glucose that was previously stored. Your body must always have glucose in the blood to keep the vital organs functioning properly. (For more information on the physiology related to diabetes, see Chapter 4.)

Alcohol goes to the liver to be detoxified, processed, and broken down into safe byproducts. While the liver is breaking down the alcohol, it may not be able to release glucose normally. If the glucose release from the liver is compromised, then the insulin (or certain diabetes pills/medications) may continue to push the blood-glucose levels lower and lower. A single drink can take two or more hours to be processed by the liver, so glucose regulation may be impaired for that amount of time or longer. The liver stays busy for two hours or more *per drink*, so the more drinks you consume, the longer you are at risk for low blood-glucose reactions. Figure 11-3 helps clarify the concept.

In Figure 11-3, the gray shaded area represents the rise and fall of the blood glucose after eating a meal. When foods are finished being digested and absorbed, the liver's job is to release glucose that had been previously stored. Alcohol impairs that process because the liver preferentially breaks down the alcohol. Hypoglycemia may ensue.

WARNING

If you drink on an empty stomach, that means there is no carb digesting, so there's no glucose supply via digestion. Your liver is supposed to release glucose between meals. If alcohol impairs the liver from releasing glucose, you cut off your only glucose supply. Your meds can make your blood glucose drop too low.

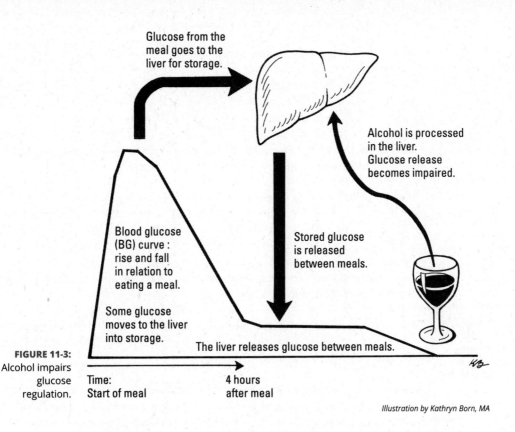

Glucose from the meal goes to the liver for storage.

Alcohol is processed in the liver. Glucose release becomes impaired.

Blood glucose (BG) curve : rise and fall in relation to eating a meal.

Some glucose moves to the liver into storage.

Stored glucose is released between meals.

The liver releases glucose between meals.

Time:
Start of meal

4 hours
after meal

FIGURE 11-3:
Alcohol impairs glucose regulation.

Illustration by Kathryn Born, MA

Looking at liquor's carbs and calories

A common misconception about alcohol is that many people assume alcohol turns to sugar, or alcohol will raise their blood–glucose levels. Actually, hard liquor doesn't have any carb, wine is very low in carb, and beer has about as much carb as a piece of bread:

>> Hard alcohol (distilled spirits) doesn't have any carbs, except for whatever it's mixed with.

>> Most wines have only 3–5 grams of carbohydrate per 5-ounce glass. The sugar from the grape juice turned into alcohol during the fermentation process.

>> Beer has roughly 13 grams of carb per 12-ounce portion. The carbs in beer come from wheat, barley, or malt.

However, if your drink comes with a cherry and an umbrella, I'm guessing it has carbs, probably lots. Mixed drinks can be especially high in calories when you consider the alcohol and the mixers. Sugary mixers, soda, or juices can lead to a rise in blood glucose, at least temporarily, because the liquid carbs get into the bloodstream fast. But blood glucose may end up plummeting later.

Insulin users may wonder whether they should "cover the carbs" in their alcoholic beverages with insulin. That may work okay at mealtime for one drink: for example, if you have a beer with a carb-containing dinner. Say the beer has 13 grams of carb and the meal has 55 grams of carb. You may be fine counting the total as 68 grams of carb and taking the appropriate dose of insulin. The food and the insulin both last about four hours. The alcohol should be done processing within about two hours. That's why you're less likely to get low blood sugar if you have your drink with a meal.

However, drinking on an empty stomach is a different story. Consider this: If you take insulin to cover the carbs in an alcoholic beverage, the rapid-acting insulin will last about four hours, but the liquid carbs in a beer or in carb-containing mixers will be digested very quickly — within 15 minutes of drinking. On an empty stomach, alcohol has a blood-glucose-lowering effect for two or more hours per drink. The carbs won't last as long as the alcohol and the insulin, which increases the risk of having hypoglycemia.

REMEMBER

Talk to your doctor about insulin and alcohol. The discussion in this book is conceptual and not meant to provide insulin dosing instructions. Medication use and adjustments must be discussed with your doctor.

Some alcoholic beverages have carbs, but all of them have calories. Alcohol has 7 calories per gram, protein and carbohydrate have 4 calories per gram each, and fat has 9 calories per gram, so fat and alcohol are the most calorically dense. Alcohol can contribute to weight gain, so it's important to account for the calories consumed. Table 11-2 lists popular alcoholic beverages and their average carb and calorie counts. Extra stout beers would have more carbs and calories than listed, and beers in general vary by brand. Mixed drinks have a wide range of carb and calorie counts — too wide to mention here — but some frou-frou drinks push upwards of 500 calories up that straw.

TABLE 11-2   **The Carb and Calorie Counts of Common Alcoholic Beverages**

Beverage	Grams of Carb	Calorie Count
80 proof spirits — 1.5 oz.	0	100
Wine (red or white) — 5 oz.	3–5	125
Beer (light) — 12 oz.	5–6	100
Beers (average) — 12 oz.	11–15	150

The numbers listed in Table 11-2 represent some averages across the categories mentioned, but there is certainly variation. Check labels, look online, or contact manufacturers for details. I talk about the calorie counts of other beverages and why it's important to know them earlier in this chapter.

Drinking safely

Drinking increases the risk of low blood-glucose levels (hypoglycemia) for anyone taking insulin or certain oral agents (pills) used to treat diabetes. Keep your meter handy and use it. Staying safe means limiting your intake of alcohol. It's very important that you *never* drink alcohol on an empty stomach. If you're going to have a drink, have it with a meal or snack that has adequate carbohydrates. And first and foremost, get your healthcare provider's approval and advice before drinking.

The following sections provide additional pointers on drinking alcohol safely when you have diabetes.

Knowing the recommended limits and portions

Healthcare experts generally recommend that adult women limit their alcoholic beverages to one drink per day and that adult men limit consumption to two drinks per day at most.

The actual alcohol content of a standard drink is 14 grams of pure alcohol. Each of the following portions count as one alcoholic beverage:

>> 5 ounces of wine

>> 12 ounces of beer

>> 1.5 ounces of distilled spirits (80 proof)

By the way, a shot glass holds 1.5 ounces.

Checking blood glucose levels and being prepared

Besides the health risks already discussed in this chapter, alcohol use with diabetes can cause a few more problems. Here are a few additional things to keep in mind:

>> Alcohol can impair your judgment, and diabetes self-care may suffer.

>> Alcohol may diminish your ability to feel the symptoms of hypoglycemia, so the lows can sneak up on you without warning.

>> If your blood-glucose levels drop too low, you may become unsteady on your feet. Other people may think you're drunk when in fact you may have low blood-glucose levels (hypoglycemia) and be in need of assistance.

The only way to stay on top of what your blood-glucose levels are doing is to take out your meter and check. (If you're on a continuous glucose monitor, check it frequently.) Carry glucose tablets or other quick-acting carbs in case you need to treat low blood glucose. Be aware that if you have had one episode of hypoglycemia, you're more likely to have another low in the coming hours.

WARNING

While one generation may be having drinks at cocktail hour, *before* dinner, and another generation may be drinking into the wee hours of the morning, which may be many hours *after* dinner, both are at risk for hypoglycemia because these drinking times tend to be on an empty stomach. Consider the need for a carb snack. Late-night drinking can be especially treacherous because blood-glucose levels can fall extremely low and go undetected by you or anyone else once you are asleep.

Consider these safety pointers:

>> Wear medical alert identification.

>> Check your blood glucose more frequently if you've had alcohol.

>> Carry carb snacks and quick carbs for treating lows.

>> Set an alarm on loud to wake yourself up to check your blood glucose in the middle of the night if you've been drinking. Keep your meter and low supplies, such as juice, by the bedside.

>> Educate family and friends on how to assist you, should the need arise.

>> Be especially careful about drinking after exercise because you're even more prone to hypoglycemia.

REMEMBER

If you're going to be enjoying a drink, be sure to do so safely. Be aware, be prepared, and pair your alcoholic beverage with a carbohydrate-containing snack or meal.

Chapter **12**

Let Me Call You Sweetie: Sugars and Substitutes

Y ears ago if you were diagnosed with diabetes, you were typically told to stop eating sugar entirely. If you were seen with a cookie in your hand, the diet police would come out of the woodwork and scold you. To this day, a lot of shaming and judgment still happens when someone with diabetes has a treat. Most often others are well-intentioned when they ask, "Should you be eating that?" But they aren't necessarily well-informed about diabetes or its treatment, or about your particular situation.

Of course it makes total sense to control sugar intake if you have diabetes. It also makes just as much sense to control sugar intake if you don't have diabetes. Getting 15 grams of carb from a small apple provides vitamins, minerals, and other nutrients, whereas getting 15 grams of carb from 4 ounces of soda just dumps sugar into your body with no nutritional benefit. Sugar-sweetened beverages should be avoided. Sugar is very concentrated in carbs and calories, and void of nutrients. Sugar intake should be limited, but there is room to fit in a treat now and then in the context of an otherwise healthy, balanced diet. Having a pudding cup with 15 grams of carb is certainly tolerated better than the corner piece from the birthday cake — you know the one I'm talking about . . . it has frosting on both sides and the big frosting flowers on top. That dessert may not go over so well with your diabetes.

Here's what the American Diabetes Association (ADA) says about consuming sugar if you have diabetes: "You can substitute small amounts of sugar for other carbohydrate-containing foods into your meal plan and still keep your blood-glucose levels on track. Consumption should be minimized to avoid displacing nutrient-dense food choices." In addition, the American Heart Association (AHA) suggests that women limit their overall sugar consumption to less than 100 calories per day, which turns out to be about 6 teaspoons of sugar. For men the limit is 150 sugar calories per day, or no more than 9 teaspoons of sugar. For perspective, a 12-ounce sugar-sweetened soda has about 10 teaspoons of added sugar, which exceeds the budget. (Find out more about this subject in the later sidebar "Sugar consumption in the United States.")

Good nutrition is fundamental to all of us. For diabetes, the focus should be understanding how to manage *all* forms of carbohydrate. That means eating reasonable portion sizes, and for many individuals it means learning to count carbs. Equally important is having a firm grasp on how different carbs affect blood-glucose levels. Did you know that eating 10 grams of carb from chocolate-covered almonds versus 10 grams of carb from jelly beans does not have the same impact on blood-glucose levels? That's because fat delays digestion, and chocolate and nuts are both high in fat. The sugar from the chocolate enters the bloodstream slowly. On the other hand, the sugar from the jelly beans digests quickly, which causes a sharper rise in blood-glucose levels.

Is one better than the other? It depends on the circumstances. If you're experiencing low blood glucose (hypoglycemia), you want to eat the jelly beans because they will raise your blood-glucose level quickly. You shouldn't use chocolate or nuts to treat lows. On the flip side, if you just want a sweet snack, a few chocolate-covered nuts won't spike your blood glucose as much as the same amount of carb coming from jelly beans or any other pure-sugar candy. In any case, dessert calories add up fast, so portion control is important.

This chapter gives you the lowdown on sugar, sugar alcohols, and sugar substitutes. For more information on the variables that affect blood-glucose responses, see Chapter 10. For details on treating hypoglycemia, see Chapter 15.

Comparing Sugars: The Sugar Showdown

Sugar, honey, and syrups all have a similar impact on blood-glucose levels. Sugar is undoubtedly concentrated in carbs, so relatively small amounts have the potential to boost blood-glucose levels considerably. If you have been abstaining from sugar, don't let the pendulum swing too far in the other direction — don't over-indulge just because the dietary advice has relaxed enough to acknowledge that people with diabetes can include modest amounts of sugar. There is a time and a place for either *inclusion* or *avoidance.* If you're getting exercise, you may find that you tolerate that piece of candy better than if you were glued to your chair in front of the computer.

WARNING

Clearly, if your blood-glucose levels are running above target, that isn't the time to have any sweets. Your blood-glucose monitor will let you know how well (or not) you tolerate a small serving of dessert. Beware of restaurant desserts in any case, though, as some pack in well over 100 grams of carb in a slice of cake, a serving of flan, or an ice cream brownie sundae.

The following sections describe the most common types of sugars, as well as natural fructose and agave nectar.

THE CASE OF THE COOKIE IN THE LUNCHBOX

Many years ago a child who was being followed in our pediatric diabetes clinic was politely confronted by an adult who worked for the school district. The offense was having a cookie in her lunchbox. The adult assumed that the parents were not properly taking care of their child who had type 1 diabetes, so she called child protective services to report the parents. The cookie had 10 grams of carbohydrate. However, also in the lunchbox were a turkey sandwich on whole-grain bread, which had 30 grams of carb; milk with 15 grams of carb; and carrots with 5 grams of carb. What the school employee didn't seem to realize was that the parents had counted the carbs in the lunch, and the insulin dose was going to be appropriately matched to that amount of carb. The lunch contained a total of 60 grams of carb, which was completely appropriate. For reference, many school lunch programs serve lunches with 60–75 grams of carb per meal because that amount is standard for a child in middle school.

We de-escalated the situation by explaining that all of the carb foods in the child's lunch would be digested and turned into glucose, and that the insulin dose would transport that glucose into the child's cells to be used for fuel. Imagine the distress the child felt and the frustration the parents endured to defend their right to include a small cookie in the context of a balanced diet.

To be singled out as the only child who is denied a cookie can lead to undue psychological distress. A cookie is not *pure sugar.* Cookies have starch (flour), protein (eggs), and fat (butter, nuts) along with the sugar, so the cookie actually takes a while to digest and can easily be managed with insulin.

Introducing the heavyweights: Sugar, honey, syrup, and other notables

REMEMBER

Most of the sugars in the following sections have a similar impact on blood-glucose levels. Sugar, honey, syrups, and other caloric sweeteners are concentrated in both calories and carbs. Use them sparingly. A single tablespoon of sugar packs in as many grams of carb as an entire cup of cantaloupe or raspberries. Most sugars have about 4–5 grams of carbohydrate per teaspoon, 12–15 grams of carb per tablespoon, and 48–60 grams of carb per quarter cup. One cup of white sugar has 200 grams of carbohydrate.

WARNING

Review labels on the containers of any sugars and syrups and check the exact carb count. Beware: These can all raise blood-glucose levels sharply, so limit the amount used. I address other calorie-containing sweeteners later in this chapter because sugar alcohols, fructose, and agave nectar have some key differences that separate them from the sugars in the following sections.

White sugar

White sugar (sucrose) is what is typically found in the sugar bowl, cube, or packet. Sugar crystals are available in varying textures, from *fine* to *ultrafine*. Bakers often prefer the finer, smaller particles. Powdered sugar, also called confectioners' sugar, is ground and sifted and has a little cornstarch added to prevent caking. There are also coarser, larger sugar crystals that are used to sprinkle on top of cookies, for example.

TECHNICAL STUFF

White table sugar comes from either sugarcane or sugar beets. The sugars are extracted, boiled, and concentrated. The brown color in raw sugar is from the natural molasses in the sugar. The molasses can be separated from the sugar crystals in a process that involves spinning the sugar in a centrifuge and washing the sugar crystals to remove the molasses. The Sugar Association explains that the sugar obtained from beets and sugarcane is "neither chemically altered nor bleached to achieve its naturally white color."

Molasses

Molasses is made from sugarcane and sugar beet syrup. After extracting the white sugar crystals, molasses is the viscous liquid that remains. It contains minerals such as iron, magnesium, and potassium, as well as trace vitamins.

Brown sugar

Brown sugar retains some of the natural molasses, which imparts color and flavor. There are several varieties in the brown sugar category, and they differ in the level of processing or in the amount of molasses retained. Besides the familiar light brown and dark brown varieties, there is also turbinado sugar, which is a partially refined, light brown sugar with larger crystals, and Muscovado or Barbados sugar, which is less refined and retains a higher amount of molasses so it's stickier.

Coconut palm sugar

This sweetener is gaining popularity. It is made from the sap of the coconut palm tree. It has a golden color and withstands high heat. The carb count is the same as white sugar.

Liquid sugar

Liquid sugar is simply white granulated sugar that has been dissolved in water. Another liquid sugar is called invert sugar. *Invert sugar* is formed by splitting sucrose into its two component sugars: glucose and fructose. (Check out Chapter 3 for more about the chemical structure of sugars.)

Honey

Bees produce honey from plant nectar. Honey contains a blend of fructose, glucose, and water. Honey has trace amounts of vitamins, minerals, and enzymes. Honey's flavor depends on the source of nectar gathered by the bees. The fructose in honey imparts a sweeter taste than white sugar.

Rice syrup

Rice syrup is made from rice starch that has been enzymatically split. The syrup is composed of single-, double-, and triple-glucose molecules.

Corn syrup

Corn is processed to make cornstarch and then further processed to break the cornstarch down into individual glucose sugars. Corn syrup is sometimes called glucose syrup.

High-fructose corn syrup

The glucose in corn syrup can be treated with enzymes to convert some of the glucose to fructose. The most common form of high-fructose corn syrup (HFCS) is 55 percent fructose and 45 percent glucose.

Maple syrup

Maple syrup comes from the sap of sugar maple trees. It contains mostly natural sucrose and water. There are small traces of glucose, minerals, and some B-vitamins.

Other sugars

On ingredients lists, names that end in -ose indicate sugar, such as maltose, dextrose, glucose, fructose, levulose, and sucrose. Maltodextrin is similar to sugar; it's a short chain of glucose molecules, which can be made from corn, rice, or potatoes.

Pointing out the qualities of natural fructose and agave nectar

Fructose is the natural sugar that is found in fruits. Vegetables also have fructose, and amounts vary, with the root vegetables having more than the other vegetables. Crystalline fructose is the powdered form that has been extracted from the plants and is packaged and sold as a sweetener.

In chemistry, fructose is a single sugar molecule. Glucose is also a single sugar molecule. Both glucose and fructose have the same chemical make-up, which is 6 carbons, 12 hydrogens, and 6 oxygens. The glucose molecule is a *hexose* because it has a six-sided form, whereas fructose is known as a *pentose* because it has a five-sided form. See Figure 12-1.

FIGURE 12-1:
Glucose and fructose molecules.

| Glucose 6-sided sugar | |
| Fructose 5-sided sugar | |

© John Wiley & Sons, Inc.

Glucose is the preferred fuel source for cells and tissues, and the only fuel source for the brain. The hexose form is readily available for the cells to use for fuel. Fructose is not processed and used in the same way as glucose. The pentose form is not quite cell ready. The fructose from a meal shuttles to the liver to await further instructions. The liver can do one of three main things with it:

>> The liver can turn the fructose into glucose and then hold on to it and store it as glycogen.

>> The liver can turn fructose into glucose and send it back out into the bloodstream for more immediate use.

>> The liver can convert excess fructose to fat. (By the way, anything with calories can be converted to fat if you eat more calories than your body needs.)

For more information on how glucose is used and stored in the body, see Chapter 4.

WARNING

Excessive intakes of high-fructose corn syrup, large intakes of crystalline fructose, or too much agave nectar can raise blood-triglyceride levels. Triglycerides are a type of fat (lipid) that circulates in your blood. Excess calories can be converted to triglycerides, which can be stored in fat cells or may accumulate in your bloodstream. People with diabetes already have a higher risk of heart disease, and high triglyceride levels further increase that risk. See Chapter 16 for more on heart-healthy eating.

Agave nectar is derived from the blue agave plant (the same plant used to make tequila). Agave is mostly fructose. That means agave nectar also goes to the liver first, and then the liver decides what to do with it. The bottom line is that both fructose and agave nectar have a less immediate blood-glucose-raising effect. Agave and fructose have about 4–5 grams of carbohydrate per teaspoon, 12–15 grams of carb per tablespoon, and 48–60 grams of carb per quarter cup. They are said to have a lower glycemic index than regular sugars and syrups. The *glycemic index* measures the impact of the sweetener on blood-glucose levels. Agave nectar is one and a half times sweeter tasting than sugar, so you may be satisfied with a much smaller amount to sweeten your tea. (Flip to Chapter 10 for more information on the glycemic index.)

TIP

A toaster waffle has about 15 grams of carbohydrate. If you eat two of them, that's 30 grams of carb. But watch out if you're thinking of dousing them in syrup. Just ¼ cup of regular pancake or maple syrup would add nearly 45–60 grams of carb. Instead of the syrup, try one of the following:

>> Use a tablespoon of agave nectar. Agave nectar also comes in maple flavor. Before going out and buying "sugar-free" syrups, read about sugar alcohols in the next section.

>> Spread ½ cup of unsweetened applesauce over your waffles. That adds only 15 grams of carb.

>> Try fruited yogurt on waffles. Read labels on the yogurt containers to choose those with fewer carbs.

>> Berries and whipped topping are another option. A couple of tablespoons of whipped topping add a couple grams of carb, and ½ cup of strawberries has about 8 grams of carb.

>> Really limit the carbs by spreading peanut butter between the two waffles for a breakfast on the go. One tablespoon of peanut butter has only about 2–3 grams of carbohydrate (after subtracting the grams of fiber). The fat in the peanut butter also slows down the digestion of the waffle, which can blunt the post-meal blood-glucose rise.

Examining Sugar Alcohols

Many candies, cookies, ice creams, puddings, and syrups claim to be "sugar free." That doesn't mean they are *carbohydrate* free or calorie free. The label claim on the front of the package doesn't necessarily tell the whole story.

Sugar is defined by its chemical structure (which I discuss in Chapter 3). If you alter that chemical structure, even just a little bit, then it isn't sugar anymore. Many products that claim to be sugar free are sweetened with a substance known as sugar alcohol (or polyol). Despite the name, sugar alcohol does not have any sugar, and it does not have any alcohol. Sugar alcohol is a modified form of carbohydrate. Hydrogen is added to various forms of carbohydrate and chemical bonds are shifted, and then voilá — you have a new form of carbohydrate known as sugar alcohol.

Because technically the sugar has been altered, the product can be labeled as being "sugar free." The resulting sweetener is renamed "sugar alcohol." When you view the Nutrition Facts on food labels (see Chapter 7 for more about reading labels), the total carbohydrate count doesn't change much, if at all. It may say "0" grams of sugar, but look below that to find the grams of sugar alcohol. Either way, the *total carbohydrate* is what you need to focus on.

WARNING

Many so called "sugar-free" sweets are still high in carbs, fats, and calories. In fact, the counts are often comparable to their regular sugar–containing counterparts. Beware: Some people experience gas, cramping, or loose stools because sugar alcohol can be difficult to digest and absorb. The portion that remains undigested is fermented by bacteria in the large intestine. Unfortunately, that can result in problems such as gas, cramping, bloating, and perhaps diarrhea. Sugar-free gum has only a small amount of sugar alcohol, so digestive complaints are rare. If you eat too much sugar-free candy or ice cream, you may end up regretting it. Tolerance is variable and dose dependent. Some people have no adverse symptoms at all.

Not all types of sugar alcohol are the same. Some are better tolerated than others. Products sweetened with mannitol or sorbitol are required to carry a label warning stating that *some users may experience a laxative effect.* The other sugar alcohols don't need to carry such a warning.

Sugar alcohol can be created from single units of sugar, double units of sugar, or chains of sugars:

>> Single sugars (monosaccharides) such as glucose and fructose are modified to make sorbitol and mannitol respectively.

>> Double sugars (disaccharides) are also used to produce sugar alcohol. For example, the lactose from milk can be turned into lactitol.

>> Starch fragments (polysaccharides) are modified to create hydrogenated starch hydrolysates.

Table 12-1 shows examples of sugar alcohols.

TABLE 12-1 ## Examples of Sugar Alcohol

Made from Monosaccharides	Made from Disaccharides	Made from Polysaccharides
Sorbitol	Maltitol	Maltitol syrup
Mannitol	Isomalt	Hydrogenated starch hydrolysates (HSH)
Erythritol	Lactitol	
Xylitol		

WARNING

While entirely safe for humans, xylitol is toxic to our canine and feline friends, so make sure your dogs and cats don't eat any products sweetened with xylitol. This particular sweetener stimulates the release of insulin in pets, which can lead to hypoglycemia, seizures, liver problems, or death. This doesn't happen to humans, so you're not at risk. Pet owners must be made aware, though.

Why do food scientists go through all of this trouble to create sugar alcohol out of sugars and starches? Well, there are a few benefits. For one thing, sugar alcohol doesn't promote cavities. Secondly, there may be a reduced effect on blood-glucose levels when using sugar alcohol rather than other caloric sweeteners. Because sugar alcohol is not well digested, fewer calories are absorbed (but with that comes the risk of gas and diarrhea). Sugar alcohol adds texture, bulk, a desirable "mouthfeel," and retention of moisture to the products that incorporate it. Nonnutritive sweeteners do not offer those properties. The sugar substitutes are covered in the next section.

If you count carbs and base your insulin dose on the grams of carbohydrate you eat, then you may consider a modified approach when eating a product made with sugar alcohol. Because sugar alcohol is not fully digestible, take insulin for only half the amount of sugar alcohol in the product. You can also deduct the grams of fiber from the total carbohydrate because fiber doesn't digest. Discuss the concept with your healthcare providers before changing the way you calculate your insulin dose. See Figure 12-2 for tips on deciphering digestible carbohydrate when reading Nutrition Facts food labels on items that contain sugar alcohol.

Nutrition Facts

Serving Size 2 cookies (32g)
Servings Per Container 16

Amount Per Serving

Calories 90	Calories from Fat 45

	% Daily Value
Total Fat 5g	8%
Saturated Fat 1.5g	8%
Trans Fat 0g	
Cholesterol 10mg	4%
Sodium 115mg	5%
Total Carbohydrate 17g	10%
Dietary Fiber 3g	16%
Sugars 2g	
Sugar Alcohol 8g	
Protein 6g	

Vitamin A	4%	Vitamin C	0%
Calcium	0%	Iron	10%

Total carbohydrate:	17 g
subtract the fiber:	− 3 g
subtract 1/2 the sugar alcohol	− 4 g
Expected amount of digestible carb =	10 g

FIGURE 12-2: Calculating digestible carb when you eat a product with sugar alcohol.

© John Wiley & Sons, Inc.

TIP

One thing to consider, especially if sugar alcohol gives you abdominal discomfort, is that you can choose to buy the regular version of the product, which in the example in Figure 12-2 happens to be cookies. If it turns out that the regular sugar–containing version has 20 grams of carb, then you would simply take the dose needed to cover the 20 grams of carb.

Opting for Alternatives: The Sugar Substitutes

Sugar substitutes are referred to as nonnutritive sweeteners because they don't contain calories or nutrients. They are sometimes called artificial sweeteners, but you may be surprised to find out that several of them are actually made out of natural substances and not chemicals. For example, aspartame isn't a chemical; it's made out of two amino acids, which are simply building blocks of proteins. Sucralose is made out of natural sugarcane, and stevia is made out of the leaves of a plant.

Nonnutritive sweeteners are added to foods to provide sweetness without adding calories, so they are popular alternatives for people trying to cut calories. Another benefit: They do not raise blood–glucose levels because they are not carbohydrates.

The Food and Drug Administration (FDA) regulates all food ingredients, including low-calorie sweeteners. The sweeteners on the market today — which I cover in the following sections — have passed rigorous safety assessments. Only very minute amounts are needed for sweetening, because the nonnutritive sweeteners are several hundred to several thousand times sweeter than sugar.

TECHNICAL STUFF

The FDA sets an Acceptable Daily Intake (ADI) for low-calorie sweeteners. The ADI is the amount of the sweetener that can be safely consumed daily, and over the course of a lifetime, without health risks. For added insurance, the ADI is set at one hundredth of the amount that has been determined to be safe. Current intake for nonnutritive sweetener on the market is far below the established ADI. The FDA has approved these sweeteners for the general population, including pregnant women and children.

SUGAR CONSUMPTION IN THE UNITED STATES

The massive consumption of sugary soft drinks, typically sweetened with high-fructose corn syrup or sugar, parallels the rise in obesity in the United States. Whether the association is causal or coincidental is a source of constant debate. No one can deny Americans consume too much added sugar. It's ubiquitous in processed foods. The United States is the world's largest consumer of sweeteners, especially high-fructose corn syrup. Health experts agree that it is time to put the brakes on sugar consumption.

The Dietary Guidelines for Americans recommend reducing calories from added sugars. The American Heart Association guidelines suggest that women limit sugar consumption to less than 6 teaspoons per day from all added sugar sources. That translates to keeping sugar intake to less than 100 calories. For men the suggestion is to limit added sugars to fewer than 9 teaspoons per day, or less than 150 calories.

According to NHANES (National Health and Nutrition Examination Survey), Americans average 20 teaspoons of sugar each day. Other sources cite 32 teaspoons per day. You may wonder how that could be possible! One reason is that sugar is one of the main food additives in processed foods. It shows up in breakfast cereals, sweets and treats, salad dressings, spaghetti sauce, and ketchup, just to scratch the surface. Sweetened beverages are a main contributor of sugar. A 20-ounce soda has about 15 teaspoons of sugar. Specialty coffee drinks are similar.

Diet soft drinks are calorie free and carb free, on the other hand — no sugar whatsoever. They are sweetened with sugar substitutes. Just because diet sodas are approved for use, though, doesn't mean you should drink them in place of water or nutrient-rich milk. For more eye-opening info on the sugar content of beverages, see Chapter 7.

Digging into the differences of the substitutes on the market

Over the years many sugar substitutes have been studied and approved for use. Commonly used sugar substitutes are shown in Table 12-2.

TABLE 12-2 ### Nonnutritive Sweeteners

Sweetener (Brand Names)	Year Approved	Retains Sweetness when Heated
Acesulfame potassium, ace-K (Sunett, Sweet One)	1988	Yes
Advantame (no brand name yet)	2014	Yes
Aspartame (Equal, NutraSweet)	1981	No
Saccharin (Sweet'N Low)	Prior to 1958	Yes
Stevia (Pure Via, Truvia)	2008	Yes
Sucralose (Splenda)	1999	Yes

TECHNICAL STUFF

Not shown in the table are cyclamates because they are not approved for use in the United States; however, cyclamates are still used in other countries. Also not shown is Neotame, which is a sweetener that gained approval in 2002 but is not currently used by manufacturers in the United States.

The majority of the sweeteners in Table 12-2 are between 200 and 300 times as sweet as white sugar. Splenda is 600 times sweeter. The newest kid on the block is Advantame, which is an impressive 20,000 times sweeter than sugar, so only minute amounts are needed to impart sweetness.

Exploring sugar-substitute safety records

Sugar substitutes are an ongoing topic of hot debate. Reams of reputable research reports assure their safety, yet some consumers remain distrustful. The media is a mixed bag. Some information is accurate, while other information is alarmist and not necessarily based on science. Be sure to stick to information from established, reputable institutions. The research is vast. You can find excellent details regarding the safety and use of nonnutritive sweeteners online. If you have any sensitivities, such as headaches, that you associate with consuming one or more of the sugar substitutes, then avoid use per your discretion. Discuss concerns with your healthcare provider.

SACCHARIN: A SWEETENER WITH A SURLY PAST

Saccharin is the granddaddy of artificial sweeteners, and its history begins in the 1870s, when it was first discovered. Its widespread use pre-dates the existence of the FDA, the agency that regulates food safety and labeling. Saccharin enjoyed its place on the GRAS (Generally Regarded As Safe) list for decades until another sweetener, Cyclamate, raised eyebrows as being potentially carcinogenic.

Under pressure to verify safety, saccharin was evaluated. Safety studies linked saccharin to bladder cancer in rats. The rats were given very high doses of saccharin. For perspective, and adjusted for body weight, a human would need to consume 800 cans of saccharin-sweetened soda to ingest an equivalent amount. Due to the study results, in the 1970s saccharin was removed from the GRAS list and was required to carry a warning label on all packages.

Subsequent scientific studies examined the mechanism by which the rats developed bladder cancer, and it was found that the risk applied only to rats and not to humans. The reason rats developed the tumors had to do with unique qualities regarding their urine, which humans do not share. In 2000, the warnings regarding saccharin use were discontinued. Nevertheless, the public saw those warnings on packaging for nearly 30 years, which likely contributes to the apprehension regarding sweetener use to this day.

TIP

Use your browser to search for a scientific statement from the American Heart Association and the American Diabetes Association. It's called "Nonnutritive Sweeteners: Current Use and Health Perspectives." It was published in the journal *Diabetes Care* and can be read in its entirety online. Here are a few more links for information on sweeteners. When you're on the website, use the search box to find info on sugar substitutes:

- » **International Food Information Council Foundation:** www.foodinsight.org. Search for "facts about low-calorie sweeteners."
- » **National Cancer Institute:** www.cancer.gov. Search for "artificial sweeteners and cancer."
- » **Mayo Clinic:** www.mayoclinic.org. Search for "artificial sweeteners and other sugar substitutes."
- » **Academy of Nutrition and Dietetics:** www.eatright.org. Search for "artificial sweeteners."

With so much information available, why are consumers distrustful? The reason likely goes back a few decades. Saccharin, which is the sweetener used in Sweet'N Low, carried a warning on its label for nearly 30 years. The label cautioned about potential cancer risk. The warning came off of the label as subsequent studies supported safe use for human consumption. There was also a sweetener called Cyclamate that the FDA banned in 1969.

Using substitutes in cooking and baking

Sugar substitutes do not impart all of the same qualities to baked goods that sugar provides. Not all of them retain their sweetness when heated at high temperatures, as shown in Table 12-2. Real sugar adds bulk to baked goods and is responsible for browning. Sugar also keeps products moister.

TIP

Many of the sugar substitutes marketed also offer blends. The artificial sweetener is blended with regular white sugar or brown sugar. These blends allow you to retain some of the desirable properties imparted by sugar but with reduced calories and reduced carbs. Follow the instructions on the package for use.

If you were to use just a nonnutritive sweetener without any real sugar when baking, here are some things to be aware of:

>> Your baked recipes won't rise as much.

>> The finished product will be lighter in color.

>> Less moisture is retained, so your baked goods may be drier.

>> Texture may be different, especially in cookies.

>> Baking time may be altered, often reduced, so keep an eye on your oven.

Most, but not all, of the artificial sweeteners can be used in baking. Results vary, so if you're going to experiment, you may want to start by cutting the amount of sugar in the recipe in half and using one of the nonnutritive sweeteners for the remainder of the sweetness needed. Read the packages so you know how much to add.

While aspartame is not recommended in baking, it can be used when making puddings or cranberry sauce after heating is complete. In other words, cook the cranberries with the desired seasonings, but do not add the aspartame until you remove the pan from the stove. Sweeten to taste and refrigerate. You can use any of the artificial sweeteners in this fashion.

WARNING

You may have noticed a warning on products containing aspartame. The warning announces that the product contains phenylalanine. Just to clarify, phenylalanine is an amino acid, a protein building block that occurs naturally in all protein foods. People with a rare disease called PKU must avoid it, but they must avoid regular protein foods as well. Their disease is managed with special formulas and a very strict diet. Babies born in the United States are tested for PKU as part of routine newborn screenings, so it is identified in infancy.

4

Embracing Whole Health and Happiness

IN THIS PART . . .

Select foods that taste good and are good for you.

Develop a fitness plan and reap its benefits.

Recognize, prevent, and treat hypoglycemia.

Discover how to eat smart for your weight and heart.

Find solutions to unique dietary challenges when managing diabetes during childhood, pregnancy, and senior years.

Identify who should be eating gluten-free and how to get started.

Chapter **13**

Eating for Health and Happiness

D iabetes or not, we all need a well-balanced intake of healthy foods in appropriate portions. Chapters 5 and 6 can help you assess your daily carbohydrate needs and how best to distribute carbs between meals and possibly snacks. You can use the plate model in Chapter 8 to plan balanced meals using foods from all food groups. This chapter explores individual food groups and their nutritional benefits, and provides tips on how to choose wisely within each group. I also address strategies for taming your sweet tooth with reasonable treats. Consult a registered dietitian if you need more tips or to have your current dietary habits assessed.

Eating a Rainbow of Fruits and Vegetables

Fruits and vegetables have a lot in common. They provide similar vitamins, minerals, and fiber. What differs is the amount of carbohydrate they contain. Fruits and starchy vegetables have higher carb counts than nonstarchy vegetables and leafy greens. In other words, most vegetables are low in calories and carbs, but starchy vegetables (potatoes, peas, corn) and legumes (dried beans and split peas) are exceptions. Because they are higher in carbs, they are in the starch group along with bread and rice (see Appendix A for details), but they still contribute the nutritional benefits of the vegetable group.

REMEMBER

All varieties should be included; no fruits or vegetables are off limits. Just eat appropriate portions that meet your carb-intake goals. See Chapters 5 and 6 if you aren't sure how much carb you should be aiming for at meals and snacks.

Fruits and vegetables are naturally low in calories and full of nutrition, so eat up. Key vitamins in the fruits and vegetables group include the following:

>> **Vitamin C:** A necessity for the development and repair of all bodily tissues and a powerful antioxidant that aids in the absorption of iron from plant foods

>> **Vitamin A:** Critical for the health of the eyes, skin, and immune system

>> **Potassium:** Helps with muscle, nerve, and heart function and aids in blood-pressure control

>> **Folate (also called folic acid):** A key nutrient in the synthesis of red blood cells and tissues

>> **Fiber (soluble and insoluble):** Beneficial for your heart and keeps your intestinal tract healthy

The 2015–2020 Dietary Guidelines for Americans encourage women to eat roughly 2–2½ cups of vegetables per day and men to consume about 2½–3 cups per day. The target daily intake for fruit is about 1½–2 cups for women and 2 cups for men. Buy fruits and vegetables that are in season to enjoy them at their peak flavor.

TIP

It pays to mix it up and eat a wide variety of fruits and vegetables to reap the spectrum of nutrients they contain. Be sure to include dark green vegetables such as broccoli, kale, and Swiss chard. Also choose items that are dark orange in color, including mangos, apricots, cantaloupe, carrots, sweet potatoes, and butternut squash. Here are handy tips for increasing your intake of all fruits and veggies:

>> Include crunchy raw carrots, celery, cucumbers, and bell pepper strips in your lunch menu. Scoop up hummus, guacamole, or low-fat ranch dressing.

>> Keep frozen vegetables or canned items (processed without added salt) on hand.

>> Start your meal with a leafy salad, and serve steamed, baked, grilled, or roasted vegetables with the meal. In fact, fill half of your dinner plate with vegetables, as doing so may make it easier to control your intake of foods that are higher in calories, carbs, and fats.

>> Enjoy fruit with your meal or between meals as a healthy snack. The key for blood-glucose control is to limit yourself to one serving of fruit at a time and skip the juice. An appropriate serving is a small piece of fruit or about a cup of melon, berries, or mixed fruits. To count the carbs more precisely, see Appendix A.

>> Keep fresh seasonal fruits on hand. For convenience, cut melons and pineapple and then refrigerate them in a sealed container.

>> If you buy canned fruits, choose those that are packed in natural juices, not syrup, and buy unsweetened applesauce.

Loading Up on Whole Grains

Grains are rich in carbohydrates, and they also contain some protein. The 2015–2020 Dietary Guidelines for Americans encourage women to eat 5–6 grain portions per day and men to consume 6–8 portions per day, half of which should be whole-grain selections. The portions they refer to are the sizes in the starch list in Appendix A. Each exchange portion provides 15 grams of carb and 3 grams of protein. Whole grains offer important vitamins and minerals needed for optimal health. They're rich in fiber, iron, magnesium, selenium, and several B vitamins (thiamin, riboflavin, niacin, and folate).

The following sections explain what to look for when you shop for whole grains and give you some ideas on different grains to try.

Identifying best-bet grains

Grains are subdivided into whole grains and refined grains. What's the difference?

>> **Whole grains** contain the kernel, bran, germ, and endosperm.

>> **Refined grains** have been milled to remove the bran and the germ. Valuable nutrients and fiber are stripped by the refining process. Refined grains are often "enriched" to add back iron and vitamins, but the fiber is gone for good.

Whole grains digest slower than refined grains, which is good news in terms of blood-glucose control. Your blood-glucose levels may be slightly lower when you choose wholesome whole grains simply because the glucose from the food doesn't speed into your system all at once. Because whole grains take longer to digest, you may feel fuller for longer. Feeling satisfied can curb the urge to snack, which in turn supports weight-control efforts.

TIP

Try to choose whole grains for at least half of your grain servings. Look for the Whole Grain Stamp on packaged foods. Read ingredient lists and choose items that list "whole grain" first. Check the Nutrition Facts food label for the fiber count. A food is a good source of fiber if it offers at least 2.5 grams of fiber per serving; an excellent source of fiber has 5 or more grams of fiber per serving. You can also review the Nutrition Facts label for the Percent Daily Value. A food that provides 20 percent or more of the Percent Daily Value is considered high in fiber; 5 percent or less is low. Aim high when it comes to fiber. See Chapter 7 for more details on label reading and to see an image of the Whole Grain Stamp.

Increasing your options and trying new grains

Start your day with slow-cooked oats or whole-grain toast for breakfast. For lunches and dinners, choose whole-wheat or whole-grain breads, rolls, tortillas, crackers, and pastas. Limit white rice; instead, choose brown, red, black, or wild rice.

Branch out and try new grains to accompany your meal. Here are some ideas:

>> Blend brown rice, wild rice, and farro and simmer in a seasoned broth to make a hearty pilaf.

>> Add barley to homemade soups.

>> Toss cooked quinoa into a mixed green or kale salad.

>> Make fresh tabbouleh with bulgur, parsley, and minced green onion tossed with olive oil and lemon juice.

Other whole grains to try include millet, amaranth, spelt, rye, buckwheat, teff, and kamut.

TIP

One complaint about whole grains is that they take a little longer to cook than white rice. One solution is to make a bigger batch and freeze the extras for future use. Whole grains freeze well.

Leaning Toward Leaner Proteins

Protein foods provide amino-acid building blocks, which in turn become the building materials we use to synthesize and repair our cells and tissues. Meats have high-quality protein and are rich in easily absorbed iron. The key to keeping it heart-healthy is to choose lean meats. Meat fats are saturated and if eaten in excess can contribute to high blood-cholesterol levels, clogged arteries, and heart disease. Fish is the exception to the rule. The fat in fish and seafood is considered heart-healthy. Fish contains omega-3 fatty acids called DHA and EPA. There are also plenty of high-quality vegetarian protein foods. Consider cutting back on meat consumption by adopting a "meatless Monday" menu.

Individual protein needs vary, but most Americans easily meet their requirements. Overconsumption can lead to excess calories, though. A simple guideline to avoid excess intake is to choose lean proteins and keep the portion size similar to the size of the palm of your own hand. If you have questions, seek the advice of your healthcare team.

The 2015–2020 Dietary Guidelines for Americans encourage women to eat 5–5½ ounces of protein per day and men to consume 5½–6½ ounces per day. To see what counts as an ounce of protein, flip to Appendix A. By varying your protein choices, as I explain in the following sections, you'll benefit from a broader variety of vitamins and minerals, including iron, zinc, magnesium, omega-3 fats, and several important B vitamins.

Choosing the healthiest options

Choosing lean protein is good for your heart, and it also helps with weight control. Table 13-1 compares the calorie counts between lean, medium-fat, and high-fat meats. For reference, 4 ounces of meat is about the size of a deck of playing cards.

TABLE 13-1

Calorie Counts Correlated to Fat Content of Meat

Serving Size	Lean	Medium Fat	High Fat
4 ounces	180 calories	300 calories	400 calories
8 ounces	360 calories	600 calories	800 calories
12 ounces	540 calories	900 calories	1,200 calories

WARNING

Take note: High-fat meat has more than twice the number of calories than lean meat. The extra calories come from fat, saturated at that. Day after day, week after week, month after month . . . those are the sorts of differences that really add up.

The Exchange Lists in Appendix A separate specific meats into the three categories. Use the lean meats and proteins list to make your grocery shopping list. Keep your protein portion at mealtime to roughly the size of the palm of your own hand and limit your intake to two portions a day.

Fish, shellfish, and skinless poultry are all lean. Certain cuts of beef and pork also fall into the lean category — for example, sirloin, tenderloin, top round, bottom round, and flank. When choosing ground beef, aim for at least 92 percent lean. Regular ground beef is 75–80 percent lean — and that isn't lean at all. Canadian bacon and ham are considered lean pork, which makes them a better choice to nestle next to your eggs than regular bacon and breakfast sausages. Canadian bacon and ham have added sodium, however, so monitor your intake if you have high blood pressure.

WARNING

Most processed meats hit you with a double whammy: salt and fat. Limit the following: sausages, bacon, bologna, hot dogs, salami, and most deli meats.

Fishing for reasons to eat more seafood

Omega-3 fats, known as EPA and DHA, are found in seafood. These fats are healthy for your brain and your heart. They reduce the risk of *arrhythmias* (abnormal heartbeats), lower blood-triglyceride levels, and have a beneficial effect on blood pressure. Some of the richest sources of omega-3 fats include salmon, herring, anchovies, sardines, Pacific oysters, lake trout, and Atlantic and Pacific mackerel. Adults are encouraged to eat at least 8 ounces and as much as 12 ounces of fish or seafood per week. Eating seafood on a regular basis may reduce your risk of heart disease. All fish and seafood are considered lean (provided you don't accidentally dredge them in batter and deep-fry them).

WARNING

Mercury is a heavy metal that can damage the nervous system and brain. Pregnant women and children should be especially cautious to avoid exposure. Some of the larger fish with longer life spans can accumulate high levels of mercury, making them unsafe for human consumption. The FDA recommends avoiding four specific types of fish due to mercury risk: swordfish, shark, king mackerel, and tile fish (specifically from the Gulf of Mexico). Orange roughy and marlin are also high in mercury. When it comes to tuna, chunk light has less mercury than white albacore. Adults should limit albacore tuna to 6 ounces per week.

You can enjoy many types of fish and shellfish without concern of mercury contamination. Low-risk fish should be enjoyed, as they offer excellent health benefits. Examples of fish and shellfish to consume weekly include salmon, shrimp, scallops, oysters, squid, crab, haddock, flounder, sole, pollock, tilapia, catfish, and cod.

TIP

The Natural Resource Defense Council has a chart distinguishing the risk of mercury in different fish. Check out www.nrdc.org/stories/smart-seafood-buying-guide.

Vegging out with meatless proteins

Legumes are unique because they count as carbs and protein. Half of a cup of cooked beans (black, garbanzo, kidney, navy, pinto, or lentils) has about 7 grams of protein and 15 grams of carb. That's the same amount of protein as one egg. The carbs need to be considered when carb counting. Legumes are naturally low in fat, high in fiber, cholesterol free, and loaded with vitamins and minerals, making them an excellent, wholesome choice.

Nuts and nut butters offer protein but are quite high in calories, so be mindful to keep the portions controlled. One-fourth cup of nuts runs you about 200 calories.

Tofu, which is made from soybeans, comes in several levels of firmness, from silken to extra firm. It's mild in taste and versatile. Vegetarian and Asian cookbooks provide recipe ideas, but these days you can also search for recipes online. Tempeh is another soy product worthy of mention.

Seitan, sometimes called "wheat meat," is made from wheat gluten. Gluten is the protein part of the grain. Chewy in texture, it is often pre-seasoned or marinated. Despite coming from wheat, it is low in carbs.

Most grocery chains offer a wide variety of vegetarian meat substitutes. You are no longer limited to veggie burgers (although they are great). Replace fatty, processed meats with vegetarian alternatives: Try veggie hot dogs, sausages, bologna, and bacon. Ground veggie meatless products replace ground beef and pick up the flavorings used in the cooking (they make a wonderful chili). Peruse the refrigerated sections (near the tofu) or look in the frozen food aisles where you just might find vegetarian versions of chicken strips, nuggets, crab cakes, cutlets, beef tips, buffalo wings, sliders, meatballs, and chicken. These packaged items all have Nutrition Facts food labels and easy cooking instructions. Popular brands include (but are not limited to) Gardein, Morningstar Farms, Field Roast, Boca, Quorn, Yves, Tofurky, and Litelife. Give them a try; you can keep them conveniently frozen until needed, and you may be pleasantly surprised by the taste.

Daring to Do Dairy

Milk naturally contains all three macronutrients: carbohydrate, protein, and fat. It's also rich in calcium and vitamin D. The 2015–2020 Dietary Guidelines for Americans encourage adults to get three portions of calcium-rich dairy foods per day. See Appendix A for examples. The following sections go into more detail on milk's nutrition and provide nondairy options that give you similar benefits.

Watching the fat content

The fat from milk can be removed and made into butter, cream cheese, and sour cream. Dairy fats are not particularly heart-healthy, though. Like the fat in meat, milk fat is a saturated fat, so full-fat versions should be limited. Choose nonfat, low-fat (1 percent), and reduced-fat (2 percent) dairy products to take advantage of the nutrients offered in this food group.

Milk and yogurt both have carbs because they contain lactose, the natural sugar in milk. Cheese is very low lactose, usually containing just a trace. Cheese is made from the fat and the protein, so it doesn't raise blood-glucose levels. However, cheese is generally high in fat. Regular cheese is made from whole milk and has 8 or more grams of fat per ounce. Reduced-fat cheeses are made from 2 percent milk, which cuts the amount of fat down to 4–7 grams of fat per ounce. Low-fat cheeses are marked as such and have between 0 and 3 grams of fat per ounce.

Packing in more protein

Meats and protein foods are discussed earlier in this chapter. Milk, yogurt, and cheese are also rich in protein. One cup of milk provides 8–10 grams of high-quality protein, and cheese provides about 7 grams of protein per ounce. Yogurt varies in carbs, calories, fats, and protein; check the Nutrition Facts food labels for details.

Boning up on calcium

It's well known that calcium is needed for bone and dental health. Calcium is also critical for normal functioning of muscles, nerves, and blood vessels. Small amounts of calcium dissolve from our bones to provide the calcium needed elsewhere in the body. Calcium can also be added to bone, provided your dietary intake is adequate. Post-menopausal women don't build bone as effectively, which is why osteoporosis becomes a risk with aging. Some plant foods offer calcium, but it isn't absorbed as readily as the calcium in dairy products. That's because the calcium in plant foods gets bound to the plant fibers and other chemical compounds, which reduces absorption. You absorb some, but not necessarily all, of the calcium in the food.

See Table 13-2 to find out how much calcium you need; it shows the Dietary Reference Intakes for calcium based on age and gender. Amounts are displayed in milligrams. To assess your calcium intake, consider that one cup of milk or yogurt provides approximately 300 milligrams of calcium. It takes about 1.5 ounces of cheese to get 300 milligrams of calcium. An ounce of cheese is about the size of a string-cheese stick. If you don't do dairy, consider a calcium-fortified nondairy alternative (see the next section).

TABLE 13-2

Recommended Calcium Intakes

Age	Male	Female
1–3 years	700	700
4–8 years	1,000	1,000
9–18 years	1,300	1,300
19–50 years	1,000	1,000
51–70 years	1,000	1,200
71+ years	1,200	1,200

TIP

If your diet is low in calcium, it pays to take a supplement. Calcium comes in tablet form or in chewables. Our bodies can absorb only so much calcium at a time. To improve absorption, take up to 500 milligrams at once. Taking calcium supplements with meals is fine.

TIP

Vitamin D is essential in helping the body absorb and use calcium. Vitamin D status is easily assessed with a blood test. The recommended intake of Vitamin D for ages 1–70 is 600 international units (IU) per day. For ages 71 and above, the target is 800 IU per day. If your levels are low, you can take a vitamin D supplement with higher dosages, and your doctor or registered dietitian can suggest the amount. Dietary sources of vitamin D include eggs, liver, fatty fish, and fortified foods. Vitamin D is also synthesized in the skin with exposure to the sun.

Checking out nondairy substitutes

If you don't drink milk, there are many nondairy beverages to choose from, including soy milk, almond milk, other nut milks (like cashew), hemp milk, coconut milk, and rice milk. Protein content varies among selections. Some milk substitutes have just 1 gram of protein, while others are comparable to milk with 8–9 grams of protein per cup. There are also nondairy substitutes for cheese and yogurt.

Look for calcium-fortified milk substitutes. The front of the package may say "enriched" or "fortified." The Nutrition Facts label provides information on the calcium content, but currently food labels only note the calcium content as a percentage of daily need. It's based on the adult target of 1,000 milligrams per day. For reference, one cup of milk provides 30 percent of the daily calcium requirement. Thirty percent of 1,000 equals 300. Therefore, one cup of milk has 300 milligrams of calcium. Fortified nondairy beverages are usually fortified to match the calcium content of milk, and they sometimes contain even more. Some beverages are boosted to provide 45 percent of the recommended calcium requirements. If your milk substitute provides a paltry 4 percent of your calcium needs, for example, that is just 40 milligrams, and the product hasn't been fortified.

TIP

Labels will be less cumbersome by July of 2018, when the revised food labels will be out in full force. The new version of the food label will list the calcium in terms of both Percent Daily Value and in milligrams. See Chapter 7 to take a look at the new food label format.

Focusing on Healthy Fats

Liquid oils and solid fats are similar in calorie counts but worlds apart when it comes to their effect on health. The fats from meats and dairy products are saturated and should be limited. Saturated fats, trans fats, and hydrogenated fats raise blood-cholesterol levels. Cut back on these artery-clogging culprits. Improve your odds by choosing unsaturated fats. They are easy to identify because they are usually liquid at room temperature. Fats add flavor and moisture to food. Fats also assist with the absorption of fat-soluble vitamins: vitamins A, D, E, and K.

Monounsaturated oils (olive, canola, and peanut) and the omega-3 fats found in fish are the heart-healthy heroes of the fat family. Polyunsaturated oils (most of the other vegetable and nut oils) are also fine; none of the unsaturated (liquid) oils damage or block blood vessels. Nuts, seeds, avocados, and olives are foods that contain concentrated amounts of fat. They contain a good type of fat, but nevertheless they are high in calories so controlled portioning is recommended. Mayonnaise and margarine are polyunsaturated and may be used in moderation. Just make sure the label says 0 grams of trans fat. Chapter 16 is devoted to heart health, so look there for more in-depth information on how to keep your heart happy with healthy food choices.

REMEMBER

Fats and oils rack up about 120 calories per tablespoon. This is one of those times when more isn't better. While oils do provide essential fatty acids that are required for health, it doesn't take much to fulfill those needs. The oils and fats occurring naturally in foods cover the bases in terms of what we actually *need* for health. To cut down on calories from fat, look for reduced-fat versions of cream cheese, sour cream, mayonnaise, and salad dressings. Fats added during cooking and at the table should be used sparingly.

The 2015–2020 Dietary Guidelines for Americans encourage women to limit intake to 5–6 teaspoons of oil (or fat equivalents) per day and for men to limit intake to 6–7 teaspoons. See Appendix A for examples and portion sizes that are equivalent to a teaspoon of oil. Chapter 16 provides guidance on choosing heart-healthy fats.

Having Diabetes and Dessert, Too

For decades, people with diabetes were told not to eat sugar. It didn't actually cure anybody. Avoiding sugar won't automatically keep blood-glucose levels in range if there are no controls on the overall carb intake. Skipping the cookie doesn't erase the carbs in the rest of the meal. Managing carbs for diabetes means all carbs in the meal need to be accounted for, not just the dessert.

Certainly, having diabetes makes it very important to limit sweets, treats, and desserts. Sugar is concentrated in carbs, and desserts can easily blow the carb budget. For example, I recently reviewed a popular restaurant's menu and noticed that the flan had over 120 grams of carb per serving. Another dessert on the menu had nearly 200 grams of carb! To put that in perspective, a cup of white granulated sugar has 200 grams of carb. Nobody with diabetes is going to tolerate a dessert like that. That particular dessert had over 1,200 calories, making it an unhealthy choice for anyone, with or without diabetes!

Estimating carbs in desserts can be tricky. Some can be deceptively high in carbs, while others may not have as much as you'd think. If you underestimate the carbs in the dessert, your blood glucose goes sailing. On the other hand, if you overestimate the carb counts and end up taking too much insulin, you can end up with hypoglycemia.

The following sections provide pointers on how to treat yourself to dessert without going overboard on carbs.

Making your own treats

One option for having dessert when you have diabetes is to make your own goodies. When baking treats at home, you can closely estimate carb counts in your recipes. For ingredients that contain carbs, use the Nutrition Facts food labels on the package (see Chapter 7 for help). If you don't have access to the package or you buy in bulk, simply look up the item online. Check www.calorieking.com (see Chapter 9 for details) or use your search engine to look up individual ingredients.

You can then calculate the amount of carb per serving in your homemade desserts (or any recipes for that matter). Tally up the amount of carb in each ingredient in the recipe. Consider these ingredients in a cookie recipe: One cup of white flour has 92 grams of carb, and one cup of white granulated sugar has 200 grams of carb. The butter, eggs, baking soda, vanilla, and salt don't have any carbs. Figure out how many carbs are in one cookie by dividing the total carbohydrate count by the number of cookies baked. When baking at home, you can make the recipe healthier by cutting down on the sugar and fat in the recipe. You can also find recipes that incorporate sugar substitutes by looking online.

Dressing up healthy fruits

Fruits are naturally sweet and satisfying, and they are a healthy alternative to dessert. Here are some tips for making outstanding fruits stand out:

» Make fruit kabobs by skewering cubes of cantaloupe, honeydew, watermelon, strawberries, pineapple, and grapes.

» Impress your guests with a fruit salad melon boat. Cut a watermelon in half and use a melon ball tool to scoop out the flesh, leaving the hollowed empty shell. Refill the empty shell with a colorful mixed fresh-fruit salad. The melon shell is the serving bowl.

» Bake apples instead of an apple pie. Core the apples, leaving enough of the core at the base of the apple to hold the filling. Fill each apple with 1 teaspoon of butter or margarine, 1 teaspoon of brown sugar or agave nectar, ¼ teaspoon of cinnamon, and 1 teaspoon of minced pecans or walnuts. Place the apples upright in a baking dish with about ½ inch of water in the bottom of the pan to prevent scorching. Bake at 375 degrees for one hour or until desired tenderness.

» Freeze grapes for a refreshing treat.

» Melt dark chocolate in the microwave. Dip fresh strawberries into the melted chocolate and then refrigerate until the chocolate is firm. You can do the same with banana chunks, sprinkling them with minced nuts.

» Use a glass parfait dish or a wine glass to layer fresh berries and nonfat yogurt. Sprinkle the top with a tablespoon of granola.

» Make sugar-free gelatin and mix in sliced fresh fruit. Refrigerate until firm. Serve with whipped topping (optional).

Enjoying dessert while controlling the carbs

Desserts can be high in calories, fats, and carbs. Choices matter, and portion control is important. Here are a few tips for enjoying dessert and controlling the impact it has on your health:

» **Sharing:** When in restaurants, consider ordering one dessert for the table and sharing it. If the restaurant is a chain, ask your server or the manager for the nutrition information so you can look up the carb and calorie counts. Another option for chain restaurants is to check their website for the nutrition facts. The website is usually easy to locate by the restaurant's name.

» **Stocking the best bets at home:** Fudgsicles are low-fat frozen delights. They contain about 40 calories, 10 grams of carb, and 1 gram of fat. Pudding cups are also appropriately portioned. Buy yogurt in tubes and freeze them. Cut the end of the yogurt tube and squeeze from below for a yogurt push-up. Sugar-free gelatin is virtually free of calories and carbs, so you can have it anytime. If you do buy ice cream, consider frozen yogurt or the lower-calorie ice creams. Read the Nutrition Facts labels to compare calories, carbs, and fats (see Chapter 7 for guidance). Limit your serving to one scoop.

REMEMBER

Don't stock up on treats at home if they are too tempting and you can't control portions.

>> **Maintaining carb control at mealtime to make room for dessert:** Maintaining control of blood-glucose levels is easier if dessert is consumed after a lower-carb meal. For example, if your meal is a salad with greens, vegetables, and protein, you have more room in the carb budget to enjoy a dessert.

>> **Having your cake and eating it too:** A thin slice of angel food cake with a couple of sliced strawberries and a spritz of light whipped cream is far lower in carbs than your typical frosted cake. If you're celebrating a special occasion that calls for cake to be served, you can opt to go mini. Boutique cupcake stores and even big-box supermarkets offer mini cupcakes, or you can buy mini muffin tins and make your own. The trick is eating just one. You can also use mini muffin tins to make mini banana bread or zucchini bread muffins that don't require any frosting. Cake pops are another alternative to a full-sized cake. Cake pops are cake balls on a stick, similar to lollipops.

>> **Walking it off:** Adding some extra exercise after consuming dessert helps burn off some of the glucose in your blood. Exercising regularly improves overall health and assists in weight management. See Chapter 14 to explore the benefits of exercise.

Trying Cooking and Serving Tips that Support Health and Weight Goals

It's best to limit the amount of fat that is added in the cooking process. When foods are deep-fried, for example, they absorb cooking oil and the calorie counts jump. Compare a large baked potato to a large order of French fries: The potato has 290 calories, and the French fries have 515 calories. The baked potato has less than ½ gram of fat, whereas the fries have nearly 25 grams of fat. The fries have absorbed 5 teaspoons of oil. The bottom-line calorie count on the baked potato depends on what *you add* to it. Adding 3 tablespoons of "light" sour cream just bumps the calories up by 60 with less than 4 grams of fat.

Limit frequency and portion sizes of fried foods for weight control. Restaurants don't always fry in the heart-healthiest oils, so that's another reason to skip the fried foods when you're dining out.

Whether at home or in a restaurant, choose lower-fat cooking and serving methods as discussed in this section.

Opting for lower-fat cooking methods

Boiling, poaching, braising, and steaming are all cooking methods that use moist heat, which helps prevent foods from drying out:

» **Boiling** typically uses enough water to cover the food, while steaming has about an inch of water in the bottom of the pan with the food cradled in a steaming basket. Steaming retains many of the nutrients in the food.

» **Poaching** is simmering food in small amounts of broth or seasoned liquid. Poaching is a flavorful way to cook boneless chicken breast or fish, and the meat remains tender and moist. Wine can be added to the poaching liquid if desired; the alcohol cooks out.

» **Braising** is a method often used for tougher cuts of beef. To braise meat, sear and brown it in a skillet on the stovetop, and then place the meat in a tightly covered baking dish with water or other liquid in the bottom of the pan. Place the pan in the oven. Alternately, you can braise in an electric skillet. Carrots, onions, and quartered potatoes can be cooked at the same time in the pan with the meat.

High-heat dry cooking methods include baking, broiling, roasting, and grilling:

» **Baking:** The oven is a versatile cooking method because you can adjust the temperature and cooking time according to the item or recipe.

» **Broiling:** The oven can do more than just bake your food. It can also be used for broiling. You need a broiler pan, which has a slotted upper tray and a pan that holds the tray. Meat fats drip away into the broiler pan. The intense heat cooks foods quickly. Brushing with a marinade is optional.

» **Roasting:** Roasting winter vegetables in a hot oven brings out the natural sweetness in butternut squash, carrots, and parsnips. Roasted Brussels sprouts are also delicious. Cube or slice vegetables to a thickness of about ½ inch. Toss with a small amount of olive oil. Spread vegetables on a cooking sheet and bake at 400 degrees for 20–30 minutes. Make kale chips by coating chopped kale leaves lightly in oil; arrange on a cooking sheet and bake until crisp.

» **Grilling:** Grilling can be done on an outside barbeque or an indoor electric grill. The fat drips away from the meat. Grilled vegetables are excellent too, so when you fire up the BBQ, be sure to skewer some zucchini, peppers, onions, mushrooms, and cherry tomatoes. Grilled pineapple is a tasty accompaniment.

Cooking methods that use a small amount of oil include sautéing and stir-frying:

>> A sauté pan with a small amount of fat works well for vegetables, shrimp, scrambled eggs, or any food that cooks quickly.

>> Stir-frying can be done in a large skillet, but a wok works best. Make sure the oil is hot before adding the food to the wok. Stir and toss while cooking over high heat.

Controlling portion sizes

You can watch your portion sizes with the help of the following tips:

>> Serve from the stove instead of placing all the cooked foods on the table. It's too easy to take second helpings when foods are served family style in serving dishes at arm's reach.

>> Use a measuring cup to scoop your potatoes, rice, and pasta from the pan. That way you are measuring at the same time that you serve yourself. (See Chapter 8 for more details on this concept.)

>> Use smaller bowls and plates. Many people like to see their plates full. If your dinner is on a salad plate, it will look full even though you are eating less. For desserts and fruits, use a small decorative parfait dish to control portions.

>> Put leftovers away promptly. Divvy up the leftovers into small containers and refrigerate or freeze for a quick reheated meal at a future date. Microwave ovens work well for reheating leftovers.

Controlling portions when eating at restaurants can be as easy as sharing an entrée. Or create your own meal with a combination of appetizers and a salad. Ask your server for a to-go box as soon as your meal arrives. Before diving in, package up part of the meal to take home. When the option exists, order the smaller portion.

TIP

A quick way to assess appropriate serving sizes when you're away from home is to look at your hand. Your starch serving (rice, pasta, potato) should be the size of your tightly clenched fist, and your protein (fish, chicken, meat) should be about the size of the palm of your own hand.

WARNING

Watch out for restaurant desserts. Decadent desserts pack in the sugar, fat, and calories. Sharing one dessert amongst the table may be the safest bet.

Chapter **14**

Reaping the Rewards of Fitness

P hysical activity offers health benefits for everyone on the planet. That pretty much sums it up. We all stand to benefit by being more active. Most of us know that, yet statistics from the Centers for Disease Control show that only 49 percent of American adults meet the physical activity guidelines for aerobic activity. When it comes to meeting the guidelines for both aerobic activity and strength training, the number drops to a mere 20.9 percent of adults.

If you aren't currently engaging in physical activity, take the first step and start modestly. It's never too late to begin healthy habits. Exercise is a critical component of overall well-being, weight control, cardiovascular fitness, and the management of insulin resistance. That's not all: Exercise is good for mental health, and exercisers tend to live longer. If you don't exercise, you miss out on the potential health benefits, but even more concerning is that the lack of exercise increases your risk of developing chronic diseases.

Most people can readily come up with a list of reasons why they don't exercise. If pressed, those same people may be able to find solutions for each of their excuses. Prioritize exercise to the status it deserves. Find activities that interest you. Figure out what time of day works best for you. Strategize ways to fit fitness into your daily routine. Find activities that your family can enjoy together. Figure out what you can do indoors when weather prohibits outdoor activities. Enlist the support of family and friends. This chapter highlights the benefits of exercise, especially for people with diabetes, and how to do it safely.

Exercising Safely

If you're a new recruit to exercise, start with something manageable. Your current level of fitness will determine what you can comfortably do. Someone who has been sedentary for years should start with a modest exercise goal. That may mean five minutes of physical activity, or it can be a walk around the block. People who have prior exercise experience but have been on an exercise hiatus may be able to jump back into their previous routines. The main thing is to get started. From there you can incrementally add more activity. The following sections explain how to proceed safely with an exercise program by checking in with your healthcare provider first and keeping essentials at your side.

REMEMBER

If you aren't sure about where to start or if you have limitations due to health issues, ask your healthcare team for guidance.

Getting the green light from your doctor

Your healthcare provider knows your medical history and thus is the most qualified person to guide you on exercise. If you use insulin, ask your doctor whether you should adjust your insulin dose when exercising to reduce the risk of hypoglycemia (which I discuss later in this chapter). If you are not at risk for lows and are generally healthy, there may not be any restrictions on increasing your level of activity.

The following sections describe the medical tests you should have before you start an exercise routine and the medical alert ID you should wear.

Undergoing medical exams

REMEMBER

Everyone needs a complete physical examination annually. Whether you need to schedule additional follow-up visits depends on your medical history. For uncomplicated diabetes, follow-ups are generally recommended at least two to four times per year. Your provider may suggest more frequent visits if your blood glucose isn't adequately controlled, if you start a new medication, or if you have diabetes complications or other significant medical issues.

Weight and blood-pressure checks should be routine at every medical visit. Your doctor should assess the health of your nerves and feet. Bring your meter and blood-glucose records to all visits and have your A1C checked every three months. Blood-glucose data drives management decisions (see Chapter 15 for more information).

Stay up to date with your diabetes checkup checklist. Take care of the following:

» The health of your kidneys and eyes should be assessed annually, and your feet at least annually. Screening for complications to your eyes requires a dilated exam. Kidney health is monitored with a blood test and a urine screening test that looks for a protein called albumin.

» Lipid levels should be monitored at a frequency determined by your provider and based on your medical history.

» Dental checkups are also important and recommended at least every six months.

REMEMBER

Discuss exercise with your healthcare provider. Find out whether you have any exercise restrictions due to medical conditions.

An exercise stress test, sometimes called a treadmill test, is used to evaluate your heart's response to exercise. An alternate method is available, which uses a medication rather than exercise to increase the heart rate. Stress tests are not done routinely for everyone with diabetes, but rather as deemed necessary by your healthcare provider based on your personal risk factors.

Wearing a medical alert ID

If you are injured during exercise (or any other time) and unable to communicate for any reason, or if you are incapacitated by hypoglycemia or a diabetic coma, the paramedics assisting you will need to know what to do. First responders look for medical alert identification. In extreme situations every minute counts. If you have insulin-dependent diabetes, it's important for paramedics to assess your blood-glucose levels. Severe hypoglycemia requires glucagon or intravenous glucose to raise blood-glucose levels quickly. Diabetic ketoacidosis requires insulin and IV fluids (see Chapter 4 for details on ketones).

REMEMBER

At the minimum, your medical alert ID should list that you have diabetes. If you use insulin, specify that. Provide your full name and the name and phone number of an emergency contact person. Some IDs allow you to create an online health profile to house all of your key information; the ID provides the access code. Some alert tags come with a USB drive that houses your personal medical history and key contact numbers.

THE IMPORTANCE OF WEARING MEDICAL ALERT IDENTIFICATION

This is a true story. When I was a student at UC Berkeley, I was at the transit station waiting for my commuter train. Near me was a woman in a business suit who suddenly slumped to her knees. I rushed to her side and asked whether she was okay. She couldn't manage to tell me what was wrong. I noticed her medical alert necklace, which said she had type 1 diabetes. It was apparent to me that she was having a low-blood-glucose reaction. I grabbed a juice from a nearby kiosk, which she was able to drink. After about ten minutes, she had recovered and thanked me. That was more than 25 years ago.

Occurrences such as these are less frequent these days because of technological advances, improved insulin options, and education. Nevertheless, they underscore the importance of wearing medical alert identification.

Medical ID bracelets, necklaces, or watchband clips offer a wide range of options. From basic to bold, there are options for the sports-minded, outdoorsy types, polished executives, and the young or young at heart. Available styles include retro, western, classy, beaded, and jeweled. Search for medical alert identification on any web browser.

Being prepared: What to keep handy

REMEMBER

With a little planning, you can engage in physical activity safely. If you take insulin or any pills that put you at risk for hypoglycemia, planning ahead and being prepared are especially important. Check out the following list of what to keep with you as you exercise:

>> **Planning for your particular activity:** Dress appropriately for your activity. For example, if you're stepping out for a walk, wear walking shoes that are comfortable and protect your feet. Use a helmet for bike riding. Apply sunscreen for outdoor activities and avoid exercising in temperature extremes.

>> **Bringing your glucose monitor with you:** Glucose monitors are compact and lightweight. Keep yours with you when exercising. It can be left poolside while you swim, or in a backpack, fanny pack, or bike pack for walking, jogging, and biking.

>> **Toting insulin:** Insulin users need access to insulin at all times; don't leave home without it. It's important to protect insulin from the elements. Keep insulin out of direct sunlight and don't leave it in a hot car. When insulin gets

too hot, it doesn't work properly and must be discarded. It can be kept cool but must not freeze. Tote bags designed for insulin storage have compartments to hold refreezable ice packs.

>> **Carrying low supplies:** If you use insulin or any of the oral medications that have the potential to cause hypoglycemia, be sure to carry glucose tablets, juice, or any other quick-digesting carb choice. Exercise can lower blood-glucose levels rapidly. For more information on the prevention, detection, and treatment of hypoglycemia, see Chapter 15.

>> **Packing snacks:** When exercise is strenuous or prolonged, you may need a snack, juice, or a diluted electrolyte drink to sustain your glucose levels.

>> **Staying hydrated:** Drink plenty of water. Exercise increases fluid requirements, especially in hot climates. Drink additional water or carbohydrate-free beverages when blood-glucose levels run above target ranges. Elevated glucose levels can lead to increased urination, and if fluid losses are not replenished, you can become dehydrated. Reserve the carb-containing beverages for treating and preventing lows. See Chapter 11 for more advice on beverage choices.

Encouraging Exercise for Everyone

I often hear people say that they would like to exercise more but they just don't have the time. Sometimes best intentions are thwarted because exercise gets bumped lower and lower on the list of things to do. Exercise needs to be higher on the priority list. As you read through this chapter, take note of the many health benefits exercise offers. Tell yourself that exercise is a "prescription," and it's as important as medicine or any other aspect of your healthcare. Continue reading for ideas on how to get started.

Developing an exercise plan

REMEMBER

There's something for everyone when it comes to exercise options. Discuss your circumstances with your healthcare team. It's important to exercise within your capabilities. Start modestly and work your way up as you build stamina and strength. Keep safety in mind at all times.

The following sections describe different types of exercise as well as frequency, intensity, and duration.

Choosing exercises that you like and can safely do

To successfully incorporate exercise into your routine, it's important to pick activities that you enjoy. Keep things interesting by including a variety of activities. For example, you may sign up for an exercise class that meets once or twice a week. On the off days, you can go for a walk (see the next section) or use an aerobics DVD or online exercise video that gets you moving in your own living room.

TIP

Look into what's available in your community. Find out when local swimming pools are open for adult lap swimming. Consider health clubs, gyms, basketball or tennis courts, golf, walking trails, bike paths, or a local YMCA. Some communities put together walking groups, tai chi gatherings, bird-watching clubs, recreational sports teams, and exercise sessions at senior centers. Consider line dancing, ballroom dancing, a spin class, or investing in exercise equipment for your home. Save on costs and buy used equipment such as a stationary bike or treadmill. Even simple hand weights can be used while watching television.

Getting off on the right foot: The wonders of walking

Walking counts as exercise. It's free, and the timing is flexible. Go for a walk whenever you can fit it in. Just be sure to take care of your feet by wearing shoes designed for walking and comfortable, moisture-wicking socks.

TIP

Add extra steps to your current daily routine. When you're shopping, simply park farther from the entrance. When you're inside a shopping mall, take a walk through it. Reserve part of your lunch break to walk around the building or the block. Take the stairs. Get off the bus one stop earlier and walk the rest of the way.

As you become more conditioned, push yourself to walk faster and farther. Consider a step counter, pedometer, or fitness tracker. Apps on smartphones track steps. Wear a fitness tracker on your wrist or on your belt. Many trackers sync with apps on your smartphone to track your progress over time. Increase your target incrementally until you're walking 10,000 steps per day.

Adding aerobic activities and resistance training

Aerobic exercise, or cardio, involves using the major muscle groups in a repetitive fashion. Aerobic activities include walking (see the preceding section), jogging, stair climbing, cycling, rowing, dancing, swimming, elliptical machines, and aerobics classes. Cardio strengthens your heart and lungs.

Resistance training is also called strength training. The goal is to strengthen the major muscle groups in the legs, hips, back, abdomen, chest, shoulders, and arms. Studies have shown that resistance training improves A1C in adults with type 2 diabetes.

Lifting weights is an example of resistance exercise. Invest in hand weights to use at home. They come in a wide variety of weights, starting as low as one pound. Keep them handy and use them at least twice a week. If you enjoy watching TV, you can do your weight-lifting exercises while viewing. Elastic stretch bands are another alternative. If you belong to a gym, reduce the risk of injury by asking a trainer to show you how to use the exercise equipment properly.

Warming up, cooling down, and stretching

Prepare your muscles for the workout. Warming up simply means engaging in activity for three to five minutes at a relaxed pace to get your blood flowing and your muscles ready for action. As you end your workout, cool down by doing your activity at a relaxed pace for a few minutes.

You can incorporate gentle stretching before or after exercise. Whether you choose to bend and stretch at home or join a yoga class is up to you. It pays to stay limber and flexible. Stretching reduces the risk of injury.

Considering frequency, intensity, and duration targets

It isn't necessary to take your pulse to rate your workout. Perceived exertion takes into account your level of fitness. If you feel like you can push yourself a little harder or go for a little longer, then do so. Do what is right and safe for you.

TIP

Consider the talk-sing test. You should be able to talk while working out, but if you can sing, you probably aren't pushing yourself hard enough. You shouldn't be breathless or gasping for air. Find the sweet spot where you feel challenged but comfortable.

You don't have to sweat to call it exercise. Exercise means moving and using your body. Consider these three aspects of a workout:

>> **Frequency:** The goal is to exercise at least five days per week. The eventual goal for aerobic activity is 30 minutes per day. Exercise can be completed in one session, or it can be split into two sessions of 15 minutes or three sessions of 10 minutes. Try not to go more than two consecutive days without exercise. Resistance exercise, also known as strength training, should be done at least twice per week.

>> **Intensity:** You aren't trying to break any records here. You are the best judge of how hard to push yourself. Start with what you are able to do and work your way up gradually. The eventual goal is to work out at a moderate intensity at least 150 minutes per week. Examples of moderate-intensity

exercise include brisk walking, water aerobics, leisurely bicycling, and gardening.

An alternate option is to exercise at a vigorous level of intensity for at least 75 minutes per week. Vigorous activities include jogging, running, swimming laps, playing racket ball, riding a bicycle uphill or at higher speeds, and playing singles tennis.

The bulk of your workout can be somewhat challenging but shouldn't lead to pain or discomfort. *Interval training* inserts short bursts of intense activity into your usual workout. For example, when walking, you can speed up and walk more briskly for one to two minutes every five minutes. The concept can be modified to fit your activity and your level of fitness.

REMEMBER

If you have medical issues, have complications, or are older, ask your doctor for advice on how much to push yourself during your exercise sessions.

WARNING

Exercise should not hurt or cause injury. Stop exercising if at any time you feel pain, discomfort, dizziness, or shortness of breath. Discuss symptoms with your doctor.

>> **Duration:** The goal is for all adults to accumulate at least 150 minutes of moderate activity per week. If weight loss is your goal or you are trying to keep off the pounds you've already lost, 60 minutes of daily exercise has been shown to be more effective. The duration of individual exercise sessions is up to you. You can break exercise up into 10- or 15-minute mini sessions dispersed throughout the day. However, longer durations of moderate-intensity exercise burn more body fat. A moderately paced walk for 45–60 minutes burns glucose *and* fat. A quick dash or a couple of flights of steps burns primarily glucose.

REMEMBER

It's all good. You can make the argument that any exercise is beneficial. Don't be discouraged if you can do only five minutes on the stationary bike or treadmill. Stick with it. Your stamina will improve and you will be able to tack on some extra time as you become more conditioned.

Enjoying the benefits

Exercise benefits the entire body: muscles, bones, joints, heart, lungs, and circulation. Good health is sometimes taken for granted — only when a problem develops do we realize how much we depend on our bodies! Exercise is an important part of keeping your bodily systems in top running condition. The list ahead highlights some of the benefits of being fit. There isn't a single "medicine" that can do all of the following things:

- » **Maintaining strength, balance, and flexibility:** Bones and muscles are strengthened through use. Walking or any weight-bearing activity reduces the risk of osteoporosis. Exercise helps to tone and build muscle. Preservation of muscle strength is important for everyone, but it's essential as we age because it helps assure safety and independence in performing daily activities.

- » **Relieving stress and sleeping better:** Who wouldn't want to feel less stressed and sleep better? Sign me up right now. Exercise helps clear the head and releases tension.

WARNING

If you use insulin or medications that stimulate insulin production, use caution if you're exercising in the evening due to the risk of post-exercise hypoglycemia. Check your blood-glucose levels before bed. If you're unusually active, you can set an alarm to check blood-glucose levels in the middle of the night. Delayed hypoglycemia is addressed in more detail later in this chapter.

- » **Reducing your risk of chronic disease:** Heart disease and stroke are two of the leading causes of death. Exercising regularly lowers your risks. Research also shows that exercise reduces the risk of developing certain forms of cancer, including breast and colon cancers. Regular physical activity helps with arthritis and other joint conditions.

- » **Improving mental health:** Exercise is good for your physical *and* mental health. Being active is associated with improved mood and decreased symptoms of depression. Exercising increases endorphins, the chemicals in the brain that improve mood and a sense of well-being.

- » **Having fun and socializing:** Exercising with family and friends builds relationships. Spending quality time together builds memories too. Don't sit back and wait for someone to ask you to be active. Take the initiative and invite someone to go for a walk or take an exercise class with you. Group fitness classes are also a great way to meet people and forge new friendships.

REMEMBER

Exercise is a foundation treatment strategy for managing type 2 diabetes because exercise helps insulin work more effectively. Exercise is also good for heart health, weight control, blood pressure, and more. Exercise adds another variable to the complex management of type 1 diabetes, but with insight and planning, everyone with diabetes can enjoy exercise safely. Specifics are covered in more detail later in this chapter.

Being mindful of medical limitations

If you have medical issues and physical limitations as I describe in the following sections, you may need modifications to your exercise plan. Certain medical conditions, or having diabetes–related complications, may dictate what exercises are safe to do. If you have heart disease, *retinopathy* (damage to your eyes), or *neuropathy* (damage to your nerves), ask your provider to help you develop an appropriate exercise plan. Discuss reasonable targets for frequency, intensity, and duration of activity.

TIP

Find out whether your community has a swimming pool that accommodates people with handicaps. Some utilize lifts to safely lower you into the water. Temperatures are often kept warmer in these pools. The bottom of the pool may be rough, so wear appropriate water shoes.

Finding activities that are friendly for your feet

If you have peripheral neuropathy, you'll need to be especially careful to protect your feet. Neuropathy is a complication that affects nerves and can lead to burning and tingling in the feet. It can also lead to decreased sensation and numbness. People with this complication are at risk for foot injury.

REMEMBER

Avoid exercises that pound the feet. Walk, don't run. Avoid the stair-climber and don't jump rope. Safe exercises include stationary biking, swimming, walking, resistance exercises, chair exercises, and other non-weight-bearing activities.

Exercising while safely seated

If you are confined to a wheelchair or unsteady on your feet, it's possible to get a good workout while seated. Moving muscles systematically improves fitness. Buy an exercise DVD or tune in to an online exercise video to learn appropriate armchair exercises. You can also follow along with a televised exercise program. Public television hosts a show called *Sit and Be Fit* that teaches armchair aerobics.

Using caution with specific complications

Having diabetic complications imposes certain restrictions on exercise, but there's usually some form of activity that's safe to do. Several specific medical conditions are addressed here:

>> **Autonomic neuropathy:** Autonomic nerves direct many bodily functions including the heart and regulation of body temperature. Avoid exercising in the heat. You may need an exercise stress test, as described in the earlier section "Undergoing medical exams"; discuss this with your doctor.

>> **High blood pressure:** Avoid heavy lifting and straining. Use caution with strenuous activity. Your best options include walking and other moderate-intensity workouts. For weight lifting, use lighter weights and more repetitions.

>> **Nephropathy:** Kidney health is affected by blood pressure, so it's prudent to follow the same advice as listed for high blood pressure. Otherwise, there are no restrictions.

>> **Peripheral vascular disease:** Fatty deposits in the arteries of the legs can reduce blood flow to the muscles and lead to pain and cramping. Avoid high-impact aerobics. Better alternatives include walking, swimming, and chair exercises.

>> **Retinopathy:** Avoid heavy weight lifting and straining. Minimize jarring activities or those that position the head lower than the torso. Choose low-impact activities such as walking, cycling, swimming, or water aerobics.

Clarifying What's Going On Behind the Scenes When You Exercise

This section explains how exercise taps into glucose, glycogen, and fat to fuel activity. In the absence of diabetes, hormones automatically regulate fuel use and control blood-glucose levels. Having diabetes alters that delicate balance. Here you also find out how to reduce the risk of exercise-induced hypoglycemia for those at risk.

Controlling blood glucose: How hormones are supposed to do it automatically

The glucose that is stored in the muscles and liver is called *glycogen*. Glycogen in the liver can be broken back down into individual glucose molecules and released into the bloodstream, where it can be transported to the muscles and tissues in need of fuel. The liver can synthesize new glucose as needed. (Chapter 4 provides details on the process.)

Hormones regulate blood-glucose levels. Several different hormones can raise blood glucose. Glucagon, epinephrine, growth hormone, and cortisol are the counter-regulatory hormones. They are responsible for mobilizing the fuels used by muscles: glucose and fat.

>> The pancreas produces glucagon. You may be familiar with glucagon because it's also available in prescription form. People with type 1 diabetes should have glucagon kits available for treating severe hypoglycemia. Glucagon is administered by injection if a person with diabetes loses consciousness due to

hypoglycemia. Glucagon drives the liver to release glucose from glycogen stores and to make glucose from scratch in a process called *gluconeogenesis.*

» Epinephrine, which is adrenaline, is the "fight-or-flight" hormone. Adrenaline surges when you are in danger (or during competitive sports). It, too, mobilizes glucose.

» Growth hormone, which is released from the pituitary gland, drives the growth of bone, muscle, and tissue. It can also stimulate the liver to release glucose.

» Cortisol is made by the adrenal glands and helps the body modulate glucose levels.

Insulin is the only hormone that lowers blood glucose. Counter-regulatory hormones assure that there is enough fuel to burn during exercise, but insulin is needed to transport glucose into the muscles where it is burned for energy. In the absence of diabetes, insulin production increases and decreases automatically in relation to rising and falling blood-glucose levels. The working pancreas is adept at giving just the right amount of insulin for the situation. Type 1 diabetes means the pancreas can't make insulin, and in type 2 diabetes, the insulin doesn't work as well as it should. Details on both types of diabetes are addressed in the next section.

Identifying how diabetes alters fuel use

The absence of insulin in type 1 diabetes leads to metabolic mayhem. Insufficient insulin leads to elevated blood-glucose levels even during exercise. Recall that counter-regulatory hormones mobilize fatty acids from body stores and stimulate the liver to release glucose. Insulin is needed in appropriate amounts to move that fuel into the muscles. Without insulin, the glucose and fatty acids keep pouring into the bloodstream and levels rise higher and higher. Exercise doesn't fix this problem. Only insulin can open the cell doors and let the glucose in. Insulin deficiency results in fatty acids that are metabolized by the liver into byproducts known as ketones (see Chapter 4). Kidneys try to reduce glucose and ketone levels through urination, which can lead to dehydration.

Type 2 diabetes causes insulin resistance. People with type 2 make insulin, but it doesn't work very well. Early in the disease process, the pancreas works harder to make extra insulin. Prediabetes is the period of time when blood-glucose levels are above normal but not yet diagnostic of type 2 diabetes. You can be sure the pancreas is working overtime trying to prevent blood-glucose levels from rising further. Years into the process, the pancreas simply can't keep up the pace, and insulin production drops. Sedentary lifestyles and obesity worsen insulin resistance. Exercise is beneficial because it improves insulin sensitivity. Losing weight, even modest amounts, also improves insulin action. That's why diet and exercise are foundational treatment strategies when it comes to managing type 2 diabetes.

Sustaining exercise by tapping into fuels

Muscles burn both glucose and fat. We don't get to pick the order in which they get used. It would be nice if we could choose to burn fat first, but it doesn't work that way. If you walk across the room, you burn a small amount of glucose. If you walk out the door, you burn more glucose. If you keep walking, eventually you'll burn fat too:

» Glucose is the muscles' preferred fuel source. Glucose travels through the bloodstream and is delivered throughout the body to the working muscles.

» Muscles store glucose as glycogen. About 80 percent of the body's reserved glucose is housed in the muscles. That convenient location means the glucose is readily available to burn when the muscles start moving. Sustained exercise relies on glycogen storage to fuel the muscles. The glycogen stored in the liver is released as needed to provide additional glucose to the muscles.

» Muscles burn a fuel mixture consisting of glucose and fat in appropriate proportions. As exercise duration increases, the amount of fat burned increases. You don't have to be a marathon runner; just sustain your exercise sessions for longer periods of time to tap deeper into fat reserves.

Understanding hypoglycemia

Exercise increases the risk of hypoglycemia for people with diabetes who use insulin or any medication that stimulates the pancreas to produce insulin. Hypoglycemia is usually defined as blood glucose below 70 milligrams per deciliter (mg/dl). If your glucose levels are dropping, have a snack to prevent hypoglycemia.

Knowledge, experience, and proper planning can reduce the risk of hypoglycemia so that exercise can be enjoyed safely. Hypoglycemia is discussed briefly here; Chapter 15 is devoted to the topic.

Preventing lows

The proper balance between insulin and carbohydrates can mitigate the risk of hypoglycemia. You may need to snack on carbs before, during, or after exercise to sustain blood-glucose levels if you use insulin or medications that stimulate the pancreas to produce insulin. Adjusting insulin for planned activity is another strategy well worth discussing with your healthcare team. Fine-tuning carbs and insulin is discussed later in this chapter. If you don't use medications that put you at risk for hypoglycemia, exercise won't cause your blood-glucose levels to drop too low.

Treating lows

When blood-glucose levels fall too low, bringing them back up swiftly is important. Treat hypoglycemia by consuming carbohydrates that digest quickly. Glucose tablets are the gold standard. Carb-containing foods that are readily absorbed include fruit juice and sugar-sweetened beverages. Sugary candies can be used provided they do not contain fat. Fat delays digestion, which means no chocolate for treating lows.

REMEMBER

The general rule of thumb is to take 15–20 grams of quick-acting carbs and recheck your blood-glucose levels in 15 minutes. If your levels have not adequately risen, take an additional 15 grams of carb. Repeat until your blood-glucose levels are within safe targets.

The next step is to consider the need for a snack to prevent recurrent hypoglycemia. A snack containing carbs, protein, and fat will digest over a sustained period of time and reduce the chance of subsequent hypoglycemia.

Looking out for delayed hypoglycemia

Hypoglycemia can occur up to 24 hours after exercise has ended. When muscle glycogen reserves are depleted during activity, storage sites refill in the hours post-exercise. Glucose is drawn out of the bloodstream and into the muscles until glycogen storage sites are filled to capacity.

REMEMBER

After vigorous or long-duration exercise, consider checking blood-glucose levels in the middle of the night. Learn how to prevent episodes of delayed hypoglycemia by making adjustments to insulin and snacks. Details appear later in this chapter.

Exercising with Type 1: Staying Safe While Having Fun

Managing blood glucose during exercise can be a challenge for a person with type 1 diabetes, but learning to do so is well worth the effort. The following sections provide exercise pointers specifically for people with type 1 diabetes.

Monitoring matters

A car idling in the driveway doesn't burn much fuel, and neither does sitting on the couch. Light activity burns more; moderate or intense activity burns even more. The fuels used by the human body are glucose and fat. Chapter 4 discusses how muscles and the liver store glucose as glycogen. Glycogen provides glucose when food isn't available. Exercise readily uses the glycogen that is stored in the muscles. Insulin is more effective when exercising. Contracting muscles suck up the glucose that is traveling through the bloodstream. Hypoglycemia can occur if medication is too strong or your carb intake is too low for the workout.

Glucose levels may rise during activity due to the mobilization of fuels, which is driven by counter-regulatory hormones. Hormones are the messengers telling the liver to make and release glucose. Competitive sports can cause an adrenaline rush that bumps up the glucose released from the liver. Intense exercise and heavy weight lifting can also result in temporary elevations in glucose if the liver lets out glucose faster than the muscles are able to use it. (See the earlier section "Clarifying What's Going On Behind the Scenes When You Exercise" for more information.)

REMEMBER

Blood-glucose monitoring provides real-time data that is crucial for exercising safely. Check your glucose levels as frequently as needed to obtain the data you need to make diabetes self-management decisions. Blood-glucose monitoring provides valuable information about how you respond to exercise. Monitor your blood-glucose levels before, during, and after exercise and use that information to learn to balance insulin, carbs, and activity. Share your glucose records with your diabetes team for their input (as I explain in Chapter 15).

REMEMBER

Knowing how to interpret blood-glucose data is an essential skill. Don't judge your numbers. It's easy to be hard on yourself when results aren't where you wish they were. Don't use that as a reason not to check. Share your glucose data with your diabetes team. Ask your doctor or a certified diabetes educator to teach you how to make sense of the numbers. After all, you are the one managing your diabetes on a day-to-day basis.

Fueling up or dialing down: Fine-tuning carbs and insulin

REMEMBER

Through glucose monitoring, you can gather the information needed to balance insulin, diet, and exercise. Ask your diabetes care team about altering insulin doses on active days. Be sure to read Chapter 6 to review insulin action times. When heading out to exercise, reflect on which insulins will be active in your system. Consider the timing and carb content of your last meal to determine whether any of the carbs will be digesting and available during exercise.

Consuming carbs to fuel your fitness

Eat carbs as needed to fuel your activity. You may need to "carb up" before or during prolonged workouts. Playing team sports may require carb snacks between races or at halftime. Nonathletic weekend warriors may need to nibble on snacks. The only ways to ascertain whether you need a snack are to check your blood-glucose levels and consider your past experience.

Considering insulin adjustments

Insulin users may need to learn to make minor adjustments to insulin dosing to reduce the risk of hypoglycemia during planned activity.

If you plan to exercise within the first hour after eating, you may be able to take slightly less insulin for that meal. Consider someone who is skiing. He takes a lunch break but then hits the slopes again. Exercise facilitates insulin action, meaning the dose works better due to muscle activity. The muscles also burn more glucose to support the exercise. The net effect is that glucose will be used up faster. Knowing this, the skier may decide to reduce his dose of insulin at lunch.

REMEMBER

Insulin requirements depend on the activity and the individual. Discuss insulin dosing with your doctor. '

If you think you may have depleted your glycogen stores during afternoon activity, you may be able to cut back slightly on the dose of insulin you take at dinnertime. An alternate way to think about it is to take insulin for 45 grams of carb but eat 60 grams of carb. The extra 15 grams of carb are a gift to the muscles to replenish glycogen reserves.

REMEMBER

Individual insulin needs and fuel usage depend on many variables. There's no one-size-fits-all insulin recipe. The concept is that you may need different insulin-to-carb ratios and correction ratios on active versus sedentary days. Or you may need some extra carbs during exercise to support your activity.

WARNING

The concepts in this section and this chapter are not a substitute for professional medical advice. Do not make any adjustments to medications without speaking to your medical providers. The information regarding adjustments to carbs and insulin during exercise is theoretical and meant only to clarify concepts.

Knowing when to postpone activity: Too high or too low, don't go

REMEMBER

Determining ideal blood–glucose targets can be tricky. If your blood–glucose levels are too low or too high, it may be a good idea to put exercise on hold and make adjustments to either carbs or insulin. Consider the following scenarios:

>> **The risk of driving on empty:** Insulin users should check blood-glucose levels prior to exercising. The risk of hypoglycemia increases if pre-exercise glucose levels are below 100–120 mg/dl. Consider the need for a snack. Your doctor can help you determine the ideal blood-glucose range for exercise.

>> **Postponing when glucose levels hit the limits:** If pre-exercise blood-glucose levels are elevated, the amount of insulin is insufficient in relation to available glucose. Well-meaning counter-regulatory hormones will drive the liver to release more glucose during exercise, even if blood-glucose levels are high to begin with. Insulin doesn't work as well when glucose levels are very elevated. A glucose level above 250 mg/dl is cause for pause when you have type 1 diabetes. Consider the need for additional insulin, but dose conservatively due to the pending activity. This is a situation that should be discussed in advance with your diabetes specialist.

>> **Avoiding exercise if you have ketones:** Ketones indicate a significant insulin deficiency. Do not exercise if you have ketones. Glucose can't enter the muscles without the help of insulin. Counter-regulatory hormones always mobilize glucose and fatty acids to fuel exercise. The lack of insulin means those fuels can't be used properly. Blood-glucose levels will continue to rise, and fats will be converted to ketone. Forcing muscles to exercise will accelerate the process and could lead to diabetic ketoacidosis.

Exercising with Type 2: Why It's Right for You

Exercise is a treatment for type 2 diabetes. Studies show that exercise along with modest weight loss is one of the most effective ways to prevent prediabetes from progressing to type 2 diabetes. If you already have type 2 diabetes, exercise is one of the best ways to improve insulin sensitivity. The following sections describe the benefits of exercise specifically for people with type 2 diabetes.

Improving glycemic control

When it comes to type 2 diabetes, exercise is part of the treatment. People with type 2 diabetes have insulin resistance, and exercise increases insulin sensitivity. Insulin is more effective when muscles are moving. The glucose-lowering effect can persist beyond the actual exercise session.

During exercise, insulin is able to transport glucose into the muscle cells more readily. Imagine that insulin is the doorman assigned the task of opening cell doors to allow the glucose passage into the cell. Envision an exercising muscle cell eager to eat glucose. It pulls at the glucose. When the insulin doorman opens the cell door, a stream of glucose molecules is drawn into the contracting muscle.

Exercise can improve blood-glucose levels for hours after the exercise has ended. It has to do with burning glycogen from within the muscles' reserves. Muscles replenish glycogen stores, so glucose from the bloodstream continues to move into the muscles until the glycogen levels are restored. The longer the duration of the exercise and the more strenuous it is, the longer the post-exercise glucose-lowering effect will last.

REMEMBER

Keep in mind that if you eat a snack before exercising, you are more likely to burn the snack and not tap into glycogen or fat stores nearly as much. You should have a snack if you are at risk for hypoglycemia or if your pre-exercise blood-glucose levels indicate the need. But if your blood-glucose levels are fine, skip the additional carbs. When glucose levels are up but you are hungry, curb your appetite with a low-carb snack. See Chapter 22 for snack ideas.

Reducing cardiovascular risks

Exercise reduces the risk of heart disease and stroke. To cash in on the benefits, strive to meet the guidelines on physical activity: Accumulate at least 150 minutes of moderate-intensity activity each week and incorporate resistance exercises with mild to moderate weights twice weekly. Exercise improves heart health in the following ways:

>> **Lowering blood pressure:** Walking, swimming, leisurely cycling, and water aerobics help lower blood pressure when done on a regular basis.

>> **Improving lipid levels:** Staying physically fit and incorporating exercise helps to improve lipid levels in three ways:

- Exercise lowers LDL cholesterol (the artery-clogging type of cholesterol).

- Exercise raises HDL cholesterol (the kind that cleans out arteries).

- Exercise lowers triglycerides (the oily fats in the bloodstream).

>> **Promoting cardiovascular fitness:** Physical activity strengthens your heart and improves circulation. Aerobic activity gets the heart pumping, which is a positive workout for the heart. The heart is a muscle; exercising helps keep it fit. Being overweight adds to the workload of the heart. Weight loss is good for your heart and good for your diabetes.

Supporting weight-control efforts

Modest weight loss has been shown to improve blood-glucose control in people with type 2 diabetes who are overweight to begin with. Losing 5–10 percent of starting weight is often enough to reap the rewards. Numerous variables affect body weight. One major influence on weight status is the balancing of calories consumed with calories burned. Individual caloric needs are determined by age, gender, genetics, body composition, and physical activity.

Staying at a steady weight indicates that calories consumed are balancing with calories burned. If more calories are consumed than actually needed, the body will convert the excess into fat. For perspective, one pound of body fat stores 3,500 calories. Your personal caloric requirements are the sum of the calories you need to sustain bodily functions along with the number of calories you need to move. Movement refers to your daily activities and exercise. You may be able to influence how many calories you burn, as discussed ahead.

Increasing your metabolic rate

Every organ uses fuel, including the brain, liver, lungs, and kidneys. Calories are used to regulate body temperature and to make new cells, tissues, and hormones. A flurry of activity happens behind the scenes even when you're at rest. The sum of these physical and chemical processes is known as *metabolism*. About 70 percent of your daily caloric requirements go to metabolism. Activity level and exercise account for the remainder of the calories needed.

You can dispose of more calories by increasing your exercise, which is addressed next. However, you may also be able to increase your metabolic rate so that you burn more calories even at rest. It boils down to how much muscle you have. Muscles use up more fuel than body fat. Body fat doesn't require many calories for upkeep. Muscles store energy in the form of glycogen (the storage form of glucose). When you exercise, the glycogen within the muscles is used. Muscles want their glycogen stores to be kept filled. It takes energy (calories) for the muscles to refill glucose stores. People who build and strengthen their muscles and who exercise regularly have a higher metabolic rate, especially those who work out at higher intensities. If you increase your metabolism, you will burn more calories even when relaxing, and that makes weight control easier.

Burning rather than storing calories

The sum of the calories consumed in a day is divvied up to feed all the body's metabolic necessities. What happens next depends on how many calories are consumed and the level of activity and exercise on any given day. After distributing the calories needed to support metabolism and activity, any surplus calories are converted to fat. It's simple math: If you eat more than you burn, you will gain weight. Any discussion about weight management should address the importance of physical activity. The more you exercise, the more calories you burn.

Keeping off the weight that's lost

Successful weight loss means being able to keep the weight off. The National Weight Control Registry (http://nwcr.ws) says that a key factor to success is to engage in at least an hour of exercise per day. The data also suggests that the other components of long-term successful weight management include controlling dietary calories and fats, eating breakfast, weighing yourself regularly, and getting back on the wagon if you slip up. I second that motion! Temporary diets and crash dieting don't work for the long haul. Skipping meals backfires too. Going long periods of time without food can slow down your metabolism and make it harder to lose weight. That's why breakfast is a critical meal.

TIP

What works best for successful weight management is to eat a healthy, balanced diet, with appropriate portions, and to do so lifelong. Record-keeping can be useful. Track your weight with a home scale. Keep food logs periodically and take a good look at what you are actually eating.

Chapter **15**

Getting a Handle on Hypoglycemia

Without diabetes, the human body does an amazing job at keeping blood-glucose levels in a fairly narrow and safe range. Fasting and pre-meal levels normally range from 70–99 milligrams per deciliter (mg/dl). Of course after eating, glucose levels rise as carbohydrates digest and enter the bloodstream. Normal post-meal blood-glucose levels range from 100 to 139 mg/dl.

Insulin, a hormone produced by the pancreas, helps the body use and store glucose. Insulin *lowers* blood-glucose levels. Other hormones, known as counter-regulatory hormones, *raise* blood-glucose levels by stimulating the liver to make and release glucose. Insulin and counter-regulatory hormones are supposed to work in orchestration to keep blood-glucose levels controlled.

When the pancreas is working properly, insulin production turns on and off as needed. Insulin that is made by the pancreas is secreted directly into the bloodstream and lasts only a few minutes before it is cleared from the bloodstream by the kidneys. The pancreas secretes insulin as needed and pauses when blood glucose drops to the lower limits of normal. Counter-regulatory hormones then get to work to raise blood glucose by stimulating the release of glucose from the liver.

When glucose levels rise sufficiently, the counter-regulatory hormones subside. Back and forth it goes day after day. Hard-working hormones are behind the scenes regulating blood-glucose levels. Diabetes, however, interferes with that delicate balance.

Hypoglycemia means deficiency of glucose in the blood. Diabetes doesn't cause hypoglycemia; some of the medications used to treat diabetes can lead to hypoglycemia if there is an imbalance between medications, foods, and activity levels. Diabetes can only cause *high blood sugar,* more accurately referred to as *high blood glucose* or *hyperglycemia.* Mild hypoglycemia is easily treated by consuming glucose or any other rapidly digesting form of sugar. Hypoglycemia is considered severe if treatment requires the help of another person or a paramedic. Low blood glucose is a complication that can lead to injuries and accidents. Severe hypoglycemia, if untreated, can lead to loss of consciousness, seizure, coma, and rarely even death. Luckily, with knowledge and preparation, you can prevent problems and stay safe.

REMEMBER

This chapter provides information for people who have diabetes and are at risk for hypoglycemia. Speak to your healthcare provider and review your medication list to find out whether or not you are at risk for hypoglycemia.

Understanding Hypoglycemia

Insulin is the main medication associated with the risk of *low blood sugar,* more accurately referred to as *low blood glucose* or *hypoglycemia*; however, some diabetes pills can also cause hypoglycemia. Type 1 diabetes results in the inability to produce insulin, so people who have type 1 must take insulin for life. Many people with type 2 diabetes also take insulin to manage their diabetes because insulin is very effective in lowering blood-glucose levels. Insulin is a lifesaving but powerful medication, so proper training and self-management education are required for safe use.

Insulin is injected under the skin into fatty tissue called *adipose.* It takes time for the insulin to make its way from adipose to the bloodstream. Timing of action depends on the type of insulin. Insulin comes in rapid-acting, short-acting, intermediate-acting, and long-acting varieties. Once insulin is injected, it will continue to lower blood-glucose levels for its full duration of action. Insulin doses must be coordinated with carbohydrate intake and with consideration to planned activity and exercise.

Some oral medications that are used to treat type 2 diabetes work by stimulating the pancreas to secrete more insulin. Those medications can also cause hypoglycemia, particularly if a meal is missed or if too few carbs are eaten. Other diabetes medications pose no risk of hypoglycemia whatsoever. Blood-glucose monitoring provides important information that can be used to make adjustments to your treatment regimen. Monitor your blood-glucose levels, keep records, and share results with your healthcare providers. If you're uncertain about your risk for hypoglycemia, speak to your doctor or a pharmacist.

This section explains what level of blood glucose is considered too low, identifies the causes and symptoms of hypoglycemia, and discusses hypoglycemia unawareness. The rest of this chapter provides information to help you treat, problem-solve, prevent, and get help with hypoglycemia.

Injected insulin and certain diabetes pills that increase insulin production can lead to hypoglycemia. The successful management of diabetes requires learning to strike the right balance between foods (particularly carbs), medications, and exercise. Discuss your personal blood-glucose targets with your healthcare provider and follow dosing instructions for all medications prescribed.

Defining a low blood-glucose level

A blood-glucose level that dips below 70 mg/dl is typically considered hypoglycemic. Young children and the elderly are at higher risk for severe hypoglycemia, so it makes sense to have a safety margin and strive to keep their blood-glucose levels safely above 90 mg/dl. Consider an elderly person who is at risk for falls. For a frail senior to take a fall and break a hip due to hypoglycemia would be a big setback. Young children are especially vulnerable because they have trouble recognizing symptoms and communicating the need for help.

Blood-glucose monitoring is an important part of diabetes management. Keeping records and learning from past experiences can improve blood-glucose control in the future. Problem-solving for prevention of hypoglycemia is addressed later in this chapter.

Identifying causes of hypoglycemia

Hypoglycemia occurs when there is an imbalance between insulin, carbs, and exercise. At times it may feel like you are walking a tightrope, trying to stay safely in the center and maintain stability without tipping too far to one side (hyperglycemia, or high blood glucose) or the other (hypoglycemia). You can reduce the risk of hypoglycemia by learning more about managing your diabetes. The most common causes of low blood glucose are discussed in this section, followed by information on how to recognize symptoms.

REMEMBER

Everyone with insulin-treated diabetes should have a medical alert bracelet, necklace, or some form of identification that says you have diabetes. Many styles can pass as jewelry. If you don't want a bracelet, consider a necklace chain with a tag that hangs inside your shirt. It's discreet but still there if needed. I've even seen several people with medical alert tattoos! Anything goes. If you ever require assistance due to severe hypoglycemia, the medical alert provides critical information to help assure that you get the treatment you need. Health issues other than hypoglycemia can be included on medical alert tags, too. A wide variety of styles for women and men are available online. Just use your favorite search engine to look up medical alert tags.

Taking too much medication

If you take more insulin than needed or double the doses of some of the diabetes pills, the excess medication could lead to low blood-glucose levels. Sometimes medication dosing mistakes happen. The following are some such examples:

>> **Taking the wrong kind of insulin:** If you ever mistakenly take your rapid-acting insulin at bedtime instead of your long-acting insulin, then you have no choice but to eat carbs. You must consume enough carbs to balance the insulin you took. Such a mistake also means you should stay awake and check your blood-glucose levels frequently in the coming hours. Prevent this error by carefully inspecting the insulin vial or pen prior to injecting.

>> **Calculating the wrong insulin dose:** If you use insulin-to-carb ratios (see Chapter 6), it is very important to count carbs correctly. Nutrition Facts food labels list the grams of carbohydrate. I'm aware of situations when the insulin dose was accidentally based on the number associated with the weight of the product or the percent daily value instead of the number of grams of carbohydrate. If you are guesstimating on carb counts, you may end up with the wrong dose. See Chapter 7 for clarification on how to read food labels correctly and Chapter 8 to find out how to count carbs in foods that don't have labels.

>> **Stacking doses:** Many people with type 1 diabetes are taught how to calculate and take insulin correction doses when blood-glucose levels are above target. For example, the insulin dose taken at mealtime consists of two parts:

- The first variable to consider is the dose of insulin needed to balance the amount of carb in the meal, which is determined using the insulin-to-carb ratio.

- The second variable to consider is the pre-meal blood glucose value.

A correction ratio is used if the pre-meal blood glucose is above target. Take for example a person with a blood-glucose level of 200 before eating 45 grams of carb. Insulin is needed for the carbs, and additional insulin is needed to bring down the elevated glucose level. Rapid-acting insulin continues to lower blood glucose for about four hours. Yet many people get impatient if an hour passes and the blood-glucose level is still elevated. It would be a mistake to calculate another correction dose so soon. Taking another correction dose within three hours of the last correction dose puts you at risk for subsequent hypoglycemia. If one dose is working on top of another dose, then the synergy can cause blood-glucose levels to drop too low.

REMEMBER

Discuss insulin correction doses with your healthcare provider. If you use an insulin pump, your pump likely has a feature called "insulin-on-board," which takes previous doses into account when calculating subsequent correction doses.

>> **Doubling doses of diabetes pills:** Have you ever second-guessed yourself and questioned whether or not you took your pills? If you end up taking a double dose, your blood glucose can drop too much. You may find it easier to keep track of doses if you organize your pills into a pill caddy.

REMEMBER

If you forget a dose, don't double up on the next dose. It's important to take all medications as prescribed. Do not increase medication doses on your own, because doing so can cause hypoglycemia and other problems. See your healthcare provider to get a tune-up on your prescriptions if your blood glucose is not well controlled.

Failing to eat enough carb

Carbohydrates provide glucose to fuel your body. If you don't eat enough carbs to meet your basic needs (as shown in the following examples), medications that are used to treat diabetes could cause hypoglycemia during the day or overnight while you sleep. See Chapter 5 for tips on setting a reasonable carbohydrate–intake goal. The following circumstances can lead to a carb shortage:

>> **Missing a meal:** Distributing carbs throughout the day into three meals helps provide batches of glucose to fuel your body. During the day some of the available glucose from your meals is shuttled into your liver and muscles to be stored as glycogen. If you miss meals or have meals that don't contain enough carb, you may not have spare glucose to satisfactorily fill glycogen storage sites. Depleted glycogen stores increase your risk of hypoglycemia.

>> **Undereating carbs at mealtime:** If you take a dose of insulin to cover your meal but then eat less than planned, you could end up with low blood glucose. Once you take a dose of insulin, you are committed to eating the

expected amount of carb. If you don't finish an entrée, you may be able to make up the carbs by eating a serving of fruit. Or perhaps you could opt to check blood-glucose levels frequently in the hours after the injection and eat more carbs only if and when needed.

>> **Ongoing carb restriction:** Carbs provide glucose to fuel vital organs, cells, tissues, and muscles. Glucose also supports physical activity. The vital organs use a sizable amount, as glucose is the preferred fuel for the brain, liver, and red blood cells. Muscles also burn glucose. You need enough carb to keep all systems running efficiently during the day and to maintain stable blood-glucose levels overnight. Carb food groups also provide important nutrients. Chapter 13 provides advice on healthy eating.

REMEMBER

If you're eating reasonable amounts of healthy foods and your blood-glucose levels are elevated, it may be time to meet with your doctor to discuss medication options.

Mismatching meals and meds

Understanding how your insulin works is critically important. See Chapter 6 to review onset, peak, and duration times for various types of insulin. Meals and injections must be timed so that the insulin is available at the same time that the food is being digested. The following list gives examples of mismatching meals and meds:

>> **Injecting off schedule:** Rapid-acting insulin is designed to be taken right before eating or within 15 minutes of the meal. If you inject too far in advance, the insulin peaks before the food digests and blood glucose can plummet. Don't inject at home and then drive to the restaurant! Regular insulin is slower to get going and is supposed to be injected 30 minutes before the meal.

REMEMBER

If you aren't sure what kind of insulin you take, be sure to review your insulin plan and dosing schedule with your doctor.

>> **Timing pitfalls with blended insulins:** 70/30 insulin is a blend of two different types of insulin. It may be an appropriate option for treating type 2 diabetes but isn't the insulin of choice for treating type 1 diabetes. It is 70 percent intermediate-acting insulin and 30 percent rapid- or short-acting insulin. When 70/30 is injected before breakfast, the rapid-acting insulin kicks in and covers the carbs in the breakfast meal. The intermediate-acting insulin will peak later to cover the carbs in lunch. If lunch is delayed or doesn't contain enough carb, then blood-glucose levels can drop. The same concept holds true for the 75/25 and 50/50 blended insulin preparations.

REMEMBER

Being regimented in meal timing and carb amounts is important when using blended insulin preparations. Plan to eat the same amount of carbs from day to day and keep the carb amounts at meals consistent. When using blended insulin (such as 70/30 or 75/25), it is important to eat lunch four to five hours after the morning injection. Taking blended insulin before dinner covers the carbs in dinner and the glucose that is released from the liver while you sleep. You do not need to eat another meal four to five hours after the dinner injection. Whether or not you should have a small bedtime snack depends on circumstances and should be discussed with your healthcare providers.

Exercising without carb compensation

Your liver and muscles hold a storage form of glucose called glycogen. When you exercise, you use glucose from the bloodstream and also tap into glycogen stored in the liver and muscles. The more you exercise, the more glucose you burn. If you don't eat enough carbs to support your activity, you could end up with low blood glucose (as you see in the following list). Eat carbs as needed before, during, or after exercise to prevent hypoglycemia. Figuring out whether or not you need to snack to compensate for exercise or how many carbs you need for your particular workout is a matter of trial and error. See Chapter 14 for more about exercise.

» **Being caught unprepared:** Monitor blood-glucose levels before and throughout exercise. Snack as needed to prevent hypoglycemia. Be prepared; carry your meter, carb-containing snacks, and glucose tablets or other quick-digesting carbs in case your blood glucose drops. Stay hydrated; carry water. Appropriate carb options for treating lows are discussed later in this chapter.

» **Depleting glycogen stores and causing delayed hypoglycemia:** Exercise can use up significant amounts of glucose. If you don't have an adequate amount of carb available to support your level of exercise, you'll burn through some of the glucose that has been stored as glycogen in your muscles and liver. Glycogen stores strive to be refilled and will draw glucose from the bloodstream until fully replenished. That means blood-glucose levels can continue to drop for hours after strenuous or long-duration exercise sessions. Delayed hypoglycemia is a result of not eating enough carbohydrate to support the exercise session. In a more extreme example, someone who skis all day could experience hypoglycemia up to 24 hours later as glucose from the bloodstream is drawn upon to refill glycogen storage sites.

Drinking alcohol

Many people are surprised to find out that alcohol doesn't turn to sugar. Wine is actually low in carbs even though it is made from grape juice. During fermentation, the yeast converts juice into alcohol. Hard liquor contains no carbs whatsoever unless you add mixers. But that doesn't mean drinking alcohol has no impact on blood-glucose levels.

WARNING

Drinking alcohol can lead to significant hypoglycemia for anyone with diabetes who uses insulin or pills that stimulate insulin production. The reason, in simple terms, is that alcohol is processed in the liver. When the liver is busy detoxifying the alcohol, it may be unable to release normal amounts of glucose. The liver is the body's key source of glucose when food is not digesting. A balanced meal may take about four hours to digest, but after that, the liver is supplying glucose between meals and while you sleep. Once the liver diverts its attention to breaking down the alcohol, it may not be able to supply adequate amounts of glucose. Blood-glucose levels can then drop because of the diabetes medications in your system.

If you become hypoglycemic after drinking alcohol, you could lose coordination and end up staggering. Anyone who may have seen you drinking could assume you are intoxicated and not realize you are in need of assistance. The following are alcohol-related causes of hypoglycemia (see Chapter 11 for more information on alcohol and other beverage options):

>> **Exceeding suggested limits:** A single drink may take two or more hours for the liver to process. That means two drinks can tie up your liver for four hours, three drinks for six or more hours, and so on. You're at risk for hypoglycemia the entire time the liver is busy breaking down the alcohol. The more you drink, the more prolonged the risk.

The American Diabetes Association and other health experts recommend limiting alcohol to not more than one drink per day for women and two drinks for men, and never on an empty stomach. Drinking in the evening can be especially treacherous as blood-glucose levels can dip dangerously low while you sleep. Late-night drinking at bars, clubs, concerts, and parties increases the risk of nocturnal hypoglycemia. It is unlikely that you or anyone around you will notice that you are low if you are sound asleep. Cocktail hour before dinner is also risky because lunch has likely finished digesting by then. Find a carb-containing snack as needed.

REMEMBER

Some people should not drink at all because of medication interactions or other health concerns. Ask your doctor to assess your health history and medication list to provide personal guidance on safe alcohol use.

>> **Drinking on an empty stomach:** It is safer to have your drink at mealtime. Be sure to eat something with carbs. The carbs from the meal will be digested and provide glucose, which leaves your liver free to devote its attention to detoxifying the alcohol. If you want an alcoholic beverage between meals, consider the need for a carbohydrate snack. Chicken wings and nuts don't count because they do not supply carbs. Pretzels or crackers may be a better choice.

Recognizing the symptoms of hypoglycemia

It is important to use your meter to verify blood-glucose levels. It's possible to perceive symptoms of hypoglycemia when your blood glucose is not actually low. If your body has grown accustomed to having persistently elevated blood-glucose levels, you may start to feel symptoms of hypoglycemia when you are actually safely in a normal range. Your body may send the signals of low blood glucose just because you are lower than you have been in a long while. If your blood glucose is not actually low, you don't need to drink juice or treat the low. Wait and recheck later.

WARNING

Some people don't have any symptoms at all even when they have critically low blood-glucose levels. The lack of symptoms is known as *hypoglycemia unawareness.* This phenomenon indicates that your body has gotten used to being low and no longer perceives hypoglycemia as unusual so it stops sending signals. I discuss hypoglycemia unawareness in more detail in the next section.

Following are some of the most common symptoms of low blood glucose:

» Sweating, clamminess

» Shakiness, tremors

» Rapid heartbeat

» Nervousness, anxiety

» Irritability, impatience

» Blurred vision

» Nausea

» Hunger

» Tingly lips, numbness

» Lightheadedness

» Confusion

» Headaches

» Sleepiness, fatigue

» Pallor (paleness)

» Unsteadiness, dizziness

» Nightmares, thrashing

» Unresponsiveness

» Fainting, seizures

Losing symptoms of lows: Hypoglycemia unawareness

When blood-glucose levels dip close to 70 mg/dl, the counter-regulatory hormones should signal the liver to make and release glucose. Those hormones may cause rapid heartbeat, shaking, and sweating. If blood-glucose levels frequently dip too low, the body gets used to it so symptoms may not kick in until blood-glucose levels are below 65 mg/dl. If you dip below that too often, your body may adjust its panic response and not send signals until blood-glucose levels hit 60 mg/dl, then 55 mg/dl, then 50 mg/dl. If your levels get too low too often, your body may simply stop sending the signals of hypoglycemia.

Impaired awareness of hypoglycemia is really dangerous. Imagine driving down the freeway with a blood-glucose level of 40 mg/dl and having no symptoms at all. You could be driving one minute and passed out the next minute. Hypoglycemia unawareness can be hazardous to you and those around you; don't drive until your body is recalibrated to sense the lows, and always check blood-glucose levels before driving.

It is possible to regain symptoms with the help of the following tactics:

>> **Reversing hypoglycemia unawareness:** The best way to reverse hypoglycemia unawareness is to diligently avoid hypoglycemia. Keep blood-glucose levels higher for several weeks or longer. That may mean running your blood-glucose levels higher than typically recommended or higher than you are comfortable with. Discuss blood-glucose targets with your healthcare provider. If you avoid hypoglycemia long enough, your body can readjust and learn to recognize hypoglycemia and provide symptoms again. Symptoms are important warning signals that can prompt you to eat carbs before your blood glucose is dangerously low.

>> **Monitoring more frequently:** Anyone with frequent hypoglycemia or any degree of hypoglycemia unawareness should monitor blood glucose with greater frequency and may benefit from a continuous glucose monitor (CGM). To use a continuous glucose monitoring system, the user inserts a disposable sensor probe under the skin; it is taped down and remains in place for about a week. The CGM checks your blood-glucose levels every few minutes around the clock. Blood-glucose readings are transmitted wirelessly, and results are displayed on a receiver or an insulin pump. Alarms can be set to alert you when your blood glucose is dropping. Setting the lower limit alarm for 80 or 90 mg/dl provides the opportunity to eat a snack before becoming hypoglycemic. The device also indicates the rate of change so you know how quickly your blood-glucose level is dropping (or rising) and can make appropriate management decisions. CGM systems can be used periodically for gathering

detailed glucose data to guide diabetes management decisions, or the user can insert a new sensor immediately after the expired sensor is removed. For more on blood glucose monitoring, see Chapter 23.

Treating Hypoglycemia

REMEMBER

Anyone at risk for hypoglycemia should be prepared by carrying carbs at all times. It isn't good enough to have glucose tablets in the car when you're out walking around the lake. The carbs always need to be with you. Not all carbs are created equal when it comes to treating low blood glucose.

This section provides details on which carbs to use and how much to take when treating mild hypoglycemia. I also discuss the management of severe hypoglycemia with glucagon.

Choosing quick-acting carbs

When treating hypoglycemia, the objective is to get your blood glucose to come back up as quickly as possible. Glucose, available in tablet or gel form, works rapidly. Other carbs also work well, such as the following:

>> Liquids get through the stomach quickly. Fruit juice and regular sugar-containing soft drinks such as soda (not diet) also have the potential to raise blood-glucose levels in just a few minutes.

>> You can use candy as a treatment for lows provided it is pure sugar and doesn't contain chocolate, fat, or nuts. Fat delays digestion, and chocolate, nuts, and butter are all high in fat. Fatty desserts, including candy bars, cookies, and pies, also won't digest as quickly as jelly beans, gumdrops, Skittles, or Starburst candies. The pure sugar candies make their way through the stomach quickly. Fat delays gastric emptying, so fatty foods are held up in the stomach for too long.

>> Fresh or dried fruit are appropriate options for treating lows. Fruit contains natural sugar, and there's no fat or protein to delay absorption.

Taking the right amount of carb

When treating low blood glucose, you need enough carb to sufficiently raise blood glucose. If you overdo it and eat too much, you can end up with elevated blood-glucose levels.

REMEMBER

The usual recommendation for treating hypoglycemia is to consume 15 to 20 grams of easily digested carbohydrate. Consider the severity of the low, however. Very low blood-glucose levels may need a more robust dose of carb. Blood-glucose levels below 50 mg/dl may need 20 to 30 grams of carb. Young children may need only 5 to 10 grams of carb to recover from hypoglycemia, due to their small body size, and their pediatric diabetes specialists should provide personalized advice.

Things to consider when deciding how much carb is needed to treat hypoglycemia include

>> **Body size:** An adult athlete needs more than a ten-year-old.

>> **Previous exercise:** You likely need more carbs if you just finished a game of tennis versus sitting in front of a computer.

>> **The timing and amount of the last dose of insulin:** Considering insulin action is covered in detail later in this chapter.

I explore managing variables related to hypoglycemia in more depth later in this chapter.

Following are some appropriate choices for treating hypoglycemia. The carbohydrate options listed are approximately 15 grams of carb per choice. All of them digest quickly, making them good options when treating hypoglycemia:

>> 4 glucose tabs (read labels to find the exact amount of carb contained)

>> 1 tablespoon of sugar, honey, or syrup

>> 4 ounces (½ cup) of fruit juice

>> 4 ounces (½ cup) of regular soda (not diet)

>> 4 Starburst candies

>> 15 Skittles candies

>> 2 tablespoons raisins (1 mini box)

>> 8 ounces (1 cup) nonfat or 1 percent milk

Here are a few additional options for 15 grams of carbs:

>> Fruit can be used to treat hypoglycemia. An appropriate portion would be an apple or orange the size of a tennis ball, half of a banana, 17 grapes, or a cup of melon. See Appendix A for a complete list of fruits with serving sizes equaling 15 grams of carb.

>> You can opt for jelly beans, gummy drops, hard candies, or any pure-sugar candy that doesn't contain protein or fat. Read labels to determine the correct portion to achieve 15 grams of carb.

Carrying candy for treating lows may be too tempting for some people. You're the best judge. If the jelly beans are going to be "calling your name" all day, you may not want them in your purse or backpack. Glucose tablets have less appeal so they tend to stay tucked away safely until actually needed.

>> Glucose gel is also available, and it's easy to consume: No chewing is needed. Read labels for carb counts. Tubes of glucose gel come in handy for surfers or people who do water sports and need to keep a carb source handy. The glucose gel comes in a waterproof tube with a screw-off cap, and the tube can be slipped into the wetsuit.

Gel should not be put in the mouth of a person who has passed out from hypoglycemia. Nothing should go in the mouth during a seizure or loss of consciousness due to the risk of choking.

Rechecking your blood-glucose level

Rechecking your blood-glucose levels 15 minutes after treating hypoglycemia is highly recommended. Don't assume 15 grams of carb was enough to fix the problem. If blood-glucose levels are still low after 15 minutes, repeat the process: Take another 15 grams of carb and recheck again in 15 minutes. Once your blood-glucose levels are back up, you can make a decision about whether or not you should eat a carb-containing snack to prevent recurrent hypoglycemia.

The rule of 15 for treating lows is as follows:

1. **Take 15 grams of quick-digesting carb.**

2. **Wait 15 minutes; recheck blood glucose.**

3. **If still low, take another 15 grams of quick-digesting carb and recheck blood glucose levels again in 15 minutes.**

Repeat these steps until the hypoglycemia resolves. Call your clinic for advice as needed.

If it will be more than 30 minutes until your next meal, you should consider the need for a snack with 10 to 20 grams of carb to reduce the chance of another episode of hypoglycemia. That snack should contain some protein or fat so it digests more slowly.

Let your doctor know if you're having frequent episodes of hypoglycemia, if hypoglycemic events aren't easily resolved, or if you notice a pattern of hypoglycemia occurring at a similar time of day. Contact your doctor to report *severe hypoglycemia,* which is defined as hypoglycemia that caused a seizure, loss of consciousness, or treatment requiring the assistance of another person (for example, you were confused or uncoordinated to the point of being unable to find and consume carbs).

Watching out for rebounds

When blood-glucose levels drop, internal hormones attempt to rescue you and raise your blood glucose. Adrenaline is the "fight-or-flight" hormone responsible for telling the liver to dump glucose into the bloodstream so you have energy to run or respond. Adrenaline is what causes your heart to pound and your hands and knees to shake if you are abruptly startled or in a precarious situation. Some of the symptoms of low blood glucose are caused by hormones such as adrenaline. Hypoglycemia can cause the heart to race and the hands to tremble. The body perceives hypoglycemia as a precarious situation.

Sometimes the liver is overzealous and lets out too much glucose, leading to hyperglycemia. It's called a "rebound" when blood-glucose levels shoot up too high after being too low. Sometimes a high blood-glucose level after an episode of hypoglycemia is simply the result of eating too many carbs to treat the low. It can be hard to stop eating after just 15 grams of carb because hypoglycemia doesn't feel good. It's tempting to keep eating everything in sight until you feel better. Keep in mind that the uncomfortable feelings associated with hypoglycemia may persist for a while. Blood-glucose levels can be rising sufficiently, and yet you may still feel shaky and panicky for several more minutes. It takes time for the fight-or-flight hormones to get the message that you are going to be okay. Remember to follow the rule of 15 when treating hypoglycemia: Eat 15 grams of carb, wait 15 minutes, and recheck blood glucose. Repeat until blood-glucose levels recover.

Requiring assistance: Severe lows and glucagon

Glucagon is a hormone that raises blood glucose by stimulating the liver to make and release glucose. Normally the pancreas makes glucagon automatically when blood-glucose levels fall too low, but with long-standing diabetes, glucagon production can become compromised. Glucagon is available by prescription and is administered by injection. Glucagon kits should be prescribed to everyone with type 1 diabetes and for people with type 2 diabetes on intensive insulin therapy.

REMEMBER

Glucagon by injection is an appropriate treatment for severe hypoglycemia — for example, if the person with diabetes cannot safely swallow, displays severe lack of coordination or combativeness, loses consciousness, or has a seizure. Glucagon needs to be administered by a family member, friend, teacher, or co-worker. Potential helpers need to be identified and trained ahead of time so they know how to respond in the event of an emergency.

Glucagon kits (which expire annually) typically contain a vial of powder and a syringe that is pre-filled with a fluid. The powder in the vial is the glucagon. The glucagon needs to be mixed before using. First the fluid in the syringe must be injected into the vial of powder. Then the vial is swirled to dissolve the glucagon powder. Once mixed, the glucagon dose is drawn back into the syringe and can be administered by injection into the thigh or upper arm. The dose for children is smaller than the dose for adults.

REMEMBER

The instructions discussed here are simply to familiarize you with the concept and are not a substitution for proper in-person training by a healthcare provider.

REMEMBER

If someone with diabetes has passed out or is having a seizure, call 911. Any person trained to give glucagon can do so but it is important to stay with the unresponsive person because glucagon can cause nausea and vomiting. It is critically important to protect the airway and prevent aspiration (vomit entering the lungs). Place the person in the recovery position by rolling him on onto his side with the upper leg bent. The knee should act as a support and prevent him from rolling. Gently tilt the chin upward to keep the air passage open. See Figure 15-1.

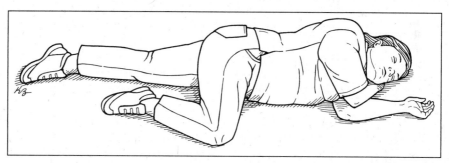

FIGURE 15-1:
The recovery position.

Illustration by Kathryn Born, MA

REMEMBER

For someone who has passed out, glucagon is the treatment of choice because you can't put any carbohydrates in the mouth of an unconscious person due to the risk of choking. Have a doctor, pharmacist, nurse, or diabetes educator review the use, procedure, and precautions of glucagon with you, then you in turn can train those who potentially may administer it.

Strategizing for Common Hypoglycemia Scenarios

Treating hypoglycemia appropriately is important. This section delves deeper into situations that call for additional considerations, such as treating lows at mealtime and bedtime. The amount of carbohydrate needed to recover from hypoglycemia depends on the amount and timing of the previous insulin injection, so that concept is also explored in more detail.

Managing mealtime lows

Without diabetes, normal fasting blood glucose ranges between 70–99 mg/dl. Striving for those levels is fine if you have type 2 diabetes and are not taking insulin or any pills that can cause hypoglycemia. Insulin treatment comes with the risk of hypoglycemia, so blood-glucose targets for people with type 1 diabetes are set a little higher to provide a margin of safety. Pre-meal blood glucose targets of 80–130 mg/dl may be more appropriate for a person using insulin.

WARNING

If you check your blood glucose before a meal and it's below 70 mg/dl, you may be tempted to simply eat your meal more quickly. That isn't the best solution. Keep in mind that hypoglycemia should be treated with quick-digesting forms of carb as discussed earlier in this chapter. The goal is to consume carbs that can raise blood-glucose levels within 10 to 15 minutes. Regular meals contain fat, protein, and fiber, which can delay the digestion of the carbohydrate. A normal meal typically takes several hours to be fully digested. When you are hypoglycemic, you need something readily digestible.

When you're hypoglycemic before a meal, you must first treat the low with rapidly digesting carbs. Once the blood glucose has stabilized, it is fine to strategize what to do about the dose of insulin needed for the pending meal.

WARNING

Keep in mind that rapid-acting insulin works very quickly. The insulin may start to lower blood-glucose levels before the meal has had a chance to digest. This is particularly true for fatty meals. It is possible to become hypoglycemic with a belly full of fatty food. Low blood glucose in this situation is harder to treat because the heavy meal blocks the passageway through the stomach. The juice or carbs being used to treat the low may end up being soaked up into the wad of food in the stomach. Read ahead for steps that can prevent this tricky situation.

REMEMBER

If you take rapid-acting insulin at mealtime (such as Humalog, NovoLog, or Api-dra), consider the following steps for treating mealtime hypoglycemia. However, before making adjustments to your insulin plan, you should talk with your doctor. Discuss potential scenarios with your doctor in advance. Ask what you should do if you are hypoglycemic before a meal or before bed.

Steps to consider if you have hypoglycemia at mealtime and take rapid-acting insulin are as follows:

1. **First treat the low blood glucose with 15–20 grams of quick-acting carbs.**

2. **Wait 10–15 minutes to allow the quick carbs to pass through the stomach.**

3. **Recheck blood glucose to assure you are no longer low.**

    If blood glucose is still below 70 mg/dl, take another 15 grams of quick-acting carbs. Recheck blood glucose in 15 minutes. Repeat the procedure until the blood-glucose level is above 70 mg/dl.

4. **Once your blood glucose is back up above 70 mg/dl, you should eat your meal.**

REMEMBER

    The carbs in the meal still need insulin. When calculating the insulin dose for the meal, *never* count the carbs that you just consumed to treat the low blood sugar. Those carbs are free and were needed to recover from the low. Do *not* give insulin for the carbs used to treat hypoglycemia.

5. **Having just been hypoglycemic before your meal puts you at risk for another episode of hypoglycemia later. *You may need a reduced dose of insulin for the pending meal.***

REMEMBER

    The actual insulin dose depends on the amount of carbs in the meal, the degree of hypoglycemia you just experienced, and previous or planned exercise. Discuss this potential situation with your doctor and find out in advance what your doctor suggests you should do.

6. **Consider the composition of the meal. If the meal is fatty, fried, or cheesy, it is likely to digest more slowly than usual. Focus on eating the carbs in the meal first.**

REMEMBER

    If you've just recovered from hypoglycemia before your meal, start your meal by eating the fruit, milk, or starch — not the salad or protein. It may not be a bad idea to eat at least part of your meal before giving the mealtime insulin dose to give your food a little head start. Discuss that option with your doctor.

If you take Regular insulin, Steps 1–5 still apply. Step 6 is specific to rapid-acting insulins.

Sleeping safely after a bedtime low

If you have an episode of hypoglycemia in the evening, it is important to make sure that you take every precaution to resolve the low and stabilize blood-glucose levels before going to bed. Don't forget to recheck blood glucose after treating the low to make sure that you have fully recovered or else you may end up with another episode of hypoglycemia while sleeping. After recovering from hypoglycemia at bedtime, you may want to aim for a blood glucose level of 120–150 mg/dl before going to sleep. Consider the need for a bedtime snack that has about 15 grams of carb, and don't take insulin for that small snack. A carb snack that has protein and fat will digest more slowly while you sleep, which may help stabilize blood-glucose levels for longer. Your snack may need to be smaller or bigger and depends on many variables, such as body size, amount of physical activity, and the timing and amount of your last insulin dose. If you want a big snack at bedtime, you will likely need insulin to cover the additional carb (but not the carb used for treating the actual hypoglycemia), and the insulin dose may need to be somewhat less than usual to reduce the risk of recurrent hypoglycemia. Discuss bedtime blood-glucose targets, snacking, and insulin dosing with your doctor.

I've known many parents who haven't had a good night's sleep since their child was diagnosed with type 1 diabetes. They are up several times per night to look in on their child and perform blood-glucose checks. One benefit of a continuous glucose monitor (CGM) is that an alarm can be set to sound when blood-glucose levels drift toward low. Parents can put a baby monitor in the child's room and a receiver next to their own bed. They sleep better knowing they will hear an alarm if their child drops too low. Continuous glucose monitors are not just for kids. Anyone can benefit from the low (and high) alarms. Some insulin pumps have a "low glucose suspend" feature. If the CGM detects low blood glucose, the pump automatically shuts off the basal insulin delivery for two hours, which helps prevent hypoglycemia. There are also service dogs that are trained to detect low blood glucose. The service dog alerts the person with diabetes or the caregiver when hypoglycemia is sensed. That's pretty amazing stuff.

Considering insulin action when treating hypoglycemia

Low blood glucose indicates an imbalance between carbohydrate and insulin. Injected insulin has a set duration of action. If hypoglycemia occurs when the insulin is at its peak effect, the blood glucose can plummet further. When treating low blood glucose, think about the insulin that is at work in your system. See Figure 15-2, which illustrates the action timing of mealtime rapid-acting insulin.

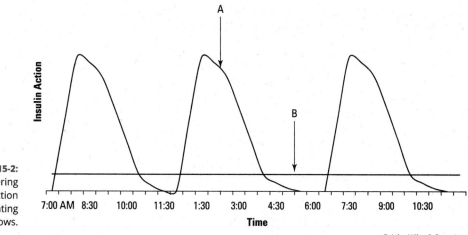

© John Wiley & Sons, Inc.

FIGURE 15-2: Considering insulin action when treating lows.

The curved lines represent the three mealtime injections of rapid-acting insulin. The horizontal line represents the long-acting insulin for someone who uses injected insulin (or may represent the pump basal rates for someone on an insulin pump). The two arrows, A and B, represent theoretical times when a person could experience hypoglycemia.

Consider a situation when hypoglycemia occurs at 2 p.m., as indicated by Arrow A. Notice that the insulin is near its peak effect. There are nearly two hours of insulin action left (when you consider that rapid-acing insulin works for about four hours). The injection given at noon will continue to lower blood-glucose levels until about 4 p.m. To adequately treat hypoglycemia at the time indicated by Arrow A, you would first require enough quick-digesting carbs to resolve the hypoglycemia, then you would need additional carbs to offset the remaining amount of insulin. As Arrow A indicates, about two hours of insulin action remain, so a snack is required to go with that insulin.

If hypoglycemia occurs at 5 p.m., as indicated by Arrow B, you would need enough quick-digesting carbs to treat the low blood sugar. There is no remaining insulin action from the 12 p.m. pre-lunch injection. At 5 p.m. the only insulin in the system is the baseline, long-acting insulin (or the pump basal rate for individuals using a pump.) You can consider whether or not you need an additional snack. If you've exercised or if your next meal is still more than a half-hour away, you may need some carbs. However, Situation A has stronger insulin action, so more carbs are needed in that situation than in Situation B.

REMEMBER

The lesson here is to always consider the insulin that is actively working in your system. There are times when more than the usual amount of carbs is needed to recover from hypoglycemia.

Preventing Hypoglycemia

So far this chapter has provided information on recognizing and treating hypo-glycemia. Better yet would be to learn how to prevent or at least minimize the frequency and severity of hypoglycemia. This section has tips on being properly prepared so that you can treat mild hypoglycemia before blood-glucose levels drop dangerously low. It also prompts you to reflect on variables that can lead to hypoglycemia and emphasizes using blood-glucose data for problem-solving. You are the most important person on your healthcare team because you can supply the information that is needed for making adjustments to your regimen.

Being prepared

The best way to stay safe is to be prepared. If you take insulin or any medications that can lead to hypoglycemia, then you should keep a few key things with you at all times:

» **Carrying your meter:** Carry your meter because it is important to verify your blood-glucose levels. Symptoms are not always a reliable indicator. After treating hypoglycemia, recheck blood-glucose levels again in 15 minutes to assure hypoglycemia has resolved (as I explain in the earlier section "Rechecking your blood-glucose level"). If you do not have your meter with you and you think your blood glucose is low, it is best to treat the suspected low.

» **Carrying snacks:** Carry carb-containing snacks you can consume as needed for preventing hypoglycemia. Keep nonperishable foods handy. Ideas include pretzels, granola bars, crackers, or any easy-to-carry snack that provides carbohydrate.

» **Carrying low supplies:** Anyone at risk for hypoglycemia must be prepared at all times by carrying appropriate carbs for treating hypoglycemia. Always have some sort of quick-digesting carbs with you. Glucose tablets, juice, or sugary candies that do not contain nuts or chocolate are appropriate choices. Fat delays digestion and slows recovery. Fruit is another good option. (See the earlier section "Choosing quick-acting carbs" for more information.) Keep something in your car's glove compartment that won't spoil or melt. Be prepared whether at work or at play.

Looking for patterns and problem-solving

Keep records and try to learn from past experiences. When you have a low, jot down a few notes related to the situation. Did you get low during exercise or have delayed hypoglycemia hours after exercise ended? Have you been having lows in the middle of the night? How much carbohydrate was needed to recover from the low? I discuss keeping records later in this chapter as well as in Chapter 23.

Share your notes and thoughts with your diabetes specialist. It's possible that the long-acting insulin dose needs to be adjusted, or it could be that the insulin-to-carb ratio or correction ratio needs to be changed. Maybe you need to count carbs with more accuracy. Hopefully you and your team can make adjustments to your routine to reduce your future risk of hypoglycemia.

Reflecting on prior exercise

Exercise increases insulin sensitivity so insulin works better when you are active. At the same time your muscles also burn more glucose when you exercise. If you don't know how to make adjustments, exercise can lead to hypoglycemia.

Keep notes related to your exercise experiences. Through trial and error you may be able to figure out how many extra carbs you need to eat before and during your exercise session, or how to reduce your insulin doses on active days. Some people with type 1 diabetes use different doses of insulin on active versus sedentary days. Enlist the help of your diabetes specialist when it comes to making insulin adjustments.

Remembering your carb intake

REMEMBER

Don't skip meals and don't eat too few carbs. Carbohydrate provides glucose, the body's preferred fuel source. You need carb for immediate use and to store as glycogen for later use — between meals and overnight. Eating too few carbs can increase your risk of hypoglycemia. Chapter 5 provides guidance on estimating your daily carbohydrate needs.

Enlisting Your Doctor's Help

If you have been experiencing episodes of hypoglycemia, speak to your doctor. Weight loss and exercise improve insulin sensitivity and are considered treatment strategies for type 2 diabetes. If you've increased your exercise or decreased your weight, you may be due for a medication tune-up. Diet, exercise, and medications sometimes need rebalancing. To resolve the situation effectively, you'll need to gather some blood-glucose data. The following sections discuss the importance of record keeping and using that data to look for trends and patterns. Blood-glucose results drive management decisions, so share your data with your doctor.

Keeping and reviewing blood-glucose logs

It's important to organize your blood-glucose data so that you can look for patterns and use the information to make diabetes management decisions. You can keep records electronically in apps, on spreadsheets, on paper, or written in logbooks. If you are computer savvy, you can create your own spreadsheet for keeping logs.

Write your blood-glucose results in columns that identify the time of the check. When you look back through your data, you can identify pre-meal and post-meal blood-glucose trends. See Table 15-1 for an example of a very basic form that would allow you to organize blood-glucose readings into columns.

TABLE 15-1   **Sample Blood-Glucose Log Form**

Date	Pre-meal	After meal	Pre-meal	After meal	Pre-meal	After meal	Bedtime

The setup in Table 15-1 doesn't mean everyone with diabetes needs to check seven times per day. Someone with type 2 diabetes who is stable and well-controlled may be checking only several times per week. Someone else with type 2 diabetes may benefit by checking one to two times per day. A person who checks twice a day can vary the test times to get a more representative picture of blood-glucose trends. For example, one day check your fasting level upon waking and again after breakfast. The next day check before and after lunch. The following day check before and after dinner, or before bed. Rotating the times of the checks and then writing the results in the proper column on the logbook is more informative than only checking fasting and before dinner day after day.

People with type 1 diabetes need to check blood glucose more frequently, perhaps up to six to ten times daily. Insulin dosing decisions are based on blood-glucose readings. Times to check blood-glucose levels include mealtimes, before driving, during exercise, before bed, any time hypoglycemia is suspected, and occasionally in the middle of the night. More detailed log forms can be created to organize data according to the specific hour that the reading was obtained and to record details on carb counts and insulin doses.

Some meters have the capability to download blood-glucose data to your computer. The meter manufacturer may offer software that can organize the data into columns by the time of day or create graphs and charts that are able to identify the percentage of your readings that are within target range, or above and below target.

Sharing your data with your doctor

Share your blood glucose records with your healthcare providers. Bring your logs and meter to every single appointment. Most meters have memories. But most doctors don't have time to scroll through the meter memory to look at the results one value at a time. The information is more useful when it's organized into logs such as the one shown in Table 15-1. Make sure that the time and date are set on your meter so the results properly reflect the time of the blood-glucose check. If you need help setting the time and date, check the owner's manual or call the 800 number on the back of the meter and ask for help.

Blood-glucose data is valuable and is used to guide management decisions. If your data shows trends or patterns above target or below target, be proactive and contact your healthcare provider for advice. It isn't uncommon to need medication dose adjustments. Try not to attach judgment to the numbers. I consider all numbers "good" numbers because all numbers provide information that is useful in managing your diabetes.

Chapter **16**

Keeping the Beat with a Healthy Heart

t's undebatable: Heart disease is the leading cause of death in the United States. Age, genetics, and gender play into the risk, but the majority of the risk factors are modifiable. You can control the following risk factors: smoking, abnormal cholesterol levels, high blood pressure, obesity, physical inactivity, uncontrolled diabetes, and stress. Four of those risk factors (including uncontrolled diabetes) are influenced by food choices.

This chapter addresses how dietary intakes affect heart-health outcomes. The good news is you can make a difference, and there are lots of great foods to enjoy while staying healthy and managing your diabetes.

Eating Smart for Your Heart

We are what we eat, as the old cliché goes. We can build heathy bodies and avoid preventable diseases with healthy lifestyle behaviors and the right foods. It takes some conviction to dodge the ever-abundant fast foods, convenience foods, junk-food snacks, sugary beverages, and processed foods. But healthy foods are there too, and with the right information, we have the power to make the right choices.

Food labels assure nutrition information is provided on packaged foods. Chain restaurants must make nutrition details available to consumers. This section provides sound guidance on selecting foods that support heart health. The diet strategies that are good for your cardiovascular system come with an added benefit: Most modifications also help with weight control (which I discuss later in this chapter).

TIP

The American Diabetes Association suggests lifestyle modifications to improve heart health. It suggests weight loss (if indicated) and increased physical activity as well as the reduction of saturated fat, trans fat, and cholesterol intake (although an upper limit of cholesterol is not specified). An additional recommendation is to increase dietary omega-3 fatty acids, soluble fiber, and plant stanols and sterols. Stanols and sterols help block the absorption of cholesterol in the intestinal tract. Plant foods naturally contain trace amounts. Some margarines are fortified with stanols and sterols and marketed for lowering cholesterol.

Getting the facts on cholesterol and fats

When cholesterol is mentioned, it's usually in relation to heart disease risk factors. Cholesterol is a waxy, fat-like substance made by the liver. Cholesterol serves a purpose in human health and has specific functions to fulfill in the body. That's right — cholesterol is actually a good thing, but *only if you don't have too much of it.* Unfortunately, some people have livers that pump out too much. Genetics plays a role in cholesterol production, but dietary choices have influence. Some foods can raise your cholesterol levels.

Every cell in the body has tiny amounts of cholesterol because cell membranes require it to function normally. Additionally, cholesterol serves as a building block to make other substances. For example, some hormones are made from cholesterol. Cholesterol is required for your skin to synthesize vitamin D and to make a digestive juice called *bile.* Bile is used to help process and absorb dietary fats. (Soluble fiber and its effects on bile are discussed later in this chapter.)

Because cholesterol is made by the liver, it follows that only animal products have cholesterol. Meats, eggs, and dairy products contain cholesterol. Some are relatively low in cholesterol, while others have concentrated amounts. Plant foods contain no cholesterol whatsoever. Fruits, vegetables, grains, nuts, legumes, and vegetable oils are all naturally cholesterol-free.

For many years, consumers were told to limit their consumption of egg yolks and organ meats due to the fact that they are high in cholesterol. Shrimp was in the same brandished boat. If you've been staying up to date on the cholesterol debate, you may be aware that eggs have been pardoned. That's right, and eggs across the country are out celebrating the news.

Every five years the Dietary Guidelines for Americans are reviewed and revised based on scientific principles. The 572-page scientific report most recently presented by the Dietary Guidelines Advisory Committee said that "based on available evidence there is no appreciable relationship between the cholesterol obtained in foods and blood cholesterol levels." Therefore "cholesterol is not a nutrient of concern for overconsumption." However, bacon and sausage are not off the hook. Dietary fats are still a concern, especially the fats in meats and dairy products; see the later section "Choosing fats wisely" for more information.

REMEMBER

Scientific opinion has shifted in terms of dietary cholesterol. The focus remains on the detrimental effects of saturated, trans, and hydrogenated fats as detailed in the next section. The cause for concern is the manner in which these specific fats are processed in the body. For one thing, they stimulate cholesterol production in your liver. The fats themselves do not contain cholesterol, but the net effect is that your internal cholesterol production ramps up in response to eating them. These fats are typically solid at room temperature and are more likely to contribute to the build-up of plaque on the interior walls of blood vessels. Envision this — what do you want flowing through your blood vessels: bacon fat or olive oil?

Acquainting yourself with types of fats

There are three main macronutrients: carbohydrates, proteins, and fats. Gram for gram, fat has more than twice the number of calories than either protein or carbohydrate. Carbs have four calories per gram, proteins have four calories per gram, and fat has nine calories per gram. Liquid oils and solid fats have the same caloric density. When it comes to your body weight, all fats are the same.

REMEMBER

Not so when it comes to heart health. Liquid oils are better for blood vessels. Unsaturated fats are healthier than saturated fats. To clarify terms, fats are referred to as *saturated* or *unsaturated.* The reference is to the chemical structure of the fat. *Saturation* relates to how hydrogen atoms are bound to the carbon atoms in the fat molecule. The degree of saturation determines whether a fat is solid, semi-solid, or liquid at room temperature. The more solid (saturated) a fat is, the more likely it is to clog arteries.

TECHNICAL
STUFF

Fats are made out of carbon atoms linked together in a chain. Each carbon atom can bind to other atoms in four places. Hydrogen atoms can bind to the carbon atoms in fats:

» **A saturated fat** holds the maximum number of hydrogen atoms. Saturated fats tend to be solid at room temperature, such as butter and lard.

» **A monounsaturated fat** has one location in the chain where two carbon atoms have formed a double bond between themselves, which leaves less room for hydrogen atoms to attach.

>> **A polyunsaturated fat** has two or more locations in the chain where double bonds have formed between carbon atoms, so even fewer hydrogen atoms can bind.

Type of Fat	Carbon Chain	Number of Double Bonds
Saturated	-C-C-C-C-C-C-C-	0
Monounsaturated	-C-C=C-C-C-C-C-	1
Polyunsaturated	-C-C=C-C-C-C=C-C-	2 or more

The term "hydrogenated" refers to the process of starting with a polyunsaturated fat (which is liquid at room temperature) and forcing the double bonds between the carbons to break apart so more hydrogen atoms can be added at those locations. *Hydrogenation* causes liquid oils to thicken or solidify. Margarine and vegetable shortening are examples of hydrogenated fats. The process of hydrogenation can cause trans fats to form. The term *trans* refers to where the hydrogen atoms bind to the carbon chain, specifically, on which side of the chain the bond forms. Don't worry; you won't be tested on the chemistry.

REMEMBER

The take-home message is easy: Trans fats are the worst. Saturated fats are a close second. The goal is to limit those two types of fat, as you find out in the next section.

Choosing fats wisely

Dietary choices influence health. When it comes to your heart, it pays to choose heart-healthy fats, as shown in the right column of Table 16-1. Minimize the fats in the left column and your heart will thank you.

TABLE 16-1 **Picking Dietary Fats to Support Heart Health**

Fats to Limit: Saturated, Hydrogenated, and Trans	Heart-Healthy Fats to Choose: Monounsaturated, Polyunsaturated, and Omega-3
Dairy fats: Butter, cheese, cream cheese, cream, sour cream, whole milk, half-and-half	**Plant oils:** Liquid at room temperature; olive, canola, safflower, sunflower, flax, grape seed, walnut, peanut, sesame, soybean, vegetable blends
Meat fats: Fatty marbled meats, bacon, ribs, sausages, salami, hot dogs, bratwurst, chicken skin	**Nuts and nut butters:** Almonds, cashews, hazelnuts, peanuts, pecans, pistachio, walnuts
Tropical fats: Coconut and palm	**Seeds:** Sesame, sunflower, pine, pumpkin, flax
Hydrogenated oils, partially hydrogenated oils, trans fats	Avocado
Lard, manteca	Fish oils (omega-3 fats)

The following sections go into more detail on researching and understanding heart-healthy fats.

REMEMBER

Do your heart a favor. Choose liquid oils rather than solid fats. Oils that are liquid at room temperature do not contribute to blocked arteries and do not raise your cholesterol.

Opting for heart-friendly fats, not cholesterol-raising culprits

Fats that are liquid at room temperature fall into the heart-healthy category. Liquid oils can't block arteries and don't raise blood-cholesterol levels. Plant-based oils, fish oils (omega-3 fats; see the nearby sidebar for more information), monounsaturated fats, and polyunsaturated fats are the heart-healthier options. Foods that are rich in the heart-healthy fats include nuts, seeds, and avocado.

WARNING

Solid fats, animal fats, trans fats, hydrogenated fats, and saturated fats should be limited. Overconsumption can increase blood-cholesterol levels and increase your risk of heart disease. Meats and dairy products contain saturated fat, so choose lean and lower-fat or nonfat versions (see Chapter 13 and Appendix A for guidance).

SPOTLIGHTING OMEGA-3 FATS

For optimal health, our bodies require omega-3 fats. These specific fats are considered essential because they must be obtained through foods and can't be manufactured within the body. Omega-3 fatty acids are especially heart healthy because they help reduce triglyceride levels, inflammation, blood clotting, and the risk of chronic illnesses including heart disease. Omega-3 fats also reduce the incidence of irregular heartbeats and help lower blood pressure somewhat.

DHA and EPA are the two notable omega-3 fats that are found in fatty fish, including salmon, mackerel, herring, halibut, and lake trout. ALA is a non-fish omega-3 option that is found in flaxseeds, walnuts, soybeans, soy oil, and canola oil. The health benefits are more pronounced when using the DHA and EPA versions found in fish. Occasionally, fish oil capsules are prescribed to treat medical issues. For more information on supplementation and appropriate dosing, talk to your healthcare provider.

Figuring fats: Reading Nutrition Facts food labels

Nutrition Facts food labels are used for carb counting as discussed in Chapter 7. Labels also make it easier to choose heart-healthy packaged items. Regulations mandate that labels identify the *total* amount of fat per serving in both grams and percent daily value. Total fat intake impacts calorie intake, which in turn affects your weight, but only certain fats are detrimental to heart health. Labels must display the details on the unhealthy types of fats. The grams of saturated and trans fats are already included in the total fat, but detailed separately. Labels aren't required to list the amounts of heart-healthy monounsaturated and polyunsaturated fats, although some do so voluntarily. Cholesterol and sodium amounts are also listed.

The American Heart Association recommends limiting intakes of saturated fat, trans fat, and sodium. When based on a 2,000-calorie diet, that equates to no more than 11–13 grams of saturated fat and up to 1,500 milligrams of sodium per day. See Figure 16-1, which identifies these sections in the shaded areas. There is no %Daily Value listed for trans fat because the goal is to avoid it entirely.

Nutrition Facts

Serving Size 2/3 cup (55 g)
Servings Per Container 8

Amount Per Serving	
Calories 230	Calories from Fat 72
	% Daily Value
Total Fat 8g	**12%**
Saturated Fat 1 g	**5%**
Trans Fat 0 g	
Cholesterol 5mg	**2%**
Sodium 160 mg	**7%**
Total Carbohydrates 37g	**12%**
Dietary Fiber 4g	**16%**
Sugars 1g	
Protein 3g	

© *John Wiley & Sons, Inc.*

FIGURE 16-1: Identifying Nutrition Facts that affect heart health.

There are several ways to interpret the information on the label. You can look at the grams (g) and milligrams (mg), or you can look at the percent daily value (%Daily Value or %DV). Just keep in mind that the percentages are based on a 2,000-calorie diet, which may not coincide with your calorie targets. A Percent Daily Value of 5 percent or less is considered low in that particular nutrient or substance, and 20 percent or more is considered high. Aim low for saturated fat, trans fat, and sodium. Aim high for fiber.

High-fat meats and dairy products are discouraged because animal fats can raise cholesterol and clog arteries. You can do a quick label check to see whether a packaged meat or dairy product is low-fat, medium-fat, or high-fat. Check the Nutrition Facts food label for the Total Fat grams. The following key holds true "per ounce" of meat or cheese, and "per serving" of other dairy products:

>> **Low fat:** 0–3 grams of fat per ounce

>> **Medium fat:** 4–7 grams of fat per ounce

>> **High fat:** 8 or more grams of fat per ounce

If you are looking for lean meats and trying to limit high-fat meats, keep this slogan in mind. It relates to the grams of total fat per ounce of meat or cheese: "3 or less is best, 8 or more stays at the store."

Adding soluble fiber to your healthy heart regimen

Fiber is found only in plant foods. That means fruits, vegetables, beans, nuts, and whole grains contain fiber; meat, eggs, cheese, and fats do not contain fiber. Dietary fiber is the nondigestible portion of the plant. For this reason, as Chapter 7 points out, the grams of dietary fiber can be subtracted from the total carbohydrate count when calculating insulin doses to cover the carbs in a meal.

There are two types of fiber: soluble and insoluble. Insoluble fiber is good for intestinal health and bowel regularity. Soluble fiber benefits your heart health by lowering your blood-cholesterol levels. It has been shown that including adequate amounts of soluble fiber, in conjunction with a diet low in saturated fat and cholesterol, may reduce your risk of heart disease. To understand how soluble fiber impacts cholesterol levels, a little background information is required first.

Foods are digested in the intestine. Digestive juices include enzymes and a substance called bile. Bile, also known as bile acids or bile salts, helps process and transport dietary fats. After the bile has completed its job, it is reabsorbed to be reused when the next meal moves through the digestive system. Bile is recycled and used over and over again. Soluble fiber absorbs water, swells, and forms a gooey gel that traps the bile and prevents it from being reabsorbed. Dietary cholesterol can also get stuck in the soluble fiber. Because fiber is not digested or absorbed, it carries the bile and some of the dietary cholesterol out with the stool. Consequently, the liver has to make new bile. The liver uses cholesterol to produce bile, which in turn lowers blood-cholesterol levels.

Oats are especially high in this beneficial type of fiber. The less-processed slow-cooking oats are higher in soluble fiber than instant processed oatmeal. Additional sources include oat bran, barley, the dried bean family (legumes), soybeans, potatoes, sweet potatoes, carrots, broccoli, apples, pears, citrus fruits, berries, bananas, almonds, and flaxseeds. Whole foods offer soluble fiber along with other nutrients. Some people boost intakes with soluble fiber supplements. Psyllium or psyllium husk is the ingredient to look for.

Creating a heart-healthy grocery list

TIP

The first step toward heart-healthy home cooking is to stock your kitchen with the right foods. Use the following tips for grocery shopping:

>> Opt for liquid vegetable oils such as olive oil, canola oil, and soy oil.

>> Buy nonhydrogenated peanut butter.

>> Try nonfat or reduced-fat sour cream and cream cheese.

>> For beef and pork, choose cuts labeled "loin" or "round," such as sirloin, tenderloin, and top round.

>> Choose "select" or "choice" cuts of meat rather than "prime." Avoid marbled meats.

>> Find margarines that are labeled "no trans fats." They are usually in tubs.

>> Choose Canadian bacon rather than strips of bacon.

>> Try tofu, soy burgers, vegetarian hot dogs, and vegetarian sausages.

>> Pick nonfat and low-fat milk and yogurts.

>> Select skinless chicken breast or remove poultry skin before eating.

>> Plan on having fish twice a week.

>> Give 2 percent reduced-fat cheeses a chance.

>> Choose unsweetened oatmeal.

>> Opt for brown rice, quinoa, millet, wild rice, barley, bulgur, farro, and any other whole grain. Limit intake of refined grains and white rice.

>> Buy breads that list "whole grain" as the first ingredient on the list.

>> Skip the breakfast pastries and muffins. Instead, enjoy a slice of raisin toast or whole-grain toast and fruit spreads with no added sugars.

>> Stock up on dried beans; if you're buying canned beans, choose a low-sodium version.

- » Select unsalted nuts and seeds. Eat in moderation due to high calories.

- » Skip the sugary soft drinks; if desired, choose diet drinks (see Chapter 11 for more on beverages).

- » Leave the fruit juices at the store and purchase fruits instead.

- » Look for low-sodium and low-fat varieties of crackers and chips.

- » Purchase cooking oil spray to use with a nonstick pan.

- » Read ingredient lists and avoid foods made with hydrogenated oils.

- » Stay away from palm oil, palm kernel oil, coconut oil, and cocoa butter.

- » Load up on fruits and vegetables of all kinds. Choose fresh, frozen, or canned varieties without added sugars, sodium, or fats.

REMEMBER

The Exchange Lists in Appendix A separate the meats and proteins into three categories according to fat content. Refer to the lean meats list when planning your protein purchases. Choose fats and oils from the heart-healthy monounsaturated and polyunsaturated sections, and limit the fats identified on the saturated fats list.

Cooking your foods the heart-healthy way

So what do you do when you get your healthy groceries home? Some cooking methods are better than others when it comes to your weight and heart. Lower-fat cooking methods include baking, broiling, roasting, braising, steaming, stewing, and boiling. You can also cook in a crockpot or microwave, or use a barbeque grill. Try a nonstick skillet sprayed with cooking oil. Sauté using controlled amounts of vegetable oil.

WARNING

The one cooking method to limit or avoid is deep-frying. Deep-fried foods absorb a lot of the cooking oil, which bumps up the calories and can lead to weight gain. If you aren't willing to give up a favorite food that's fried, then cut back on quantity and frequency of consumption. If you normally have fried chicken once a week, limit it to once a month. If you usually have a large order of fries, switch to a small order. Also keep in mind the quality of the oil used for frying. Some restaurants use hydrogenated oils in their deep fryers, which is not a heart-healthy type of oil. You have more control over the type of oil used if you fry at home. At least you can fry your fish in a liquid vegetable oil that won't clog arteries.

REMEMBER

All fats and oils are equally high in calories. If weight control is a concern, reserve fried foods for special occasions.

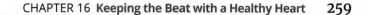

Handling the (Blood) Pressure

High blood pressure, which is also called *hypertension*, is known as the silent killer because symptoms are not always obvious. Elevated blood pressure is tough on the blood vessels. Uncontrolled diabetes can also jeopardize the integrity of the blood vessels. When hypertension damages the large blood vessels in the body, the risk of heart disease and stroke goes up significantly. Hypertension can also accelerate the risk of diabetic complications affecting the small vessels in the eyes and kidneys.

About one-third of American adults have high blood pressure. The sobering warning is that 90 percent of adults are expected to eventually develop hypertension within their lifetimes. You can improve your blood pressure and reduce your risks by controlling your weight, managing stress, exercising, avoiding tobacco, and limiting alcohol intake. I cover many of these strategies later in this chapter, but here, I focus on the well-known dietary culprit: salt.

The link between dietary salt intake and high blood pressure is well known. Salt is made from two minerals: It's 40 percent sodium and 60 percent chloride. Sodium has important roles in the body, such as regulating fluid balance and assisting in nerve and muscle function. Only minute amounts of sodium are needed, though. Small amounts of sodium occur naturally in many foods. The big problem is the amount of sodium being consumed in processed and packaged foods. The kidneys have to work at removing excess sodium from the bloodstream to dispose of it in the urine.

Excess salt intake raises blood-sodium levels, which in turn draws more fluid into the blood vessels. The extra fluid exerts more force on the blood vessels, causing them to stretch. Injured blood vessels are more likely to accumulate gunky plaque that could lead to blood-vessel blockages. When fluids accumulate due to excess dietary sodium, the heart muscle has to work harder. Excess fluid in the blood vessels isn't something you can see or necessarily feel. Some people, but not all, have additional side effects caused by fluid retention, such as puffiness, swelling, or weight gain. If you make a deliberate effort, you can reduce the sodium (salt) intake in your diet. The next sections walk you through how to do that.

Taking a look at the DASH diet

The DASH diet, which stands for Dietary Approaches to Stop Hypertension, has been shown to improve blood pressure. The diet is rich in fruits, vegetables, low-fat dairy products, fish, poultry, lean meats, beans, nuts, seeds, whole grains, and heart-healthy fats. The diet plan was developed by the National Heart, Lung, and Blood Institute, which is part of the National Institutes of Health. More

information may be found online at the following site: www.nhlbi.nih.gov/
health/health-topics/topics/dash.

The DASH diet encourages eating foods rich in potassium, a mineral that is necessary for health. Adequate potassium intake is important because it counteracts the
effects of sodium by relaxing blood-vessel walls. Most people do not reach the
recommended intake targets for potassium. Foods rich in this mineral include
potatoes, sweet potatoes, greens, spinach, kale, tomatoes, mushrooms, okra,
winter squash, legumes, avocados, cantaloupe, oranges, apricots, bananas, milk,
yogurt, fish, poultry, and beef.

WARNING

Certain medical conditions, such as kidney disease, require potassium restriction.
Damaged kidneys can cause potassium to accumulate in the bloodstream, which is
dangerous. If you have kidney disease or take medications that cause your body to
retain potassium, speak to a dietitian about planning a low-potassium diet. Some
salt substitutes are made from potassium chloride rather than sodium chloride,
and those products should be avoided by anyone restricting potassium.

Shaking the salt habit and opting for alternate seasonings

The Dietary Guidelines for Americans recommend limiting daily sodium intake to
2,300 milligrams (mg). The American Heart Association says the ideal limit is
1,500 mg per day. One single teaspoon of salt is 2,300 mg. Clearly, salting your
food racks up the sodium.

REMEMBER

Don't be fooled. Sea salt and regular table salt have the same amount of sodium.
Ditto for rock salt, kosher salt, pink salt, or any other variety. Salt is salt.

Take the salt shaker off the table. Don't add salt during cooking. There are many
ways to add flavor without compromising your health. Here are some ideas:

>> Choose any herb or spice provided it isn't a salt blend. If you aren't sure where
to start with individual seasonings, try a pre-mixed blend or a salt-free
seasoning shaker.

>> Incorporate fresh garlic or garlic powder, not garlic salt.

>> Add onions, cilantro, ginger, lemon, limes, and peppers (white, black, and red).

>> Flavored vinegars add zip.

>> Wine used in cooking adds flavor, and the alcohol cooks off.

>> Soy sauce is high in sodium, so use it sparingly. One teaspoon of soy sauce has nearly 300 milligrams of sodium. Low-sodium soy sauce has less. Brands vary, so compare the Nutrition Facts food labels.

There's no need to add salt to the cooking water for pasta, rice, or grains. In restaurants, ask for your dishes to be prepared without salt.

Identifying hidden sodium suspects

It's estimated that Americans eat well over 3,000 milligrams of sodium per day. About 12 percent is naturally occurring in foods. You may be surprised to hear that roughly 75 percent of the sodium consumed comes from eating processed foods, not from the salt shaker. Here are some common hiding places for sodium:

>> Salt is a preservative. The reason beef jerky can sit in your cupboard for weeks without spoiling is because it is so high in sodium that bacteria don't find it palatable and they move on. Processed meats are salted too. Bacon, sausage, hot dogs, bologna, salami, and many other processed lunch meats are loaded with sodium. Choose fresh lean meats, fish, and poultry instead.

>> Soups are notoriously high in sodium. Read the food labels and check the sodium counts as discussed earlier in this chapter. Look for lower-sodium versions of soups and broths. By the way, bouillon cubes are salt cubes.

>> Convenience foods such as frozen appetizers and entrees rack up the sodium quickly. Look for those that boast being heart healthy or reduced in sodium.

Keep in mind the daily total budget. If you are allotting yourself 1,500 mg of sodium per day, you can afford to spend 500 mg on one meal. If your daily target is 2,300 mg of sodium, adjust mealtime budgets accordingly. If you choose a processed entrée for one meal, make sure your other meals and snacks are low in sodium.

>> Canned goods often come in a no-salt-added version. If you have a pantry full of canned vegetables and legumes that do have salt, at least drain and rinse the product before eating.

>> Choose low-sodium versions of tomato juice and low-sodium V8. Add a dash of tabasco and lime to boost flavor.

>> Snack foods can pack a double punch with excess fat and salt. Choose lower-fat and reduced-sodium crunchy munchies.

>> Fast foods are notoriously high in sodium (and fat). Most chain restaurants post their nutrition information online. Compare menu options and choose wisely. Limit the frequency of fast-food forays.

>> Any meal that allows you to peel back the lid, add hot water, and wait a few minutes before it is ready for consumption is likely high in sodium. Read labels so you know what you are in for.

>> Rice pilaf, cups of noodles, instant ramen, and other side dishes with flavor packets are likely high in sodium. Look for versions that cut the salt. Another option for those items already in your cupboard is to use just half of the flavor packet instead of the whole packet of seasoning.

>> Curb the condiments. Use smaller portions of the higher-sodium items.

Deciphering label claims related to sodium

TIP

Label claims on food packages are regulated. When you're looking to limit sodium, you'll encounter numerous claims. Here's what they mean:

>> **Sodium free:** Less than 5 mg of sodium

>> **Very low sodium:** 35 mg or less of sodium

>> **Low sodium:** 140 mg or less of sodium

>> **Reduced or less sodium:** At least 25 percent less sodium than the regular product

>> **Light or lite sodium:** At least 50 percent less sodium than the regular product

Embracing Heart-Healthy Habits

Eating right pays off. It's also important to incorporate physical activity, manage stress, work toward weight control, and kick the habit if you're a smoker. This section focuses on other important variables affecting heart health.

REMEMBER

Small steps in the right direction add up. Prioritize what to focus on first. Making progress in one area often helps you find success in another. For example, exercise helps manage stress, and it also benefits weight-control efforts. Managing stress makes it easier to make the right food choices.

Managing stress

Chronic stress can take a toll on your physical and mental health. Finding healthy ways to manage your stress is important. Exercise is one way to release tension (as you find out later in this chapter). Exercise increases endorphin levels. *Endorphins* are natural chemicals that improve mood. Other mechanisms shown to reduce stress include meditation, yoga, recreational activities, creative expression through arts and crafts, and other techniques you can learn in stress-management classes.

Working with a mental-health specialist or a good counselor can be invaluable. If left unchecked, stress can sabotage your diabetes self-management efforts and increase your risk of heart disease.

Avoiding tobacco and secondhand smoke

Smoking is the most preventable cause of premature death in the United States. Besides causing cancer and raising blood pressure, smoking increases the risk of blood vessel disease, coronary heart disease, and stroke.

If you smoke, seek advice from your doctor on how to quit. Find a smoking cessation program. Nonsmokers should avoid secondhand smoke. Exposure to other people's smoke can increase your risk of having a stroke by 20–30 percent.

Staying active

The American Heart Association (AHA) encourages at least 150 minutes of physical activity per week. The suggestion is to get 30 minutes per day, five days per week. Moderate activity is fine. If you exercise more vigorously, you can aim for 75 minutes per week — for example, 25-minute sessions three days per week.

There are many options for adding physical activity, such as joining a gym, taking an exercise class, getting exercise equipment for the home, swimming, cycling, using an exercise DVD to guide your workout, or simply walking more. Walking is an excellent way to improve fitness. It's free and can be done outdoors when the weather permits or indoors if space permits. Halls, corridors, and malls offer sufficient space in a protected atmosphere.

Break up periods of sedentary time by getting up to stretch and move around every 30 minutes.

Chapter 14 provides more details on exercise.

Controlling weight

Obesity is contributing to the health crisis we face as a nation. Close to 80 million Americans are classified as *obese*, which is defined by a body mass index (BMI) of 30 or higher. (Use the chart in Chapter 5 to assess your BMI.)

Losing weight lowers your risk of heart attack and stroke. Weight loss does more than reduce cardiovascular risks; it's also a foundation strategy for treating type 2 diabetes. Weight loss improves insulin sensitivity and blood–glucose control for people with prediabetes and type 2 diabetes. Studies show that combining weight loss with exercise is an effective intervention that decreases the chance of prediabetes progressing to type 2 diabetes. Losing weight if you're overweight can also reduce blood pressure, improve sleep apnea, and lower triglyceride levels.

You don't have to achieve a normal body weight to reap health benefits. Any amount of weight loss helps. A reasonable goal is to lose about 5–10 percent of your starting weight at a rate of one pound per week. To achieve weight loss, you need to eat fewer calories than you burn. Here are some guidelines to help you do just that:

REMEMBER

>> **Reduce calories.** The heart-healthy shopping tips earlier in this chapter also help cut calories and make weight loss easier to achieve.

>> **Control portions.** At mealtimes keep your protein portion about the size of your own palm and your starch serving the size of your own clenched fist. Increase your intake of nonstarchy vegetables and salads. Cut excess calories from alcohol, junk foods, and desserts. Use smaller bowls and plates to cut portion sizes. Cook using lower-fat methods. See Chapter 8 for more details.

>> **Be active.** Make exercise (discussed in the preceding section) a priority. Find something you enjoy doing or you probably won't stick with it. Aim for 30 minutes of physical activity per day at a moderate rate of exertion. Do it all at once or split the sessions into 10- to 15-minute blocks of activity. Start with whatever works for you, and you will gradually gain stamina. In time, you will be able to increase the duration or intensity of your activity. See Chapter 14 for more on exercise.

>> **Change unhealthy behaviors.** If you reach for food, cigarettes, or alcohol as methods for coping with stress, you're headed down a slippery slope. Identify what triggers your stress and come up with a plan for handling the situation without sabotaging your health. Consider discussing issues with a counselor or therapist who can help you come up with behavior modification strategies that work for you.

Chapter **17**

Living with Diabetes throughout the Life Cycle

U nited States data compiled in 2015 estimates that more than 23,000 American children are diagnosed with diabetes annually — over 18,000 with type 1 diabetes and over 5,000 with type 2 diabetes. All told, 30 million Americans (adults and youth) live with diabetes, and the number is rising.

Diabetes management is important throughout all stages in life. This chapter begins with a look at the challenges encountered when parenting a child with diabetes. Following the pediatric particulars, you find a section on managing diabetes during pregnancy. The population is aging; this chapter concludes with a look at the special diet and fitness needs of seniors.

Raising a Child with Diabetes

A new diagnosis of type 1 diabetes can be overwhelming, especially when it's your child. Everyone in the family feels the impact. The onset of type 1 diabetes is often sudden, dramatic, and frightening, and it usually takes everyone by utter surprise.

Grief, anger, fear, and guilt are common emotions. It isn't your fault your child developed type 1 diabetes. (Read that line again.) While life won't be exactly the same as it was before, you can learn to manage diabetes, and your child will be okay. It's important to *believe that* and to make sure *your child knows that.*

Type 2 diabetes can run in families, so children who are at risk for developing diabetes should be screened. The key strategies for preventing and treating type 2 diabetes are weight control, exercise, and healthy eating habits. Everyone in the family stands to benefit from following the same healthy habits.

The following sections provide guidance on helping your child with diabetes from diagnosis through adolescence and beyond.

REMEMBER

Establish care with a team of healthcare providers who specialize in managing pediatric diabetes (see Chapters 1 and 2 for details on building a diabetes team). Intensive diabetes self-management education is crucial. Education is empowering and provides families with the necessary tools to take on the daily management of diabetes. Diabetes education also should be ongoing and continue throughout adolescence into adulthood. Tools and tips change and evolve to meet the needs of the child through the various stages of physical and emotional development. Knowledge brings hope, strength, and resolve. Now more than ever, people with diabetes have the tools needed to safely manage their condition. Diabetes shouldn't prevent children from reaching their dreams. While the road isn't always easy, it can lead children with diabetes wherever they're determined to go.

REMEMBER

All children with type 1 diabetes must take insulin, but some children with type 2 diabetes take insulin to treat their condition. Many of the diabetes pills used to treat type 2 diabetes in adults aren't approved for use in children. Your child's healthcare provider can answer your questions about your child's medical management.

Beginning with basic pointers

Parenting a child with any chronic disease requires training and education to properly manage the condition. As children with diabetes grow and mature, they can take on age-appropriate tasks and responsibilities. Caregivers should stay closely involved through all stages of the child's development. Even high-achieving, independent teens still need support and supervision from the adults in their lives. Most of the following tips apply to managing children with either type 1 or type 2 diabetes.

REMEMBER

Children model the behaviors of the adults in their lives. Parents who eat well, exercise, and engage in healthy behaviors lead their children by example.

Viewing glucose results as data

Adults involved in diabetes management must approach blood-glucose results nonjudgmentally. Glucose numbers can't possibly be in target ranges all the time. There will be blood-glucose excursions. If your response to the glucose result shows disappointment, your child is likely to feel sad or guilty.

WARNING

Children are adept at reading their caregivers' emotions. It's critical that parents keep their own emotions in check. Children sense fear and anxiety, and they react in kind. It isn't uncommon for kids to tell their parents that a blood-glucose reading was lower than it actually was. They may make up numbers after they've noticed that their parents appear happier when glucose readings are in the "normal" range. Feeling judged discourages checking. Blood-glucose numbers are simply data that should be used for problem-solving and decision-making.

Meeting your child's nutritional needs

Children with diabetes have the same nutritional needs as their nondiabetic peers. Kids must have adequate intakes of carbohydrate to support growth and physical activity. Over-restricting carbohydrate foods can skew balanced nutrition. Carb-containing food groups such as whole grains, legumes, vegetables, fruits, milk, and yogurt all contain important vitamins, minerals, and nutrients (see Chapter 13 for more information). Cutting carbs potentially cuts nutrition. Low-carb diets also increase the risk of hypoglycemia for children treated with insulin or the diabetes pills that stimulate insulin production. (Chapter 15 has details on handling hypoglycemia.)

REMEMBER

Adults are responsible for providing healthy foods and assuring that insulin doses match carbohydrate intakes. A registered dietitian can help you understand how to meet the changing nutritional needs of your child and how to assure adequate carbohydrate intake. Your child's endocrinologist, pediatrician, or other qualified medical specialist can provide guidelines on insulin dosing and blood-glucose targets.

Fitting in favorite foods

Reasonable treats can be included in the meal plans of children with diabetes. Desserts tend to be concentrated in carbohydrates, fat, and calories, so portion control is important. Insulin doses can be adjusted to account for the sweet treat. Studies have shown that sugar-containing foods can be safely consumed in the context of a healthy meal plan as long as the carbohydrates are accounted for.

Children with diabetes shouldn't be singled out as the only ones who aren't allowed to partake in the treat at a party or celebration. Children aren't under your watchful eye at all times, and those who are over-restricted tend to find and consume treats on their own. If they feel like they have to "sneak" the treat, they won't get the insulin coverage they need to compensate for it. (Flip to Chapter 13 for more about safely including desserts in your diet.)

Supervising, sharing tasks, and staying involved

As children get older and gain more independence, they still need supervision on diabetes care. All involved adults need adequate training in diabetes management. That includes, to varying degrees, parents, grandparents, relatives, coaches, baby-sitters, and teachers.

Children shouldn't be overly burdened with tasks related to managing a complex condition. Caregivers and children should communicate and work together so the kids learn the concepts and skills needed to eventually launch safely into adulthood. Families can review blood-glucose results together, measure foods, count carbs, calculate insulin doses, and problem-solve high and low glucose readings.

Besides diabetes, kids have a lot of other things going on: peer relationships, school, and outside activities such as clubs and sports. If they are saddled with too much responsibility, children can get overwhelmed and discouraged. Sometimes it may seem like they are pushing you away, but deep down they very much want and need your support.

Plan to meet with school personnel prior to each new school year. Set up a conference with the teacher, principal, and school nurse. Find out about the lunch program and whether carbohydrate information is available. Children with diabetes need a 504 plan and a Diabetes Medical Management Plan to delineate responsibilities and assure safety at school; for more information, visit the homepage of the American Diabetes Association (www.diabetes.org) and use the search box to look for "504 plan" and "diabetes medical management plan." The child's healthcare provider assists in filling out the forms. Children with diabetes can't be discriminated against, and the school must make appropriate accommodations.

Maneuvering through adolescence safely

The teenage years can be tricky with or without diabetes. It's natural for teens to gravitate toward peers and spend less time with the family. It's also a time when kids try to blend in and don't want to be different. They shouldn't have to share the diabetes diagnosis with close friends and schoolmates until they're ready to do so. Yet, at the same time, teens must manage to check blood-glucose levels and take insulin while they're at school. Kids can't take a vacation from diabetes, but some end up trying. If children with type 1 diabetes stop taking their insulin, they could land in the hospital with potentially life-threatening diabetic ketoacidosis (which I describe in Chapter 4).

At diagnosis, caregivers are completely in charge of diabetes management, but over time, skills shift to the young adult with diabetes. By the time kids head off to college, they must have a solid command of how to self-manage their diabetes. Letting go can be nerve-racking for parents. It's like watching your teen learn to drive a car. You know learning to drive is important, but handing over the keys is somewhat frightening.

WARNING

Most adolescents encounter peer pressure. Teens with diabetes face significant consequences if they drink alcohol or experiment with drugs. (See Chapter 11 for an explanation of the risk of severe hypoglycemia due to insulin and alcohol.) Involve your diabetes team in the discussion of teen safety, including measures to assure safe driving. Keep the lines of communication open.

Finding support

REMEMBER

Emotional well-being can't be overlooked. Counseling — for the individual or the family — can help. Diabetes burnout, anxiety, fear, and depression can become roadblocks to wellness unless properly addressed. Ask your doctor to refer you to an appropriate mental-health specialist. Look for diabetes support groups in your community too. Summer camps for kids with diabetes are immensely empowering. One-day, weekend, or weeklong camps immerse children with diabetes in a safe environment where they can enjoy summer camp fun while surrounded by people who have diabetes just like them. Ask your healthcare providers for information about diabetes camps in your area. You can also search online for diabetes camps in your state. The American Diabetes Association lists some options. See www.diabetes.org/in-my-community/diabetes-camp/camps/.

Addressing type 2 diabetes in youth

Type 2 diabetes was once considered "adult-onset" diabetes. Unfortunately, the nomenclature is no longer accurate. More and more adolescents are developing prediabetes and type 2 diabetes. Risk factors include having a family history of type 2 diabetes, being overweight, and lack of physical activity. Interventions hinge on healthy eating and exercising regularly. Diabetes can go unnoticed for years, which is why screening at-risk youth is so important. Prompt treatment reduces the chance of developing serious health problems.

Knowing the risk factors

The obesity crisis in the United States is a major contributing factor to the increasing incidence of type 2 diabetes in youth. The diagnosis is rare among children in the normal weight range who exercise regularly. Type 2 diabetes often presents with other *comorbidities* (diseases or conditions that occur simultaneously). *Metabolic syndrome*, for example, includes insulin resistance, obesity, hypertension, lipid abnormalities, and sometimes polycystic ovarian syndrome.

REMEMBER

Overweight children who have at least two additional risk factors should be screened for diabetes every three years. The definition of overweight in children is a body mass index (BMI) over the 85th percentile for age and gender. Ask your child's healthcare provider to assess your child's weight status and risk factors. Screening for diabetes requires a blood test and should begin at age 10 or at the first signs of puberty if the onset of puberty is before age 10. Risk factors for developing type 2 diabetes include the following:

>> Having a family history of type 2 diabetes

>> Belonging to a high-risk ethnic group: African American, Asian American, Latino, Native American, or Pacific Islander

>> Having high blood pressure

>> Having abnormal lipids (cholesterol and triglycerides)

>> Having polycystic ovarian syndrome

>> Having *acanthosis nigricans* (a darker shade of skin on the back of the neck)

>> Having been a low-birth-weight baby

>> Having a mother who had diabetes during pregnancy

Eating right and exercising as a family

Children with type 2 diabetes need the opportunity to eat right and exercise, and they shouldn't be the only ones in the family doing so. Ensuring success requires a whole-family approach to engaging in healthy habits. Children with type 2 diabetes often have a parent with type 2 diabetes. It's hard to convince an adolescent to take care of his diabetes if he has a parent who drinks sugary beverages and won't check her own blood-glucose levels. Everyone in the family benefits from healthy food choices, weight control, and exercise.

REMEMBER

The recommendation is that all children should accumulate at least an hour of exercise each day. Exercise improves insulin sensitivity and helps with weight management, making it especially important for children with type 2 diabetes. Kids with type 2 diabetes are also at risk for developing cardiovascular disease, which underscores the importance of lifestyle interventions as well as the avoidance of smoking.

TIP

The American Diabetes Association has a free 32-page booklet dedicated to explaining the diagnosis of type 2 diabetes in youth. Intervention strategies, diet tips, and exercise targets are outlined in plain terms. Go to www.diabetes.org and type "Be Healthy Today; Be Healthy for Life" in the search box.

Managing Diabetes in Pregnancy

With proper planning, women with diabetes can have safe pregnancies and healthy babies. Blood-glucose control is critical *before* and *throughout* pregnancy. The first step for any woman who has type 1 or type 2 diabetes is preconception counseling and a full medical assessment.

Pregnancy hormones can interfere with insulin action so some women develop diabetes during pregnancy, which is called *gestational diabetes,* and it typically resolves after delivery. Dietary management is a critical part of prenatal care for all women who have diabetes during their pregnancies.

Planning for pregnancy when you have type 1 or type 2 diabetes

The American Diabetes Association (ADA) states in its 2017 *Standards of Medical Care in Diabetes* that to reduce the risks of birth defects, women with type 1 or type 2 diabetes should achieve blood-glucose control as close to normal as is safely possible — ideally an A1C below 6.5 percent — before becoming pregnant. Pre-pregnancy planning should include health screenings. Once pregnant, women should be followed by a team of healthcare providers who specialize in diabetes and pregnancy. The key to minimizing risks is pregnancy planning.

REMEMBER

Maternal glucose control is critical because elevated glucose levels increase the risk of serious birth defects that can affect the baby's brain, spine, and heart. Many women don't realize they are pregnant until eight weeks or later, and by then the baby is fully formed. That's why it's crucial for women with pre-existing diabetes to tighten blood-glucose targets prior to conceiving. Meet with your healthcare team for a diabetes tune-up. Brush up on carb counting, eat a healthy diet, and work on weight control. Check your blood-glucose levels more frequently, or consider transitioning to a continuous glucose monitor if you have type 1 diabetes. See Chapter 23 for more on glucose monitoring.

A physical exam should include blood tests, eye and kidney screenings, and assessing for complications or potential medical issues. Some complications, such as retinopathy, may worsen during pregnancy. Dietary adequacy and the need for vitamin and mineral supplementation should be assessed by a registered dietitian. Taking a daily supplement of 400 micrograms (mg) of folic acid prior to conception reduces the risk of some birth defects. Medication lists should be reviewed for safety, as many medications used to treat blood pressure, cholesterol, and type 2 diabetes are not safe to use in pregnancy and need to be discontinued. Women who use diabetes pills may need to transition to insulin injections because most diabetes meds can pass through the placenta and reach the fetus. Injected insulin is a safe and effective choice while trying to conceive and during pregnancy.

Developing gestational diabetes

Pregnancy hormones interfere with insulin action, so blood-glucose levels can rise during pregnancy. Women are standardly screened for gestational diabetes mellitus (GDM) between 24 and 28 weeks of pregnancy. Anyone with risk factors for type 2 diabetes (which I list earlier in this chapter) should be screened for diabetes prior to conception due to the risk of undetected, uncontrolled diabetes in the first trimester.

Once a woman is diagnosed with GDM, the first step in treatment is to implement the diet strategies outlined later in this chapter. Blood-glucose monitoring four times daily is standard for GDM (women with type 1 diabetes should check more frequently). Check fasting blood glucose and one hour after each main meal. Keep records. If strict dietary adherence doesn't control blood-glucose levels adequately, the next step is medication, usually insulin. Women with GDM should be screened for type 2 diabetes 4 to 12 weeks after delivery to assure glucose levels are back to normal.

REMEMBER

Insulin is the preferred medication for treating hyperglycemia in GDM because it doesn't cross the placenta to the baby. While glyburide and metformin have been used in pregnancy, both agents cross the placenta, and long-term safety data isn't available.

Women who have had GDM have an increased risk of developing type 2 diabetes in the future. GDM isn't the reason for the risk; the risk is already there, or GDM likely wouldn't have occurred in the first place. Family history of diabetes, obesity, and sedentary lifestyles are strong predictors. You can minimize your risk through lifelong weight control, exercise (see Chapter 14), and healthy eating habits (see Chapter 13). It is important to be screened for diabetes regularly — every 1–3 years — and certainly before becoming pregnant again.

When maternal glucose levels are high during pregnancy, extra glucose is passed on to the baby. The baby converts the excess calories to fat; birth weight goes up and so do the risks. Uncontrolled maternal glucose levels can lead to fetal weights above 9 pounds. Big babies are harder to deliver and increase the risk of complications during delivery (to both baby and mom). Exposure to excess glucose during gestation also increases the child's chances of developing type 2 diabetes or obesity in adolescence or adulthood. Be sure to let your child's pediatrician know that you had diabetes during your pregnancy.

Understanding blood-glucose targets and fluctuations in pregnancy

Maternal hyperglycemia (a high blood-glucose level) has different risks in the early versus later part of pregnancy, as outlined in the following sections.

Addressing blood-glucose targets during pregnancy

Blood-glucose levels during pregnancy should be as close to normal as possible without causing hypoglycemia. The American Diabetes Association recommends fasting glucose levels during pregnancy be kept below 95 milligrams per deciliter (mg/dl) and below 140 mg/dl one hour after eating. Blood-glucose targets may be adjusted according to individual circumstances and should be discussed with your healthcare team.

Women with type 1 diabetes often have reduced insulin needs in the first trimester. Week by week, pregnancy hormone levels rise and eventually interfere with the way insulin works. By the second trimester, blood-glucose levels begin to rise and insulin doses need to be adjusted. It isn't uncommon for insulin requirements to double or triple by the end of the third trimester. More insulin is needed to counter the effects of the pregnancy hormones.

Minimizing risks during the first trimester

When maternal blood-glucose levels are elevated during pregnancy, the extra glucose readily passes through the placenta to the fetus. Elevated blood-glucose levels in the first trimester increase the risk of birth defects and miscarriage. First-trimester diabetes-related risks are unique to women with preexisting type 1 and type 2 diabetes. Gestational diabetes doesn't develop until the second trimester, and by then the baby is already fully formed.

First-trimester blood-glucose control reduces the risk of miscarriage and birth defects. Blood-glucose control must be established prior to becoming pregnant because fetal development occurs before most women even know they are pregnant.

Controlling risks during the second and third trimesters

Later in pregnancy, excess glucose increases birth weights, possibly to greater than 9 pounds. Bigger babies can be more difficult to deliver, which may lead to birth trauma to both mom and baby. Elevated maternal glucose levels in the second and third trimesters also increase the following risks to the fetus: neonatal hypoglycemia, jaundice, and respiratory distress syndrome. Uncontrolled diabetes in pregnancy also increases the risk of stillbirth.

Maternal risks associated with poor glycemic control include *preeclampsia* (swelling and edema, protein in the urine, and high blood pressure). Preeclampsia is dangerous for mom and baby and may require an emergency caesarian delivery. Consequently, the baby may be born prematurely, which imposes other risks on the baby.

Controlling blood-glucose levels is important throughout the entire pregnancy. Blood-glucose control in the second and third trimesters reduces the risks discussed in this section.

Taking care after delivery

As I explain earlier in this chapter, if maternal glucose levels are elevated, too much glucose goes to the fetus. The baby's pancreas has to produce extra insulin to deal with the excess glucose. After delivery, when the umbilical cord is cut, the maternal glucose supply abruptly stops. The baby's pancreas may continue pumping out extra insulin. The newborn's blood-glucose level can then drop too low.

Women with type 1 diabetes usually find that insulin requirements drop back to pre-pregnancy levels shortly after delivery. Breastfeeding is recommended; however, blood-glucose levels can drop during lactation as glucose is pulled out of the bloodstream to produce milk. Lactating mothers who use insulin may need a carb-containing snack while nursing and should always keep quick carbs handy in case blood-glucose levels drop.

Women with type 2 diabetes who were switched to insulin during pregnancy typically return to the same medications that they used prior to becoming pregnant. Women who developed gestational diabetes usually find that their glucose levels return to normal shortly after giving birth.

Employing eating tips for diabetes during pregnancy

Pregnancy is a time when nutritional needs increase. A woman requires additional calories and carbohydrates to support pregnancy. Blood-glucose levels are easier to control if carbs are distributed throughout the day into smaller, more frequent feedings. Carb budgeting and other dietary tips for improving tolerance are addressed ahead.

Controlling carbohydrates: Not too much, but not too little

It's important to meet the demands of pregnancy by adhering to the established guidelines set by the National Institutes of Health. Carbohydrate intake targets are 175 grams per day while pregnant and 200 grams per day while lactating. Carb-containing foods such as legumes, grains, fruits, milk, and yogurt supply important vitamins and minerals needed by mom and baby. Carbohydrate foods also supply glucose, which is vitally important. The baby relies on glucose to fuel growth and development. Glucose is needed for maternal vital organs and tissues, and to fuel mom's physical activity. If insufficient amounts of carbohydrate are consumed, the mother's liver is forced to convert protein into glucose and fat into ketones. (See Chapter 4 for details.)

Meals that are too high in carbohydrate are likely to raise blood-glucose levels above pregnancy targets. Yet adequate carbohydrate intake is important. During pregnancy, distributing carbs among three meals and three snacks helps stabilize blood-glucose levels. Wait at least two hours between carb-containing meals and snacks. Noncarbohydrate foods can be consumed as desired, provided that weight gain is appropriate.

Morning hormonal surges often lead to glucose intolerance at breakfast, so some women need to limit breakfast to about 30 grams of carb. Don't skip breakfast. Have at least 15 grams of carb at the morning meal. Breakfast may include up to 45 grams of carb if tolerated. Eat 45–60 grams of carbohydrate at lunch and at dinner. Snacks should have 15–30 grams of carb each. Choose a mid-morning snack, a mid-afternoon snack, and a bedtime snack. (Check out Part 5 for meal and snack ideas.)

TIP

The baby requires glucose around the clock. Mom's liver stores glucose during the day and releases it overnight. Bedtime snacks help assure an adequate amount of glucose is available to the baby while you sleep. Try to limit the overnight fasting period to less than ten hours.

Implementing other tips to achieve the best outcome

Insulin resistance imposed by pregnancy hormones can be challenging. Foods that digest quickly tend to cause a sharper post-meal blood-glucose spike. To reduce your glucose levels, try these tips:

>> Limit to one serving of fruit at a time (see Appendix A for servings equal to 15 grams of carb).

>> Limit to one serving of milk or yogurt at a time (see Appendix A for servings equal to 15 grams of carb).

>> Choose whole grains, legumes, and fiber-rich foods. Limit refined grains. (See Chapter 13 for tips on choosing wholesome foods.)

>> Avoid juice, smoothies, and liquid forms of carb (except milk).

>> Pair carbohydrates at meals with protein foods and modest amounts of fat to slow digestion and blunt blood-glucose response. (Find menu ideas in Part 5.)

>> Avoid eating fruit, milk, yogurt, and refined cereals for breakfast if your blood-glucose levels are difficult to control at that time.

>> Strictly limit sweets, desserts, added sugars, honey, and syrups.

Keep in mind that even if you are following the dietary advice, diligently counting carbs, and implementing the diet tips provided, there is still a chance that your blood-glucose levels will exceed targets. The solution is not to eat less or over-restrict healthy foods. You must eat well. Blood-glucose levels tend to rise week by week throughout pregnancy due to increasing hormone levels. Women with gestational diabetes sometimes need to take insulin during pregnancy to achieve control. Women with type 1 and type 2 diabetes likewise can expect glucose levels to rise as pregnancy progresses and should expect their insulin doses to be adjusted frequently.

TIP

Physical activities such as walking, swimming, and prenatal yoga are encouraged during pregnancy unless your doctor says otherwise. Besides improving fitness, walking and other forms of gentle exercise can blunt post-meal blood-glucose levels.

Keeping the Golden Years Golden When You Have Diabetes

Diabetes management during the senior years is as important as any other time in the life cycle. People with diabetes should be able to enjoy healthy, long lives. One out of every four Americans aged 60 and above has type 2 diabetes. It isn't uncommon to be dealing with more than one medical condition. Many seniors take multiple medications to treat diabetes, hypertension, cholesterol, or other medical issues. The heart-healthy diet tips in Chapter 16 can help you manage your blood lipids, weight, and blood pressure; all tips are consistent with dietary management principles for diabetes.

There's a common thread to the management of most conditions affecting seniors: the importance of a balanced diet and incorporating regular physical fitness. Seniors may need fewer calories than they once did, but they don't need less nutrition. (Assess your calorie and carbohydrate targets in Chapter 5.) This section touches on nutrition and fitness for seniors.

Evaluating seniors' dietary concerns

Metabolism slows with age, so caloric requirements drop for most seniors. Vitamin and mineral needs don't necessarily go down and in some cases actually go up. For example, seniors need extra vitamin D and calcium. Fortified nonfat or low-fat milk and yogurt are excellent options. Lactose-free versions are available if dairy products cause gas or upset stomach. Another vitamin that seniors may need to increase is vitamin B12.

For blood-glucose control and adequate nutrition, eat three balanced meals per day, include small snacks if needed, and remember to take diabetes medications as prescribed. If you take insulin or pills that may cause hypoglycemia, be prepared by keeping quick-digesting carbs with you at all times (as well as near your bedside).

REMEMBER

Discuss blood-glucose targets with your healthcare provider. It's important to avoid hypoglycemia, especially if you live alone. Low blood glucose may cause dizziness or result in a fall. For more information on hypoglycemia management, see Chapter 15.

Plan balanced meals using simple portioning tools as shown in Chapter 8. Serve up lunch and dinner with the plate model and hand method in mind. For example:

>> Fill half the dinner plate with nonstarchy vegetables.

>> Use one-fourth of the plate for lean protein (the size or your own palm).

>> Devote one-fourth of the plate to starch (about the size of your own clenched fist for cooked rice, pasta, or potatoes).

>> Add a cup of milk and a small serving of fruit as desired.

Follow heart-healthy diet principles to cut artery-clogging fats and excess calories. Choose lean proteins and reduced-fat dairy products. Choose heart-healthy fats, wholesome whole grains, fruits, and vegetables. Cut sodium; use herbs, spices, and salt-free seasonings. Need some menu ideas? See Part 5.

REMEMBER

A registered dietitian can review your diet and determine whether you should be taking any vitamin or mineral supplements. Your healthcare provider can check vitamin levels in your blood. A multiple vitamin geared toward seniors may be added insurance that your needs are met, but supplements don't replace the importance of a balanced diet. Over-supplementation can be dangerous, and certain substances interfere with prescription drugs. Be sure to let your healthcare providers know about any over-the-counter supplements that you take.

TIP

Some seniors don't feel inspired or may be otherwise unable to prepare daily balanced menus. Isolation, loneliness, depression, financial constraints, dental issues, and mobility problems can be barriers to eating well. Here are some tips to try:

>> Stock your cupboards with canned vegetables without added salt and canned fruits without added sugars; they're easy to chew and convenient.

>> Keep frozen meals advertised as heart-healthy or low in fat handy for times when cooking isn't possible.

>> Consider using grocery and meal delivery services to fill in the gaps.

>> Enlist the support of family and friends or hire help to do some of the shopping and cooking.

>> Prepare enough food for several meals and freeze leftovers to reheat in the future.

WARNING

The sense of thirst diminishes with age. Dehydration is all too common and completely preventable. High blood glucose leads to increased urination, which compounds the risk of dehydration. Keep water and other carbohydrate-free beverages handy and drink fluids throughout the day. Some medical conditions require fluid restriction, so discuss your daily fluid targets with your doctor.

Keeping physically fit

Engaging in regular exercise helps assure independence and reduces the risk of falls. Exercise strengthens muscles and bones, and improves balance and flexibility. Exercise also helps with weight control, blood-glucose management, and blood-pressure control, and reduces the risk of heart disease. Review exercise goals, tips, and safety by reading Chapter 14. Discuss exercise with your healthcare provider. There may be exercise restrictions depending on your health history or the presence of diabetes complications.

Unless restricted, seniors should accumulate a daily total of 30 minutes of aerobic activity at least five days per week and engage in strength training exercises at least twice weekly. Incorporate stretching to maintain flexibility. The activities you choose should reflect your individual ability. Here are some ideas:

>> **Take a walk.** Walking is an excellent form of exercise for many. Some seniors choose to walk inside the local mall before the stores open.

>> **Join a class.** Some community senior centers offer scheduled exercise classes. In particular, water activities offer relief when aches, pains, or excess body weight limits other forms of activity. Local pools usually set aside some time for adult swimming. Water aerobics classes are fun and effective.

>> **Work out at home.** You can use exercise DVDs, online videos, and television programs in your home. Public television (PBS) airs an exercise program geared to seniors called *Sit and Be Fit*. For other options, use your browser to search for exercise videos.

TIP

Some health insurance plans will pay for gym memberships for seniors because they know how much exercise can improve health outcomes! Check to see whether yours is one of them.

Chapter **18**

Going Gluten-Free (Or Not): Does the Batter Matter?

People with type 1 diabetes have an increased risk of developing celiac disease because both conditions are autoimmune disorders. *Celiac disease* is a disorder in which eating gluten-containing grains results in damage to the intestine. Having diabetes isn't a reason for going on a gluten-free diet, so if gluten isn't a concern for you, feel free to skip this chapter.

Gluten is a protein found in wheat, barley, and rye. A gluten-free diet eliminates those three grains and all ingredients derived from those grains. Going gluten-free is the only treatment for celiac disease. In the case of celiac disease, exposure to even minute amounts of gluten can lead to a long list of serious medical problems and nutrient deficiencies.

Food allergies also impose the need for dietary diligence and avoidance of the offending food. Wheat allergies affect children more so than adults, but anyone with a medically diagnosed wheat allergy should avoid eating gluten. Food intolerances are less medically severe; however, if certain foods produce unpleasant side effects, it pays to steer clear of those foods.

Gluten-free diets have gained popularity in recent years. People go gluten-free for various reasons. In fact, many of the gluten-free foods flying off the supermarket shelves are being consumed by choice, not medical necessity.

Avoiding gluten can be a challenge because wheat is the most predominant grain in the United States. Quitting gluten eliminates many foods, so diets need to be carefully constructed to assure adequate nutrition. Whether going on a gluten-free diet has been medically prescribed for your or is simply your personal preference, this chapter provides information on which foods to choose and which to avoid.

Weighing In on the Gluten-Free Debate: Fad or Fact?

Gluten-free diets have become very trendy in recent years. Increased demand has resulted in an explosion of new gluten-free products. It's easier than ever to walk into a supermarket and find gluten-free breads, snacks, crackers, pizza crusts, frozen waffles, and even name-brand baking mixes. Stores are stocking a wider array of wholesome grains that are naturally gluten-free. Unfortunately, an abundance of gluten-free snack foods and baked goods are refined, low in nutrients, and high in calories, and they're no healthier than their gluten-containing junk-food counterparts.

With the right information and a lot of attention, a properly designed gluten-free diet can be healthy, well-balanced, and nutritionally complete, and it can be consistent with diet recommendations for managing diabetes. The following sections take a closer look at the reasons people go gluten-free.

Avoiding gluten fastidiously when you have celiac disease

Celiac disease is a genetic autoimmune disorder affecting 1 out of 100 people. If someone in your immediate family has celiac disease, your risk jumps to 1 in 10. People with one autoimmune disease are more likely to develop other autoimmune diseases. Type 1 diabetes is an autoimmune disorder, and up to 10 percent of those with type 1 diabetes also develop celiac disease. If you have type 1 diabetes, ask your doctor about being screened for celiac disease. Screening involves a blood test that detects antibody markers associated with celiac — specifically, anti-tissue transglutaminase or tTG. A positive tTG lab result is followed by a tissue biopsy for definitive diagnosis.

If you suspect you may have celiac disease, it is critical to be screened *before* going on a gluten-free diet. Once you've been eating gluten-free for a while, the screening tests are less likely to detect the disease.

When people with celiac disease eat gluten, their immune systems produce an antibody. The antibody triggers immune cells within the intestine to release chemicals, which in turn damage and flatten the linings of the intestine. Normally, the small intestine is lined with tiny fingerlike projections called *villi*. This lining is also called "the brush border" because it resembles a brush. Vitamins, minerals, and nutrients are absorbed into the bloodstream through the tips and sides of the intestinal villi. In people with celiac disease, gluten exposure flattens out the villi, which reduces the ability to absorb key nutrients.

Many of the long-term consequences of undiagnosed or untreated celiac disease are the result of ongoing malnutrition. For example:

>> Poor absorption of iron, folate, and B12 leads to anemia.

>> Impaired absorption of calcium and vitamin D can cause osteoporosis.

>> Vitamin and mineral deficiencies contribute to nerve problems, improper blood clotting, bone and joint pain, dental issues, headaches, depression, impaired concentration, dementia, fatigue, infertility, and an increased risk of intestinal cancer.

Symptoms of malabsorption may include gas, bloating, diarrhea or constipation, oily stools, nausea, and vomiting. Some people with celiac develop an itchy skin rash. Celiac disease can cause poor growth and delayed puberty in children. It may lead to weight loss in adults; however, many people with celiac disease are at normal weights or may be overweight. Gastrointestinal symptoms drive some individuals to seek medical attention, which leads to the diagnosis of celiac disease. Celiac disease may go undiagnosed for many years because some people have no obvious symptoms until they are in the middle of a health crisis. Lack of symptoms does not mean lack of damage to the intestine, however, which is why screening is important for anyone with type 1 diabetes or a family history of celiac disease.

If you've been diagnosed with celiac disease, it's imperative to follow a strict gluten-free diet lifelong *even if eating gluten doesn't produce any obvious discomfort.* Small exposures to gluten can lead to damaged intestinal villi and malabsorption of nutrients, which increases your risk of developing serious medical conditions. Strict avoidance of gluten allows the intestine to heal; villi eventually regenerate, but it takes time. Even an occasional dietary slip-up or that "once-in-a-while" intake of a gluten-containing food could result in ongoing atrophied, poorly functioning villi.

Forgoing gluten if you are allergic or have an intolerance

It's estimated that up to 15 million Americans have food allergies, with an uptick in new cases in the past two decades. Roughly 1 in 13 children have a food allergy. Some, but not all, outgrow their allergy by adulthood. Eight foods account for over 90 percent of all food allergies: peanuts, tree nuts, milk, fish, shellfish, eggs, soy, and wheat.

Having diabetes doesn't increase your risk of having food allergies or food intolerances. The following sections cover both allergies and intolerances.

REMEMBER

Proper diagnosis by a qualified medical professional is important. Self-diagnosis isn't reliable and may lead to improper treatments and unnecessary food restrictions. A registered dietitian can provide in-depth education and additional resources if you need to avoid gluten or wheat for medical reasons such as celiac disease, food allergies, or food intolerances. This chapter covers just the basics.

Food allergies

The immune system is supposed to protect us from viral and bacterial invaders. Fighter cells travel through the bloodstream, patrolling the body in search of germs. A food allergy occurs when the immune cells react to a food rather than a germ. This case of mistaken identity results in a battle that should have never taken place.

The immune system mounts its attack by making an antibody called IgE, short for immunoglobin E. The IgE antibody binds to the surface of immune cells called mast cells and basophils. IgE is like a detective that has been trained to recognize the food allergen. Exposure to the food causes the immune cells to release histamines and other chemicals that are responsible for the allergy symptoms. Symptoms usually occur within 30 minutes to a few hours after exposure to the food. Symptoms can be mild to severe and include swelling, itching, hives, watery eyes, cramps, nausea, diarrhea, congestion, shortness of breath, dizziness, loss of consciousness, or, in the rarest but most severe reaction, anaphylaxis, which is life threatening.

The treatment for the food allergy is complete avoidance of the problem food. Mild symptoms may be treated with the appropriate antihistamines, oral steroids, or steroid creams. Severe reactions are treated with injected epinephrine; people at risk carry an epi pen.

Food intolerances

The main difference between food allergies and food intolerances (also called food sensitivities) is that food intolerances don't involve the immune system. Food intolerances may elicit some of the same milder symptoms associated with a food allergy, such as gastrointestinal upset, but an intolerance doesn't lead to severe reactions such as anaphylaxis.

Lactose intolerance is an example of food intolerance. Lactose, the natural sugar in milk, is made from two sugar molecules bonded together — specifically, glucose and galactose. Digestion of lactose requires an enzyme in the intestine called lactase. Lactase enzyme cleaves the double sugar into its two individual sugar molecule components. People who lack sufficient amounts of lactase enzyme are unable to digest lactose. Symptoms of lactose intolerance are cramping, bloating, gas, and diarrhea. Lactose-free milk has been treated with the enzyme lactase so the double sugar molecule has already been split into the two individual sugars before you drink it. Lactase enzyme is also available in liquid drops or tablets to minimize symptoms when lactose-containing foods are consumed.

Choosing to go gluten-free for personal reasons

Gluten-free diets have increased in popularity in the past decade or so. The diet is portrayed as being healthier and solving a rash of maladies, which isn't necessarily true. Some people with digestive issues, fatigue, or other physical complaints try gluten-free diets to see whether they'll feel better or have more energy. Others go gluten-free in hopes of losing weight. Weight loss isn't guaranteed but can occur due to the number of foods on the "do-not-eat list." When you eliminate a whole category of foods, it follows that you may lose weight. You may also lose the vitamins, minerals, and fiber typically obtained from the foods you are avoiding.

REMEMBER

If you're thinking of going gluten-free due to physical symptoms, you should first speak to a medical specialist for evaluation and proper diagnosis. If you go gluten-free for nonmedical reasons, be mindful to eat a balanced diet, as I explain later in this chapter. Going gluten-free eliminates many foods, some of which are quite wholesome while others do fall into the junk-food category. A gluten-free diet is healthy only if efforts are made to assure a balanced intake of vitamins, minerals, and other nutrients.

Against the Grain: Beginning a Gluten-Free Diet

If you have diabetes and celiac disease, you need to manage both conditions. A gluten-free diet is the only treatment for celiac disease. Many gluten-free grains can be safely included; just remember the importance of carb counting and the other diabetes management principles in this book.

A person with celiac disease requires a more restrictive diet than a person with an allergy or food intolerance to wheat. A gluten-free diet not only eliminates wheat, barley, and rye, but it also banishes a long list of products derived from those grains. People with celiac disease must avoid even traces of gluten or they may suffer medical consequences. Someone allergic or intolerant to wheat, on the other hand, may still be able to eat other gluten-containing grains and byproducts. If you follow a gluten-free diet for personal choice rather than medical necessity, there are no medical consequences to adding gluten-containing foods into your diet as desired. The following sections focus on how to start a gluten-free diet.

Avoiding grains that contain gluten

The Food Allergen Labeling and Consumer Protection Act requires common food allergens to be clearly identified on food labels. Allergens must be noted within the ingredient list or in a callout below the ingredient list. Wheat falls into the group of the eight most common food allergens, so if a product contains wheat, it must be clearly identified. Barley and rye don't fall into the list of risky food allergens and therefore don't require an allergen warning. See Chapter 7 for more details on food labeling and how to assess the presence of food allergens.

Labels are allowed, but not required, to identify gluten-free products. The FDA states that a food can be advertised as gluten-free provided that food has less than 20 parts per million (ppm) of gluten. Restaurants that use the term "gluten-free" are expected to comply with the federal definition.

A gluten-free diet eliminates wheat, barley, and rye. If only it were that simple. Many terms indicate wheat without actually saying wheat. Durum, for example, means wheat. Triticale is a hybrid of wheat and rye. For starters, giving up gluten requires learning a few new vocabulary words. Here are the names of gluten-containing grains and some of their aliases:

- Barley
- Bran
- Bulgur
- Couscous
- Cracked wheat
- Dinkel
- Durum
- Einkorn
- Emmer
- Farina
- Farro
- Flour
- Germ
- Gliadin
- Gluten
- Graham
- Groats
- Kamut
- Malt
- Pearl barley
- Rye
- Semolina
- Spelt
- Sprouted wheat
- Tabbouleh
- Triticale
- Wheat

WHAT ABOUT OATS?

While oats themselves do not contain gluten, they may become contaminated by coming in contact with gluten. When farms grow, harvest, and store gluten-containing grains, the contamination of gluten-free grains, such as oats, is nearly inevitable. Harvesting machines and grain silos used for processing and storing wheat, rye, or barley end up harboring residual amounts of gluten. When oats come into contact with that gluten during harvesting, production, or storage, they are cross-contaminated.

Farms that are dedicated solely to growing oats produce uncontaminated oats, which are usually well-tolerated by individuals with celiac disease. Oats labeled gluten-free are available in some stores and can be purchased online. Several brands advertise gluten-free, uncontaminated oats.

Eliminating gluten-containing foods

Many foods are made from gluten-containing grains. Wheat shows up more often than rye or barley. Most people on a gluten-free diet easily identify that bread products and foods made from wheat flour, such as baked goods, need to be avoided. However, some gluten-containing items are not so obvious. For example:

>> Beers and ales are made with barley, hops, and malt. Some beers are made with wheat.

>> Many processed foods have starch and fillers that may be wheat-based.

>> Standard soy sauce is made from fermented soy *and wheat.* That means many soy-based sauces, including teriyaki sauce, must be avoided.

The following list identifies some obvious and not-so-obvious sources of gluten, but note that it's not an all-inclusive list. (The next section goes a layer deeper and looks at where else gluten may be lurking.)

>> Ale	>> Graham crackers
>> Bagels	>> Granola
>> Baked goods	>> Licorice
>> Beer	>> Macaroni
>> Biscuits	>> Malt
>> Bread	>> Matzo
>> Brewer's yeast	>> Muesli
>> Cake	>> Muffins
>> Cereals	>> Noodles
>> Cookies	>> Orzo
>> Crackers	>> Pancakes
>> Crepes	>> Pasta
>> Croissants	>> Pastries
>> Croutons	>> Pita bread
>> Crust	>> Pizza crust
>> Filo dough	>> Pretzels
>> Food coloring	>> Ramen
>> Gnocchi	>> Roux

- » Sauces
- » Scones
- » Seitan
- » Soups
- » Spaghetti

- » Stuffing
- » Tempura
- » Tortillas (flour)
- » Waffles

Finding hidden gluten

Processed foods often contain fillers, food coloring, and flavor enhancers that may contain gluten. If something has modified starch, thickeners or stabilizers, texturized vegetable protein (TVP), hydrolyzed plant proteins, or any other ingredient you are unsure of, contact the manufacturer for clarification and to make sure it's gluten-free.

TIP

Some stores have done the research for you. Several supermarket chains have compiled lists of the gluten-free products that they carry. Inquire at your local stores or look on their websites.

Here's just a sample of some unusual items that may have gluten:

- » Fillers added to processed meats and deli meats may contain gluten. Beware of hot dogs, sausages, bologna, and salami. Self-basting turkeys and plumped hams are injected with broth solutions that may contain gluten. Meatballs and meatloaf often incorporate breadcrumbs.

- » Malt vinegar and any condiment made with malt vinegar should be avoided.

- » Be especially careful with sauces, marinades, and products that contain soy sauce. Typical soy sauce contains wheat, but wheat-free versions are available. Miso may contain barley. Flour is often used to thicken gravies, soups, and sauces. Roux is flour-based and used in the preparation of sauces and many Cajun dishes.

- » Communion wafers may contain gluten.

- » Candies, bouillon, and imitation crab are surprise sources of hidden gluten.

- » Many vitamins, over-the-counter medications, and prescription drugs contain gluten. Your pharmacist should be able to identify which ones. People with celiac disease are encouraged to take gluten-free multivitamins.

- » Lipstick and lip balms, play dough, stamps, and gummed envelopes are nonfood items that may have gluten.

If in doubt, check it out by contacting the company.

Avoiding cross-contamination

Individuals with celiac disease need to avoid exposure to gluten, which is hard to do unless the whole household goes gluten-free. Wheat flour used in baking may result in airborne particles of gluten, which contaminate kitchen surfaces. If a household doesn't go entirely gluten-free, a separate cupboard and counter should be reserved for gluten-free products only.

Extra precautions need to be in place to prevent accidental exposure. Here are some additional tips to reduce cross-contamination:

>> Invest in a new toaster and reserve it for gluten-free products. Using the same toaster for wheat-containing bread is not acceptable.

>> Buy condiments in squirt bottles. Double-dipping a knife into a jar of peanut butter, jelly, ketchup, or mayonnaise contaminates the remaining product once the knife has touched wheat bread.

>> Get rid of wooden cutting boards and wooden spoons. When used to prepare gluten-containing foods, traces of gluten can seep into the grain of the wood and then leach back out later when preparing a gluten-free item. Sanitize plastic spoons and cutting boards in the dishwasher or with hot soapy water after exposure to gluten.

>> Use separate sponges for cleaning up surfaces that have come into contact with gluten. Sponges not only harbor bacteria but are also a source of gluten cross-contamination.

>> Grill or deep-fry gluten-free foods first. Once oil has been used to fry breaded items, such as nuggets or onion rings, it will contaminate subsequent foods. Fryers and grills are key sources of gluten contamination in many restaurants. Although potatoes are naturally gluten-free, making French fries in the same oil that was used for breaded items ends up contaminating the potatoes.

>> Consider the cross-contamination that can happen during food manufacturing. Corn tortillas are gluten-free, but if a conveyer belt runs flour tortillas prior to corn tortillas, the corn tortillas may become contaminated.

>> Bulk bin scoops may be contaminated with gluten if customers switch scoops or use the same scoop for various bins.

>> The meat slicer used in a deli may harbor hidden gluten.

Restaurant dining can be tricky. If you order your salad without croutons, for example, the server may not think twice about picking off the croutons before serving you a pre-made salad. The fact that croutons touched the salad could cause a reaction for a person with celiac disease. Consider also that some restaurant kitchens reuse woks and skillets over and over again. Scraping out the wok doesn't remove the soy sauce used in preparation of the previous dish.

TIP

It's best to plan in advance and find out whether the restaurant can accommodate your dietary needs. Call or stop by during nonpeak hours to meet with the chef to discuss the diligence needed in preparing foods that are truly gluten-free and free from cross-contamination. Many restaurants are trying to meet the needs of their gluten-free customers. Some mark the menus to identify gluten-free dishes, while others have a separate gluten-free menu. It doesn't hurt to ask.

Staying Gluten-Free Without Nutrient Deficiencies

Maintaining a gluten-free diet requires diligent avoidance of many foods. It's important to choose a variety of gluten-free whole grains along with foods that are naturally gluten-free. While planning a nutritionally complete, gluten-free diet is entirely possible, some people tend to do what's easy and eat the same limited selections over and over. Lack of variety can lead to nutrient deficiencies. Eating a wide variety of foods from all food groups helps assure adequate intakes of all key vitamins and minerals.

Slipping up and ingesting gluten damages the capacity of the intestine to digest and absorb nutrients. It can take quite a while for the gut to heal. Impaired absorption of vitamins and minerals can lead to nutritional deficiencies.

After hearing all about what you *can't* eat on a gluten-free diet earlier in this chapter, you may be wondering whether there is anything left that you *can* eat! This section identifies foods that are naturally gluten-free, introduces the numerous gluten-free grains that you can enjoy, and discusses nutrients at risk if you stick with a gluten-free diet.

Embracing foods naturally free of gluten

Any food that has been packaged and processed could potentially have additives that contain gluten. For example, corn is gluten-free, but canned creamed corn may have flour added. Read all packaged food labels carefully. Keep in mind that many wholesome, natural foods are completely free of gluten. In their natural, unprocessed state, the following foods are gluten-free:

>> Fresh fruits and vegetables

>> Legumes, dried beans, split peas, lentils, soybeans, and tofu

>> Nuts (unseasoned) and nut butters

>> Fish and seafood (with the exception of surimi and imitation crab)

>> Unprocessed meats and poultry

>> Eggs

>> Vegetable oils and butter

>> Milk and plain yogurt (check labels on flavored yogurt)

>> Cheese (not necessarily processed cheese spreads)

>> Cottage cheese, buttermilk, cream, cream cheese, and sour cream

TIP

The list of gluten-free products is continuously growing. Check your local super-markets for gluten-free flours, baking mixes, pastas, crackers, breads, cereals, waffles, baked goods, pizza crusts, bagels, frozen entrées, canned foods, snack foods, and more. If you aren't satisfied with their offerings, check online for products you can order. Gluten Free Mall has a wide selection of gluten free products. See www.glutenfreemall.com/catalog/.

Incorporating gluten-free grains

If you're going to be gluten-free, it's time to branch out and try some new grains. The following list identifies gluten-free grains as well as other starches that can be used when planning meals. Choose "whole" grains when possible. You don't have to have celiac disease to enjoy these foods:

>> Amaranth

>> Arrowroot

>> Buckwheat

>> Cassava

>> Corn

>> Corn taco shells

>> Corn tortillas

>> Cream of rice cereal

>> Grits

>> Hominy

>> Kasha

>> Legumes

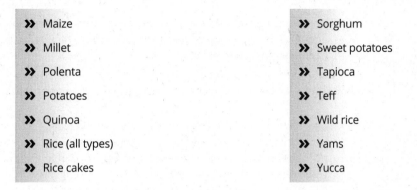

- » Maize
- » Millet
- » Polenta
- » Potatoes
- » Quinoa
- » Rice (all types)
- » Rice cakes

- » Sorghum
- » Sweet potatoes
- » Tapioca
- » Teff
- » Wild rice
- » Yams
- » Yucca

See Appendix A to locate the gluten-free grains and starches in the starch list. Serving sizes on the list provide approximately 15 grams of carbohydrate.

Watching out for nutrient deficiencies

Eliminating foods and food groups potentially limits the nutrients provided by those particular foods. Restricting gluten is not a treatment for diabetes, so I don't recommend eliminating gluten unless you have a medical reason for doing so. It takes careful planning to find those nutrients elsewhere. Whether diet restrictions are medically necessary or self-directed, it is important to eat a variety of foods that provide a wide spectrum of vitamins, minerals, and fiber.

REMEMBER

Celiac disease requires lifelong avoidance of gluten. Exposure to gluten leads to intestinal damage, which results in impaired absorption of numerous vitamins and minerals. Ongoing nutrient deficiencies may lead to malnutrition with serious medical consequences. The best prevention is persistent dietary diligence. Blood tests can determine whether you are currently low in any particular vitamins or minerals. Bone density scans are used to assess bone health. Restrictive diets may necessitate vitamin and mineral supplementation. Discuss your situation with your healthcare provider. A registered dietitian is the medical professional best suited to assess your dietary intake and provide nutritional guidance.

For healthy blood cells and to reduce the risk of anemia, focus on eating foods rich in these three critical nutrients, all of which are vital to blood-cell formation:

- » **Vitamin B12:** Food sources rich in this vitamin include meat, poultry, seafood, eggs, milk, and yogurt.
- » **Folate (folic acid):** Choose leafy green vegetables, legumes (dried bean family), and gluten-free grains and cereals that have been fortified with this nutrient.

>> **Iron:** Meat, poultry, fish, and seafood are rich in iron. Other sources include eggs, nuts, leafy green vegetables, and gluten-free grains and cereals that have been enriched with iron.

Bone health relies on adequate intakes of these two key nutrients:

>> **Calcium:** Calcium is needed for healthy bones and teeth. Focus on getting at least three servings per day from milk, yogurt, cheese, or calcium-enriched nondairy milk substitutes such as enriched soy, rice, or almond milk. Dark green vegetables, legumes, almonds, and sesame tahini also offer calcium, as do fish canned with bones such as sardines and salmon.

>> **Vitamin D:** Vitamin D is needed for the absorption of calcium. Adequate intakes of both calcium and vitamin D help reduce the risk of osteoporosis and fractures. Food sources of this fat-soluble vitamin include fatty fish, egg yolk, fortified milk and yogurt, and gluten-free grains and cereals that have been enriched with this nutrient.

The following vitamins and minerals are also important for the critical roles they play in staying healthy:

>> **Vitamin A:** Required for cell growth, healthy skin, vision, and fighting infections. Food sources include cod liver oil, leafy green vegetables, dark yellow-orange vegetables, egg yolks, and vitamin-fortified milk.

>> **Vitamin E:** Necessary for nerve health and tissue repair. Foods that contain this vitamin include avocados, nuts, vegetable oils, margarine, and leafy green vegetables. Vitamin E is also found in gluten-free "whole" grains.

>> **Vitamin K:** Critical for normal blood clotting. Sources include leafy green vegetables, broccoli, asparagus, Brussels sprouts, and spinach.

>> **Magnesium:** Plays a role in muscle, heart, and nerve function. To increase your intake of this mineral, choose nuts, gluten-free "whole" grains, meats, dairy products, and leafy green vegetables.

5

Sampling Menus Complete with Carb Counts

IN THIS PART . . .

Manage carbs in your breakfasts, lunches, and dinners.

Select menus with carb consistency; choose from 30–45 grams of carb, 45–60 grams of carb, or 60–75 grams of carb per meal.

Tweak recipes to boost nutrition while lowering fat and sodium.

Personalize your meal plans to please your preferences.

Choose snacks ranging from 0–30 grams of carb.

Chapter **19**

Beginning with Breakfast Menus

B reakfast is an important meal. During sleep the liver releases glucose that was previously stored. By morning, the glucose reserves are low and it is time to "break the fast." You need nutrition to function at your best. The menus in this chapter are designed to illustrate how to achieve variety in breakfast food choices, yet consistency in carb intake. You also find tips for customizing a healthy breakfast even more to your liking.

Starting Your Day Right with Breakfast

In this section, you find seven menu choices for breakfasts, each with three carb-range options. Carb and calorie counts are noted for each menu. The main carb-containing foods are identified in **bold** font, and the grams of fiber have been subtracted from the total carb count. The portion sizes in the base menus provide 30–45 grams of carb per meal. Tips for incremental carb portion add-ons boost the carb count to achieve 45–60 grams of carb and 60–75 grams of carb. (If you aren't sure how many carbs you need in a day, see Chapter 5. For insight on how to distribute carbs between meals, see Chapter 6.)

TIP

If you aren't much of a breakfast person, at least have one portion of a carb-containing food, roughly 15 grams of carb, such as a container of yogurt, a small piece of fruit, or a slice of toast. People who skip breakfast are at risk for overeating later in the day. Blood-glucose control is improved by distributing carb intake between three main meals, roughly four to six hours apart (small snacks are optional).

REMEMBER

Just as eating too little in the morning can be detrimental, so is eating too much. Before overeating in the morning, consider this: Natural hormonal surges known as the "dawn phenomenon" can increase insulin resistance in the morning, causing some people with diabetes to wake up with a higher fasting blood-glucose level than desired. The morning meal choices matter, because if you eat too much carbohydrate, your blood-glucose levels will likely spike, and that is especially true if the carb choices are sweet or refined. Picking healthy foods helps. (So does a walk after breakfast!)

| Breakfast Menus | BASE MENU | | | Healthy Tips and Options |
	30–45 Grams Carb per Meal	45–60 Grams Carb per Meal	60–75 Grams Carb per Meal	
Monday *Old fashioned oats*	**1 cup cooked oatmeal** **1 tablespoon raisins** **4 ounces 1% milk** 1 egg, any style Total: 37 grams carb 310 calories	To the base menu add: **1 tablespoon raisins** Total: 45 grams carb 342 calories	To the base menu add: **1 tablespoon raisins** + **1 slice whole-wheat toast** with 1 teaspoon butter Total: 61 grams carb 466 calories	Avoid sweetened versions of oatmeal. Use plain, old-fashioned, or steel-cut oats. The more fiber, the better. It's okay to add sugar substitute and cinnamon. If desired, add 4 walnut halves (adds 52 calories and no carbs).
Tuesday *On-the-go*	**1 slice whole-wheat toast** 1 tablespoon almond butter or peanut butter **1 extra-small banana or ½ average-size banana** Total: 33 grams carb 246 calories	To the base menu add: **1 cup 1% milk** Total: 45 grams carb 351 calories	To the base menu add: **1 cup 1% milk** + **1 slice whole-wheat toast** + 1 tablespoon almond butter or peanut butter Total: 63 grams carb 537 calories	You can use any nut butter: soy, cashew, sesame, or sunflower. Optional: Use calcium-fortified, nondairy milk replacements, including soy or rice milk. Check labels for carb and calorie info. Take the toast to-go, making a peanut-butter/banana toasted sandwich.

Breakfast Menus	BASE MENU			
	30–45 Grams Carb per Meal	45–60 Grams Carb per Meal	60–75 Grams Carb per Meal	Healthy Tips and Options
Wednesday *Keeping it simple*	**½ cup 2% cottage cheese** **¾ cup cut pineapple** **½ whole-grain English muffin** with 1 teaspoon butter Total: 30 grams carb 260 calories	To the base menu add: **½ cup 2% cottage cheese** + **½ whole-grain English muffin** with 1 teaspoon butter Total: 45 grams carb 463 calories	To the base menu add: **½ cup 2% cottage cheese** + **½ whole-grain English muffin** with 1 teaspoon butter + Latte made with **10 ounces 1% milk** Total: 60 grams carb 582 calories	Choose nonfat or low-fat cottage cheese. 1 cup melon, cantaloupe, or honeydew can be used instead of pineapple.
Thursday *Breakfast burrito*	**1 medium 8-inch whole-wheat flour tortilla** **½ cup beans** 1 egg, scrambled 2 tablespoons salsa 1 tablespoon light sour cream Total: 40 grams carb 349 calories	To the base menu add: **½ cup diced potato, cooked** Total: 55 grams carb 417 calories	To the base menu add: **½ cup diced potato, cooked** + **Small orange** Total: 64 grams carb 462 calories	Use beans of your choice, such as pinto or black. Add chopped jalapeño peppers or green chilies if desired. Add chopped lettuce if desired. Check labels for carb and calorie info as tortillas vary.
Friday *Broiled bagel breakfast*	**½ large whole-grain bagel, lightly toasted** 1 slice tomato 1 slice of cheese (about an ounce) 1 slice Canadian bacon (about an ounce) Total: 30 grams carb 306 calories	To the base menu add: Just double all portions in the base menu using **both halves of the bagel.** Total: 60 grams carb 612 calories	To the base menu add: Just double all portions in the base menu using **both halves of the bagel.** + 1 small apple, sliced Total: 75 grams carb 672 calories	Assemble the ingredients with the cheese on top; bake or broil until melted. Replace the Canadian bacon with smoked salmon, if desired. Use low-fat cheese to cut fat and calories. Switch the apple for any fruit on the Exchange List in Appendix A.

(continued)

(continued)

| Breakfast Menus | BASE MENU | | | Healthy Tips and Options |
	30–45 Grams Carb per Meal	45–60 Grams Carb per Meal	60–75 Grams Carb per Meal	
Saturday *Weekend brunch*	**1 whole-grain toaster waffle** **½ cup sliced strawberries** **4 ounces low-fat vanilla yogurt** 1 slice Canadian bacon (about an ounce) 1 egg, any style Total: 31 grams carb 328 calories	To the base menu add: **1 whole-grain toaster waffle** + **½ cup sliced strawberries** Total: 51 grams carb 445 calories	To the base menu add: **1 whole-grain toaster waffle** + **½ cup sliced strawberries** + **4 ounces low-fat vanilla yogurt** Total: 66 grams carb 541 calories	You can use vegetarian bacon or sausage in place of the Canadian bacon. You can lower fat further by using nonfat yogurt. Plain yogurt is also an option. Top the waffle with the yogurt and fruit instead of syrup.
Sunday *Savory scramble*	1 egg scrambled with the following chopped items (spinach, onions, mushrooms, and cheese) cooked in the oil **½ cup spinach** **¼ cup onions** **4 mushrooms** 1 ounce cheese 1 teaspoon cooking oil **1 slice whole-grain toast** **1 tablespoon no-sugar-added fruit spread (jam)** Total: 30 grams carb 374 calories	To the base menu add: **½ cup potato** + 1 egg Total: 45 grams carb 513 calories	To the base menu add: **½ cup potato** + 1 egg + **1 whole-grain slice toast** + **1 tablespoon no-sugar-added fruit spread (jam)** Total: 71 grams carb 643 calories	Use reduced-fat cheese to lower the fat and calories. Substitute crumbled tofu for the egg, if desired. Add shredded zucchini, chilies, and chopped tomato, if desired.

Personalizing Your Breakfast Meal Plan

When looking through the menus in this chapter, feel free to personalize them. Check out the following tips to modify your breakfast menus and stay healthy at the same time:

>> **Switching carbs:** It's okay to swap carb choices. For example, if the menu calls for two slices of whole-grain toast, you can swap for both halves of a whole-wheat English muffin. You can replace oatmeal with a different whole-grain cooked or dry cereal; just check Nutrition Facts labels for carb counts. You can also change the fruit selection; choose small-sized fruits, about the size of a tennis ball or baseball. For melon and berries, aim for about a cup.

TIP

Once you've made a few meals in your desired carb range, it becomes easier to develop similar menus of your own. Read labels on any packaged items that you use. For foods without labels, refer to the Exchange Lists in Appendix A to identify carb foods, portion sizes, and carb counts to assist in planning your own menus.

>> **Keeping selections healthy:** Healthy food options are encouraged. Consider the following:

- Choose whole-grain breads and cereals.

- Pick natural peanut butter without hydrogenated oils.

- Your margarine should be entirely free of trans fats. You can reduce saturated fat and hydrogenated oils by opting for soft tub margarines. Some versions are lower in calories and fat.

- If you enjoy meat at breakfast, choose lean selections such as ham or Canadian bacon rather than bacon and sausage. If you're buying sausages, compare labels and buy the lower-fat versions. Better yet, try vegetarian sausages; they are quite tasty, low in fat, and cholesterol free.

>> **Controlling carbs:** Seek out cereals with less added sugars. Compare cereal labels for carb counts and consider the amount of sugar in the cereal before you make your purchases.

When it comes to jams and jellies, look for no-added-sugar or simply fruit versions. There will still be naturally occurring sugars from the fruit.

Look at the labels on yogurt containers. You'll find some with a mere 8 grams of carb and others that have well over 40 grams of carb. It varies depending on the type of yogurt and especially on the type of sweetener used. Plain yogurts or those sweetened with a sugar substitute have less carbs than those with added sugar or honey.

Beware of syrup. One-quarter cup of pancake syrup has almost 60 grams of carb. Sugar-free syrup may not be what you're expecting. Look at the label for the *total grams of carb, not the grams of sugar*. Sugar-free syrup often contains sugar alcohol, and that's still carb. For more information on sugars and sweeteners, see Chapter 12.

» **Reconsidering your beverages:** Skip the sugar in your morning brew or opt for a packet of sugar substitute. Think twice about reaching for juice or smoothies, too, as they are both very concentrated in the amount of carb they contain. Liquids digest quickly so the carbs in juice, smoothies, and sugary specialty coffee drinks raise blood-glucose levels sharply. The evidence is in the blood-glucose reading on your meter. Those beverages can be high in calories, too. You can find more information on what you plan to sip or swig in Chapter 11.

Chapter **20**

Looking for Lunch Menus

L unch is an important midday meal. Lunch breaks can help keep your energy levels up. It's not a good idea to skip lunch, especially when you have diabetes, because doing so may lead to overeating at dinner. The menus in this chapter provide a framework to guide you when you're making your own lunches. After you've made a few meals in your desired carb range, it becomes easier to develop similar menus of your own. You also find a few tips on eating out in this chapter.

Loving Your Lunch Options

The menus in this section are designed to illustrate how to achieve variety in food choices, yet consistency in carb intake. You find seven themes for lunches with three carb-range options. Carb and calorie counts are noted for each menu. The main carb-containing foods are in **bold** font, and the grams of fiber have been subtracted from the total carb count. The portion sizes in the base menus provide 30–45 grams of carb per meal. Tips for incremental carb portion add-ons boost the carb count to achieve 45–60 grams of carb and 60–75 grams of carb. If you choose to eat more than 75 grams of carb, you can add items as needed. Appendix A indicates portion sizes that provide 15 grams of carb from starch, fruit, and milk food groups. If you aren't sure how many carbs you need, see Chapter 5.

TIP

Healthy food options are encouraged, such as choosing lean proteins and lower-fat cooking methods. When portioning your proteins, aim for a serving size that is about the same size as the palm of your own hand. If you desire bigger lunches, start your meal with a leafy green salad with your choice of cut, crunchy vegetables. If you're cutting down on your intake of fats, you can opt for reduced-fat salad dressings. Spritzing on salad oil with a spray bottle is another easy way to control how much oil you use. You can purchase separate bottles for vinegar and oil, or you can blend the two in the same bottle. Use herbs and spices as desired, but little or no salt (especially if you have high blood pressure).

| Lunch Menus | BASE MENU | | | Healthy Tips and Options |
	30–45 Grams Carb per Meal	45–60 Grams Carb per Meal	60–75 Grams Carb per Meal	
Monday *Middle Eastern falafel sandwich*	**½ whole-wheat pita bread** **2 falafel patties** **1 tablespoon hummus** Chopped lettuce, as desired 1 tablespoon diced tomato 1 tablespoon diced cucumber 1 tablespoon chopped onion Drizzle with tahini dressing (see the far-right column) Total: 32 grams carb 282 calories	To the base menu add: **¾ cup tabbouleh** Total: 46 grams carb 406 calories	To the base menu add: Double the ingredients in the base menu to make 1 whole pita. Total: 64 grams carb 564 calories	Recipe for tahini dressing: 1 tablespoon tahini 1 tablespoon lemon juice 1 tablespoon water ¼ teaspoon garlic (minced or dry) Use warm water to assist in blending. Read labels for carb and calorie info as brands of tabbouleh vary. This example is ½ cup bulgur, ⅓ cup parsley, 1 teaspoon oil, and 2 teaspoons lemon juice.

Lunch Menus	BASE MENU 30–45 Grams Carb per Meal	45–60 Grams Carb per Meal	60–75 Grams Carb per Meal	Healthy Tips and Options
Tuesday *Nicoise salad*	3 cups lettuce 1 hard-boiled egg ½ cup tuna **½ cup cooked green beans** **½ cup boiled red potatoes** **1 small tomato** 4 black olives Dressing: Blend 1 tablespoon olive oil, 2 teaspoons vinegar, herbs of choice, and black pepper **1 slice whole-grain bread (about 1 ounce)** Total: 35 grams carb 510 calories	To the base menu add: **17 small grapes (or 1 small peach)** Total: 50 grams carb 570 calories	To the base menu add: **17 small grapes (or 1 small peach)** + **½ cup garbanzo beans** Total: 66 grams carb 675 calories	Place the lettuce on a dinner-sized plate, cut up the remaining vegetables into bite-sized pieces and arrange them on top of the lettuce, add the tuna and egg, and then drizzle with the blended vinegar and oil, herbs, and black pepper. Optional: Add sliced red onion, bell pepper, and radishes. Optional: Add ¼ teaspoon mustard to the dressing. Buy tuna packed in water; drain before using.
Wednesday *Turkey wrap*	**1 medium 8-inch whole-wheat flour tortilla** 2 tablespoons light cream cheese, softened 6 thin slices of deli turkey (2 ounces) **½ cup shredded carrot** 2 lettuce leaves **¼ cup minced tomato** 1 green onion, sliced Total: 32 grams carb 276 calories	To the base menu add: **2 clementines** Total: 47 grams carb 346 calories	To the base menu add: **2 clementines** + **½ cup canned three-bean salad** Total: 62 grams carb 426 calories	Spread the cream cheese over the entire tortilla. Arrange the turkey and vegetables on top. Roll tightly. Slice in half. Opt for spinach leaves rather than lettuce. If desired, add sliced mushrooms or thinly sliced cucumber. If you want to make three-bean salad at home, the ratio is about ¼ cup kidney beans, ¼ cup garbanzo beans, and ¼ cup cooked green beans with 1 tablespoon of Italian salad dressing.

(continued)

| Lunch Menus | BASE MENU | | | Healthy Tips and Options |
	30–45 Grams Carb per Meal	45–60 Grams Carb per Meal	60–75 Grams Carb per Meal	
Thursday *Rice bowl*	**⅔ cup cooked brown rice** Stir-fry using: 1 tablespoon oil 4 ounces lean meat or tofu **½ cup broccoli** **¼ cup onion** 6 mushrooms ½ teaspoon garlic ¼ teaspoon pepper Finish with ¼ cup low-sodium broth and 1 teaspoon low-sodium soy sauce. Heat to simmer and serve over the rice. Total: 38 grams carb 438 calories	To the base menu add: **¾ cup pineapple** Total: 53 grams carb 500 calories	To the base menu add: **¾ cup pineapple** + **⅓ cup cooked brown rice** Total: 68 grams carb 567 calories	You may substitute green beans or bok choy for the broccoli. Optional: Add 1 tablespoon wine or 1 teaspoon peanut butter to the simmer sauce. Optional: Top with sliced green onion. Optional: Drizzle with toasted sesame oil or chili oil.
Friday *Pasta salad*	**1 cup cooked pasta** Chop and mix: **¼ cup yellow bell pepper** **¼ cup zucchini** **1 small tomato** **1 tablespoon onion** 6 black olives 2 ounces cubed, fresh mozzarella 2 tablespoons Italian salad dressing Total: 42 grams carb 468 calories	To the base menu add: **1¼ cups strawberries** Total: 55 grams carb 534 calories	To the base menu add: **1¼ cups strawberries** + **½ cup white kidney beans (cannellini)** Total: 70 grams carb 644 calories	Any pasta shape will work; I recommend small shells. Try whole-wheat pasta. Optional: Add cut cucumber, broccoli, or mushrooms. Onions may be red, yellow, or green, and bell pepper can be any color. Mix the beans into the pasta salad. You may substitute red kidney beans for white beans.

Lunch Menus	BASE MENU 30–45 Grams Carb per Meal	45–60 Grams Carb per Meal	60–75 Grams Carb per Meal	Healthy Tips and Options
Saturday *Beef burgers*	**Whole-wheat hamburger bun** 3-ounce beef patty, 95% lean 1 slice cheese Lettuce leaf Sliced tomato Sliced onion Sliced dill pickle 1 teaspoon mayonnaise 1 teaspoon ketchup ½ teaspoon mustard 1 ounce baked potato chips Total: 45 grams carb 471 calories	To the base menu add: **1¼ cups diced watermelon** Total: 60 grams carb 521 calories	To the base menu add: **1¼ cups diced watermelon** + **⅓ cup baked beans** Total: 75 grams carb 600 calories	You may substitute a chicken breast, salmon patty, or veggie burger for the beef. Opt for reduced-fat cheese or reduced-fat mayonnaise. Add a leafy green side salad if desired.
Sunday *Soup and sandwich*	Grilled cheese sandwich: **2 slices whole-wheat bread** 2 slices cheese (sandwich size, 1.5 ounces total) 2 teaspoons light margarine or light mayonnaise Assemble sandwich with cheese inside and spread on outside. Grill in pan until golden on both sides. **1 cup light-sodium tomato soup** Total: 45 grams carb 435 calories	To the base menu add: **1 small apple** Total: 60 grams carb 495 calories	To the base menu add: **1 small apple** + **⅓ cup cooked white or brown rice** (Add cooked rice to the soup to make tomato rice soup.) Total: 75 grams carb 565 calories	Optional: Add 2 ounces lean ham to the sandwich. Opt for reduced-fat, 2% milk cheeses. Optional: Thinly slice tomatoes and onions and insert into sandwich prior to grilling. Add a leafy green side salad if desired.

Personalizing Your Lunch Meal Plan

You can get creative and personalize these menu ideas in a variety of ways. Check out the following list for ideas, whether you're making your own lunch or eating out:

>> **Swapping out carb choices:** For example, if the menu calls for rice, you can swap the rice for other grains that have the same carb count. You can replace rice with quinoa, millet, farro, or couscous.

>> **Choosing different fruit:** Swapping is also permissible for the fruit group. Choose the fruits you prefer and keep the portion size to about 15 grams of carb. If you aren't having a serving of fruit with a meal, fruit makes a healthy in-between-meals snack. Refer to the Exchange Lists in Appendix A to find comparable items.

>> **Going vegetarian (or not):** Make any meal vegetarian by using tofu or a meat substitute. Likewise, if you don't want falafel patties, use lean meat instead.

>> **Drinking the right stuff:** Add a carb-free thirst quencher to your meal. For more information about beverages, see Chapter 11.

>> **Incorporating pre-made, packaged meals:** There's nothing wrong with keeping lunch simple when you don't have the time or the energy to make your own meal. Many packaged and frozen entrées are available to help you stay in your carb and calorie targets. Read the Nutrition Facts labels on packages (see Chapter 7 for help). Check the carbs and the calories. Compare fats and sodium too.

TIP

Once you've picked your entrée, you can add a side of vegetables or a green salad. For convenience, keep a bag of frozen broccoli or green beans on hand. Baby carrots, celery, cucumbers, and bell peppers stay fresh in the refrigerator for over a week. If you buy canned vegetables, you can opt for no-added-salt versions. Lettuce and salad greens can be purchase pre-washed for convenience. Some stores offer packaged salads with lean proteins and plenty of vegetables. Add carbs by adding a whole-wheat dinner roll or some whole-grain crackers.

TIP

When you do have time to make a meal at home, make a larger batch and freeze a serving for a future lunch.

>> **Eating in restaurants:** If you find yourself heading to a restaurant for lunch, strive to make healthy choices most of the time. If you choose to order an item that you know isn't so healthy, such as a side of fries, choose the *smallest* size. When the server delivers your meal to the table and the portion size is bigger than you expected (or bigger than you need), ask the waiter for a to-go box and package up half of the meal *before* you start eating.

If you frequent any chain restaurants, you can find and print the nutrition information for their menu items by visiting their web page. The web address is usually www.insert-the-name-of-the-restaurant.com (for example, www.subway.com). Some restaurants provide brochures with the nutrition facts, while others mark the calories, fat, and carbs on the menu. Ask your server or the manager for more information.

TIP

If you do dine out during your lunch break, take the opportunity to fit in a 10–15 minute walk.

>> **Packing it up:** Consider packing your lunch a couple days per week. You can brown-bag-it with a sandwich, raw crunchy veggies, and a serving of fruit, or if you have access to a microwave, you can do a healthy heat-and-eat. Bringing lunch can save you money and gives you more control over what you eat.

Chapter **21**

Delving into Dinner Menus

D inner replenishes the fuels you've used up during the day and establishes reserves to last you through the night. The dinner meal should be about four to six hours after lunch. Aim for a balanced meal; Chapter 8 provides information on the plate method of meal planning to incorporate foods from the various groups in appropriate portions. Healthy food options for dinner are encouraged, such as leaning toward lean proteins and choosing lower-fat cooking methods rather than deep-frying. This chapter gives you menu ideas and shows you how to customize your dinner plans.

Determining What's for Dinner

The menus in this chapter are designed to illustrate how to achieve variety in food choices, yet consistency in carb intake. You find seven themes for dinner with three carb-range options. Carb and calorie counts are noted for each menu. The main carb-containing foods are in **bold** font, and the grams of fiber have been subtracted from the total carb count. The portion sizes in the base menus provide 30–45 grams of carb per meal. Tips for incremental carb portion add-ons boost the carb count to achieve 45–60 grams of carb and 60–75 grams of carb. If you choose to eat more than 75 grams of carb, you can add items as needed. Appendix A indicates portion sizes that provide 15 grams of carb from starch, fruit, and milk food groups. If you aren't sure how many carbs you need, see Chapter 5.

Dinner Menus	BASE MENU 30–45 Grams Carb per meal	45–60 Grams Carb per meal	60–75 Grams Carb per Meal	Healthy Tips and Options
Monday *Meat-free meal*	3 ounces baked tofu ½ teaspoon soy sauce 1 teaspoon toasted sesame oil **⅔ cup cooked quinoa** **10 spears asparagus** with 1 teaspoon olive oil, lemon juice 2 cups lettuce 2 teaspoons salad dressing Total: 33 grams carb 388 calories	To the base menu add: **1 cup baked or roasted butternut squash** made with 1 teaspoon oil or butter Total: 48 grams carb 510 calories	To the base menu add: **1 cup baked or roasted butternut squash** made with 1 teaspoon oil or butter + **Small apple** Total: 63 grams carb 570 calories	Add slices of radish, onion, cucumber, or purple cabbage to your salad. Trade out the apple for any fruit portion in Appendix A. Cook grain in vegetable broth for added flavor. Opt for flavored vinegar rather than salad dressing if desired. Low-sodium soy sauce is an option.
Tuesday *South of the border*	4 ounces grilled skinless chicken (sliced) **1 small 6-inch corn tortilla** **½ cup chopped stir-fried onions and bell pepper** 1 tablespoon grated cheese 1 tablespoon guacamole 2 teaspoons low-fat sour cream **½ cup diced mango** Total: 30 grams carb 420 calories	To the base menu add: **½ cup black beans** Total: 45 grams carb 535 calories	To the base menu add: **½ cup black beans** + **1 small 6-inch corn tortilla** Total: 60 grams carb 605 calories	You can use fish or lean beef rather than chicken. Spice it up as desired using garlic, chilies, and hot sauce. If you're watching your fats, opt for fat-free sour cream and reduced-fat cheese. 1 cup of papaya has the same carb count as ½ cup mango, so you can swap.

Dinner Menus	BASE MENU 30–45 Grams Carb per meal	45–60 Grams Carb per meal	60–75 Grams Carb per Meal	Healthy Tips and Options
Wednesday *Asian cuisine*	4 ounces lean beef or pork, sautéed with garlic, 1 sliced green onion, and **1 cup chopped broccoli** **⅔ cup cooked brown rice** 1 teaspoon soy sauce 1 teaspoon sesame oil 1 teaspoon chili paste Total: 34 grams carb 400 calories	To the base menu add: **1 medium orange** Total: 47 grams carb 460 calories	To the base menu add: **1 medium orange** + **⅓ cup cooked brown rice** Total: 61 grams carb 540 calories	Trade out the orange for any fruit portion in Appendix A. Try bok choy or Chinese greens rather than broccoli for variety. Add mung bean sprouts. Low-sodium soy sauce is an option.
Thursday *Italian inspired*	**⅔ cup cooked whole-grain spaghetti** **½ cup marinara sauce, no sugar added** 3 ounces turkey meatballs (check labels to see whether the product contains any carb) 1 tablespoon grated parmesan cheese **¾ cup steamed green beans** Total: 45 grams carb 450 calories	To the base menu add: **⅓ cup cooked whole-grain spaghetti** Total: 60 grams carb 530 calories	To the base menu add: **⅓ cup cooked whole-grain spaghetti** + **17 small grapes** Total: 75 grams carb 590 calories	Add a leafy green salad with olive oil and balsamic vinegar. You can try vegetarian meatballs.

(continued)

Dinner Menus	BASE MENU 30–45 Grams Carb per meal	45–60 Grams Carb per meal	60–75 Grams Carb per Meal	Healthy Tips and Options
Friday *Catch of the day*	4 ounces cooked salmon **Kale salad** with **2 cups chopped kale** and **⅔ cup cooked farro grain,** 2 teaspoons olive oil, and 1 teaspoon vinegar Total: 41 grams carb 514 calories	To the base menu add: **Dinner roll** (whole wheat, small) with 1 teaspoon butter Total: 56 grams carb 634 calories	To the base menu add: **Dinner roll** (whole wheat, small) with 1 teaspoon butter + **1¼ cups cut strawberries** Total: 71 grams carb 694 calories	Salmon may be baked, grilled, or poached. You can switch to any type of fish. Lemon juice may be used as desired. You can add minced bell pepper, celery, and onions to the kale salad if desired (they add minimal carb). You can swap the kale for any leafy greens and season the salad as desired with pepper, herbs, and garlic. You can have watermelon instead of the strawberries. You can substitute quinoa or brown rice for the farro.
Saturday *Southern comfort*	4 ounces cooked chicken breast or thigh (skinless) **½ cup mashed potatoes** 2 tablespoons gravy **2-inch cube of cornbread** (1½ ounces) with 1 teaspoon butter **½ cup boiled or steamed collard greens** Total: 35 grams carb 450 calories	To the base menu add: **½ cup black-eyed peas** Total: 42 grams carb 540 calories	To the base menu add: **½ cup black-eyed peas** + **1 medium peach** Total: 60 grams carb 600 calories	Roast or bake chicken instead of frying. You can cook it with the skin on, but remove skin before eating. Try reduced-fat margarine or a "light" version. Skim fat before making gravy or buy low-fat, premade gravy.

Dinner Menus	BASE MENU 30–45 Grams Carb per meal	45–60 Grams Carb per meal	60–75 Grams Carb per Meal	Healthy Tips and Options
Sunday *Stuffed peppers*	1 large **bell pepper**, seeded, steamed but firm ½ cup cooked lean ground beef or turkey Stir in ⅓ cup water, **2 tablespoons of tomato paste**, and ½ teaspoon Italian seasoning. Add in **⅓ cup cooked brown rice.** Simmer all; stuff into pepper. **1 slice of bread** (whole wheat) with 1 teaspoon butter Total: 36 grams carb 397 calories	To the base menu add: **½ cup legumes such as navy beans or kidney beans** Total: 50 grams carb 509 calories	To the base menu add: **½ cup legumes such as navy beans or kidney beans** + **1 cup melon such as honeydew or cantaloupe** Total: 65 grams carb 569 calories	Swap the meat for vegetarian crumbles if desired. Chop celery, onion, and garlic and simmer with the ground protein. Adjust seasonings as desired. Add a leafy green salad if desired, with balsamic vinegar.

Personalizing Your Dinner Meal Plan

When looking through the menus in this chapter, feel free to personalize them with the help of the following tips:

>> **Swapping out carb choices:** For example, if the menu calls for rice, you can swap for other grains that have the same carb count. You can replace the rice with quinoa, millet, polenta, couscous, pasta, or stuffing. Refer to the Exchange Lists in Appendix A to find comparable items. Every choice in the starch group is listed in a portion size that provides approximately 15 grams of carb, so you may *exchange* one choice for any other.

>> **Mixing it up with fruits and veggies:** The same holds true for the fruit group. Mix it up and vary the vegetables too. If you aren't a fan of broccoli, you can trade for snap peas, green beans, okra, zucchini, or any other vegetable on the list. Serve up a leafy green side salad, if desired. Vegetables are highly encouraged, and most are pretty low in carbs. Vary the options in these basic menus, and you'll be on your way to planning carb-controlled menus of your own.

TIP

If you aren't having a serving of fruit with a meal, fruit makes a healthy snack. Choose small-sized fruits, about the size of a tennis ball or baseball. For melon and berries, aim for about a cup.

» **Adding a carb-free thirst quencher to your meal:** For more information about beverages, see Chapter 11.

» **Picking your protein portions:** "Eating smart for your weight and heart" means selecting lean proteins. Lean cuts of beef include sirloin, flank, and tenderloin. Pork tenderloin and ham also fall into the lean category. Skinless poultry, fish, and shellfish are excellent lean options. If you want to go veggie, feel free to use vegetarian meat replacements. There are many vegetarian meat substitutes that mimic the texture and taste of real meat (and most have little or no carb). If a meal suggests beef or pork and you want to switch to fish or skinless chicken (or tofu), that's fine because the protein choices won't affect the carb counts in the menus.

TIP

A good simple guideline for protein portioning is to aim for the same size and thickness as the palm of your own hand. So go ahead and tweak the menus with your choice of lean protein.

WARNING

» **Keeping an eye on your condiments:** Condiments can be hidden sources of fats, carbs, and sodium. Read labels carefully. Barbeque sauce and ketchup have some carbs; however, when used in modest amounts they shouldn't have much impact on blood-glucose levels. Large portions may contain a significant amount of carb. When it comes to blood pressure, it's the sodium you should be trying to cut down on, so skip the salt shaker and limit the soy sauce. Beware, many other sauces used in Asian cooking are also high in sodium. To limit fat, consider nonfat or light versions of salad dressing, sour cream, and mayonnaise.

» **Seasoning sensationally:** Feel free to season to satisfy, focusing on salt-free seasonings. Season your wok favorites with ginger, garlic, and chili paste. Add a dash of toasted sesame oil and a splash of flavored rice vinegar. If you like it spicy, try a squirt of Vietnamese chili sauce. Add zing to your Mexican meals with diced green chilies, jalapeños, or salsa. Bake your fish with some white wine and garlic and a squeeze of lemon juice. Break out the basil and oregano for your Italian food (of course garlic goes well here too!). Use pepper (black, white, and red), herbs, salt-free spices, and flavored vinegars to enhance your meals as desired. Enjoy.

Chapter **22**

Surveying Snack Ideas

I f you face a long time between meals, sometimes a healthy snack is just what you need to keep your energy levels up. An afternoon snack may curb your appetite enough to make portion control at dinner easier to achieve. If you go into dinner too hungry, it is easy to overeat.

However, too much snacking can sabotage blood-glucose and weight-control efforts. Afternoon snack attacks can lead to elevated blood-glucose levels before dinner, which then climb even higher after dinner. Evening is when many people kick their feet up and relax, which means elevated blood-glucose levels are slower to come back down. Late-night snacking can compound the problem. Effects can be lasting and result in elevated fasting blood-glucose levels the next day.

TIP

One fairly common reason for excessive afternoon snacking, or overeating at dinner, is skimping or skipping breakfast or lunch meals. It's better to have three main meals roughly four to six hours apart to better distribute carbs and help regulate appetite. Chapters 19, 20, and 21 provide carb-controlled menu ideas for breakfasts, lunches, and dinners.

On the other hand, sometimes a snack is needed to prevent the blood-glucose levels from dropping, especially in relation to exercise. Blood-glucose monitoring is a critical component of diabetes management. Checking blood glucose will help you determine whether you need a snack, and if so, how much. Monitoring can also show how you respond to snacks. This chapter provides ideas on planning snacks in various carb ranges and tips for choosing packaged snacks.

It's important to be mindful about what you eat. Shop for and stock up on healthy snacks for the home and the workplace. Don't go shopping when you're hungry because it's much harder to resist temptation, and the wrong things may end up in your cart. When hungry, people tend to want to satisfy hunger quickly. Making the right choices in the moment is easier if you have planned healthy snacks in advance. Pack your own snacks when possible. Prepare and portion appropriately. If you do find yourself buying a packaged snack, take the time to read and compare labels.

If you use insulin, consider the need to cover the carbs in your snacks. Have a discussion with your healthcare provider regarding insulin dosing decisions related to snacking.

Choosing Carb-Controlled Snacks

Many foods are naturally low in carbs or have no carbs at all. For example, meat, fish, chicken, cheese, eggs, nuts, tofu, avocado, leafy greens, nonstarchy vegetables, and olives are all examples of foods with few or no carbs, so these foods don't have much effect on blood-glucose levels.

Beware, though; some low-carb foods are high in calories and fat. Although meat and cheese don't have carbs and don't raise blood-glucose levels, you should be mindful of the fact that they can be significant contributors of calories and saturated fat depending on portions consumed. For example, bacon won't raise blood-glucose levels, but that doesn't mean it's a healthy choice. There are best-bet options within the low-carb foods. Lean meats are better for you than fatty meats when it comes to heart and hips.

This section provides snack ideas. Snack options may be single food items, such as string cheese, or easy-to-assemble snacks, which incorporate a few foods. Each of the snack ideas in this section lists the amount of total carb, fiber, and calories. One table each is devoted to snacks in the following carb ranges: 0–10 grams, 10–20 grams, and 20–30 grams. The following tips can help you choose the best carb range for a given snack:

>> If your blood-glucose levels are above target but you are hungry, choose a snack with few or no carbs; see the list with 0–10 grams of carb per snack.

>> If you need a bit more carb to tide you over between meals, consider a snack with 10–20 grams of carb.

>> For active days, or when you need a carb boost, choose from the list of snacks with 20–30 grams of carb.

REMEMBER

The tables provide the total carb count and the amount of fiber. Because fiber does not digest, you can subtract the grams of fiber (in the second column) from the total grams of carb (in the first column). Doing this is especially important if you use insulin-to-carb ratios in order to calculate a more accurate dose of insulin. (Check out Chapter 6 for more about these ratios.)

TIP

There may be variability in some ingredients used in the snack ideas, so when indicated, be sure to compare labels to verify pertinent nutrition information such as carbohydrates, fiber, fat, and calories.

Snack Ideas, Each with 0–10 Grams of Carb	Total Carb Grams	Fiber Grams	Calories
1 hard-boiled egg	0	0	78
1 ounce part-skim or reduced-fat string cheese	0.5	0	80
1 ounce fresh mozzarella cheese on 2 sliced tomatoes	2	1	82
½ teaspoon olive oil and fresh basil leaves	0	0	20
Total	**2**	**1**	**102**
½ cup 1 percent low-fat cottage cheese	3	0	80
25 pistachio nuts	4.8	1.8	100
20 raw pea pods (snow peas or sugar snap peas)	5.2	1.8	29
½ avocado, Hass-California type	5.8	4.6	114
1 tablespoon lemon juice	1	0	4
Total	**6.8**	**4.6**	**118**
6 ounces nonfat Greek yogurt (read labels)	7	0	100
3 ounces cooked shrimp	0	0	84
2 tablespoons cocktail sauce (read labels)	7.5	0.5	30
Total	**7.5**	**0.5**	**114**
1 stalk raw celery — 12 inches long	2.1	1	9
2 tablespoons natural peanut butter (no added sugars)	6	2	210
Total	**8.1**	**3**	**219**

(continued)

(continued)

Snack Ideas, Each with 0–10 Grams of Carb	Total Carb Grams	Fiber Grams	Calories
5 baby carrots, 1 cup raw veggies such as sliced bell peppers and celery	6	2	30
¼ cup light ranch salad dressing	3	0	80
Total	**9**	**2**	**110**
¼ cup canned pink salmon or tuna, drained	0	0	90
4 whole-wheat crackers (check labels)	9	0.5	48
Total	**9**	**0.5**	**138**
½ cup shelled cooked edamame (green soybeans)	**9**	**4**	**100**
2 cups microwave light-butter popcorn	**10**	**2**	**70**

Snack Ideas, Each with 10–20 Grams of Carb	Total Carb Grams	Fiber Grams	Calories
¼ cup hummus	8	2	140
10 baby carrots	4	1	20
Total	**12**	**3**	**160**
6 ounces nonfat yogurt; plain or sweetened with sugar substitute (read labels)	**13**	**0**	**95**
1 small apple (4 ounces — the size of a tennis ball)	14	2	60
1 ounce part-skim or reduced-fat string cheese	0.5	0	80
Total	**14.5**	**2**	**140**
3 cups of microwave light-butter popcorn	**15**	**3**	**105**
6 round crackers such as whole-wheat Ritz	13.2	1.2	84
¾ ounce slice of reduced fat cheese, cut in 6 pieces	1	0	70
2 large pitted olives, sliced	1	0	15
Assemble olives and cheese on crackers.			
Total	**15.2**	**1.2**	**169**

Snack Ideas, Each with 10–20 Grams of Carb	Total Carb Grams	Fiber Grams	Calories
1 medium orange	**15.4**	**3.1**	**62**
2 graham cracker squares (1 rectangular sheet)	12	0.5	65
1 tablespoon softened light cream cheese, blended with	1	0	35
1 teaspoon fruit preserves	3	0	12
Spread cream cheese and preserve mixture on crackers.			
Total	**16**	**0.5**	**112**
½ whole-grain English muffin, plain or toasted	12.5	0.5	60
1 tablespoon natural peanut butter (no added sugars)	3	1	105
Total	**16.5**	**1.5**	**155**
1 cup cubed cantaloupe	13.7	1.4	53
½ cup 1 percent low-fat cottage cheese	3	0	80
Total	**16.7**	**1.4**	**133**
2 rice cakes (4-inch diameter)	14	0	70
1 tablespoon almond butter	3	2	95
Total	**17**	**2**	**165**
½ cup marinated three-bean salad (read labels)	**18**	**3**	**80**
1 slice of whole-wheat bread (read labels)	18	2	90
Egg salad: 1 hard-boiled egg, 1 teaspoon mayo, minced celery/onion to taste	1	0	105
Total	**19**	**2**	**195**

Snack Ideas, Each with 20–30 Grams of Carb	Total Carb Grams	Fiber Grams	Calories
4 cups microwave light-butter popcorn	**20**	**4**	**140**
1 ounce baked tortilla chips	22	2	120
2 tablespoons guacamole	2	2	50
Total	**24**	**4**	**170**
6 ounces nonfat yogurt; plain or sweetened with sugar substitute (read labels)	13	0	95
¾ cup blackberries	11	5.7	46
Total	**24**	**5.7**	**141**
⅔ cup cooked mini pasta shells	23.4	1.4	120
1 tablespoon basil pesto sauce	1	0	70
Total	**24.4**	**1.4**	**190**
20 mini pretzels (1 ounce)	**25**	**0.5**	**110**
15 dry-roasted peanuts	3.2	1.2	88
1 ounce raisins (mini box)	22	2	90
Total	**25.2**	**3.2**	**178**
2 slices whole-grain "thin-sliced" bread	24	6	120
2 ounces sliced roasted turkey breast	0	0	60
1 teaspoon mustard, lettuce leaf, 2 slices tomato	2	1	11
Total	**26**	**7**	**191**
½ whole-wheat pita bread (1 ounce) filled with:	15	2	80
¼ cup hummus	8	2	140
4 cucumber slices, 2 tomato slices, lettuce leaf	3	2	15
Total	**26**	**6**	**235**
1 whole-wheat English muffin	23	3	120
2 tablespoons marinara sauce	2.5	0.5	15
1 ounce shredded part-skim mozzarella cheese	1	0	80
Spread sauce and sprinkle cheese on English muffin, and broil until bubbly.			
Total	**26.5**	**3.5**	**215**

Snack Ideas, Each with 20–30 Grams of Carb	Total Carb Grams	Fiber Grams	Calories
1 whole-wheat flour tortilla (8-inch size, read labels)	26	3	130
1 ounce 2 percent reduced-fat shredded cheese	1	0	80
2 tablespoons tomato salsa	3	1	10
Sprinkle tortilla with cheese; heat in oven at 350 degrees or heat in pan until cheese melts. Top with salsa.			
Total	**29**	**2**	**240**

Picking Packaged Snacks

When it comes to pre-packaged snack foods, picking wisely is critical. Read the Nutrition Facts food labels. Chapter 7 provides label-reading guidelines on how to identify portion sizes, calories, carbs, fiber, sugar, protein, fat, sodium, and cholesterol.

REMEMBER

Label claims on the front of the package don't always tell the truth, the whole truth, and nothing but the truth! An item that claims to be "carb smart" may end up being high in calories and fat. Something promoted as "low fat" may be a salty or sugary carb catastrophe. The front of the package is designed to hook you and reel you in. Check the Nutrition Facts label for *how much* you're going to be eating in terms of portion size and grams of carb. Consider other pertinent information such as calories, fiber, and fat. Read through the ingredients list to see *what* the product is made of.

One package isn't necessarily one portion. However, it can be more economical to buy in bulk. The down side of buying the larger container is that it may be harder to limit yourself to eating just one serving. Take, for example, a big bag of pita chips that says there are "seven servings per container." If you pop the bag open in the car and nibble while driving, it isn't hard to imagine that the bag could easily be empty by the time you arrive at your destination. One serving of pita chips isn't a bad choice at all. But seven servings of pita chips could end up being over 900 calories and more than 130 grams of carb. That's a problem.

TIP

If you buy packages that hold multiple servings, divvy up the container into separate portions and put individual servings into small zip-lock bags or appropriate reusable containers. Snacks will be ready to go and portion controlled. Anyone in the household can do this for the person with diabetes. When learning to count carbs, it helps to write the carb count in felt-tip marker on the zip-lock bag, or on a sticky note or label. After seeing the carb count for the portioned amount several times, everyone gets better at estimating carbs.

6

The Part of Tens

IN THIS PART . . .

Pick up a few pointers on blood-glucose monitoring.

Plan ahead and implement tips to solve carb conundrums.

Zero in on reputable online resources.

Chapter **23**

Ten Tips for Monitoring Your Blood Glucose

One of the most important advances in diabetes management came in the early 1980s: home blood-glucose monitors. These amazing devices provide critical information that can be used to drive management decisions, improve blood-glucose control, and reduce risks. Monitoring blood glucose reveals how diet, exercise, and medications influence glucose levels, enabling you to take action to avert dangerously high or low levels. In this chapter, I give you ten tips related to blood-glucose monitoring.

REMEMBER

Discovering that your numbers are out of range doesn't mean that you did something wrong or that you are a bad person. Try to have the mindset that all numbers are data and data is good. Don't personalize the numbers; use the data you collect to problem-solve and improve your future. Keep records and share them with your healthcare team, as data provides key details needed to fine-tune your care.

Picking a Meter for Your Needs

The first step in purchasing a blood-glucose monitor is to ask your insurance company which supplies it covers. Insurance companies often limit coverage to a couple of different meters. If your insurance plan covers more than one meter, you can ask your healthcare provider or local pharmacist for advice on which meter to pick. Some meter manufacturers keep the costs low enough to be affordable without insurance. Test strips end up being the biggest expense with any monitoring system.

Things to consider when picking a meter include the required blood sample size, ease of use, size of the meter, and size of the display screen. Most meters have a memory and store results. Some come with a USB port to download data so you can organize results and generate reports using software provided by the manufacturer. Certain meters have Bluetooth capability for wireless data transfer to an insulin pump or to an app. A few have bolus calculators to help with determining insulin doses. If you're visually impaired, choose a meter with a larger display screen or audio for spoken cues. If you do need a special meter due to loss of vision, ask your doctor to write a letter of necessity to your insurance company. A couple of meters have the ability to check blood-ketone levels. People with type 1 diabetes need to be able to check ketone levels, but this can be done with urine ketone test strips or a meter that checks blood-ketone levels.

REMEMBER

Refer to the instructions that come with the meter if you get an error message, have trouble using your meter, or need to set the time and date. Most companies provide a phone number for technical support. Your local pharmacist may be able to show you how to use your meter if you ask.

Safely Obtaining a Blood Sample

WARNING

Your hands need to be clean and dry before you obtain a drop of blood. Soiled hands lead to inaccurate readings. A common source of error is the residue from handling carbohydrate-containing foods. Touching fruit or eating finger foods can leave residue on your skin. When you prick your finger, the drop of blood picks up the sugar and your meter reads it as extra glucose. Don't forget to wash your hands before checking your blood glucose, especially if you've previously peeled a banana or an orange! If you aren't near a sink, you can use alcohol gel or swabs, but make sure your finger is completely dry before you poke it.

Lancing devices have adjustable depths. To decrease discomfort, set the device at the gentlest depth that still provides an adequate sample. Fewer nerves are on the sides of the fingertips, so try poking there rather than on the pads. It's all in how you squeeze too. When obtaining a sample from your fingertip, squeeze from below with the opposite hand and apply pressure while sliding up toward the fingertip. If the drop of blood is too small, you will get an error message, so make sure it is adequate before applying it to the test strip.

It goes without saying that you should never share your lancing device with anyone else.

Acknowledging Error Issues

Home blood-glucose readings are not exact. You're unlikely to get an identical reading even if you check on the same finger within seconds of a prior check. Regulations require meters to provide results that are accurate within a plus or minus 20 percent margin of error. However, many are accurate to within 10–15 percent. Regulations are more stringent for accuracy in low ranges, with readings below 75 milligrams per deciliter (mg/dl) required to be accurate to within plus or minus 15 mg/dl. If you question the accuracy of your meter or strips, run a test using control solution, which can be obtained from the manufacturer.

Some blood disorders, such as sickle cell anemia, can lead to erroneous results. High altitudes and low temperatures can also alter accuracy, so checking blood glucose outdoors while skiing is a bit tricky. Light and humidity can affect test strips too, so keep strips in their original container with the lid closed. Review the meter manual for error messages and variables affecting reliability.

Assuring as Much Accuracy as Possible

Test strips have an expiration date, which is printed on the container. Don't use expired strips. Strips need to be carried in their original container and stored away from heat, light, and moisture. Don't store your supplies in a steamy bathroom.

Some meters have test strips that allow for alternate site testing, which means you can obtain the drop of blood from your arm or hand rather than your fingertip. The blood sample from the arm is not as accurate as the blood obtained from the fingertip because blood flow to the surface of the arm is delayed in comparison to perfusion of the fingertips. When blood-glucose levels are in flux, such as when they're rising after a meal or dropping after exercise, you should use your fingertips. This is especially important if you suspect low blood glucose or are rechecking levels after treating hypoglycemia.

Bring your meter with you to all medical visits. Your healthcare provider can observe your technique and offer suggestions as needed. Use your monitor to check blood glucose at the same time you have blood drawn at a lab, and then compare results to see how your meter measures up to the lab's standard.

Disposing of Lancets and Needles Properly

WARNING

Lancet companies recommend that you put in a new lancet each time you check your blood glucose. Most people reuse lancets several times before changing them. Lancets that are overused can become dull, bent, and hurt more. Used lancets, pen needles, and syringes are considered biohazards. They all need to be disposed of properly in a sharps container. If you typically collect sharps in a plastic jug or jar, don't dispose of that in the garbage can or recycle bin. Used needles can't go in the regular garbage because they carry the risk of transmitting serious diseases. Recapping needles or lancets is not good enough. Caps can be dislodged, and workers in the waste disposal industry could be accidentally poked. Call your waste disposal company and find out how to properly dispose of sharps in your community.

TIP

Ask your local pharmacy for a sharps container for home use. Insurance may cover the cost, but if it doesn't, containers are fairly inexpensive. Some cities have a needle exchange program whereby they offer free sharps containers and take them back when they're full.

Varying Your Test Times

How often you should monitor your blood glucose depends on your type of diabetes, current level of control, health history, medications, and risk of high or low blood glucose:

>> If you have well-controlled type 2 diabetes and no risk for hypoglycemia, you may check only several times per week.

>> If you usually check once or twice daily and typically at the same time of day, such as fasting or pre-dinner, then you know results only for those specific times of day. Mix it up a bit to find out what is going on at other times. Rotate when you check to capture data about blood-glucose patterns before meals, after meals, at bedtime, and overnight.

>> Periodically check before and after the same meal to see how certain foods affect your levels.

>> If you have type 1 diabetes, it is important to check more often. Pre-meal glucose checks provide info needed for making insulin dose decisions. Other times to check include before driving; when you suspect or treat hypoglycemia; before, during, or after exercise as needed; before bed; during illness; or anytime you think you need to.

Knowing Your Blood-Glucose Targets

Speak to your healthcare team about your blood glucose (BG) target ranges for fasting, pre-meal, one to two hours after a meal, before exercise, and before bed. Goals depend upon whether or not you are at risk for hypoglycemia. Targets also depend on age and complexities of other health conditions. Here are some general guidelines:

>> Fasting BG under 115 mg/dl and post-meal BG below 160 mg/dl may be appropriate targets for someone with type 2 diabetes who is not at risk for hypoglycemia.

>> Insulin users are at risk of hypoglycemia, so fasting and pre-meal BG targets are generally 80–130 mg/dl, and post-meal targets are generally below 180 mg/dl. Clarify with your doctor.

>> Pregnancy requires tighter control, so women with gestational diabetes typically aim for fasting BG below 95 mg/dl and one hour post-meal BG below 140 mg/dl.

TIP

The United States uses milligrams per deciliter (mg/dl) when assessing blood-glucose levels. If you reside elsewhere and prefer to think in millimoles per liter (mmols/L), simply divide mg/dl by 18.

Keeping a Log and Reviewing Your Data

Just like a detective needs clues to crack a case, you and your healthcare team need blood-glucose data to figure out how to best manage your diabetes. Doctors aren't magicians who can conjure up an effective medication plan just by looking at you. They need clues. The more clues, the better.

Record your blood-glucose results in a logbook and write the numbers in the column that corresponds to whether the reading was before or after a meal, before or after exercise, before bed, or in the middle of the night. If you count carbs, jot down how many grams you ate. If you took insulin, note how many units you took. Details about your day provide clues to the cause and effect of different variables. Note the time and duration of exercise. If you were hypoglycemic, list how many grams of carb you took to treat it. Recheck glucose levels 15 minutes after treating a low to confirm that blood-glucose levels have returned to a safe level.

TIP

Some meter companies have software for downloading and organizing blood-glucose data. Find out whether your clinic has the capacity to download your meter, or call the meter manufacturer and ask about getting the software for yourself. You can generate and print logs to bring to your medical visits so your healthcare team can use that information to guide you.

TIP

If you don't typically keep written logs, do so for least a couple of weeks prior to each medical visit. Recent data allows your doctor to make appropriate intervention suggestions.

Getting Your A1C Done Regularly

The A1C lab test provides details about your "average" blood-glucose control over the past three-month period. Glucose and red blood cells travel together side by side through the same vessels to deliver fuel and oxygen. Glucose can attach itself to blood cells and other proteins in the body. The A1C test measures how much glucose has attached to the hemoglobin protein in the red blood cells in the previous three months. The significance is that glucose may be attaching at similar levels to other places in your body, such as your eyes, nerves, and kidneys, which can lead to complications.

Ask your doctor about the best target level for you. The typical A1C targets for people with diabetes are as follows:

>> **For most non-pregnant adults:** Below 7

>> **For most kids and teens:** Below 7.5

>> **For some medically complex patients:** Below 8

The A1C test is also used to diagnose diabetes. Results are determined as follows:

>> **Normal:** Less than 5.7

>> **Pre-diabetes:** 5.7–6.4

>> **Diabetes:** 6.5 or higher

Understanding how A1C numbers correlate to blood glucose is helpful in interpreting your results and seeing where you stand. Table 23-1 shows the estimated average glucose level over the previous three-month period based on A1C.

TABLE 23-1

A1C and Estimated Average Glucose

A1C	Estimated Average Glucose in mg/dl
5	97
5.5	111
6	126
6.5	140
7	154
7.5	169
8	183
8.5	197
9	212
9.5	226
10	240
10.5	255
11	269
11.5	283
12	298
12.5	312
13	326
13.5	341
14	355

Aim to get your A1C checked every three months. You don't need to be fasting for this test.

WARNING

Having your A1C checked doesn't replace the need for using your home glucose monitor. Even if your A1C is in the "target range," you may still have very high blood-glucose levels and very low blood-glucose levels that end up averaging out.

Considering Continuous Glucose Monitoring

A continuous glucose monitor (CGM) is a device that checks blood-glucose levels approximately every five minutes. A water-resistant sensor is inserted under the skin and remains in place for six to seven days, depending on the brand. Blood-glucose readings are transmitted wirelessly to a receiver or to an insulin pump. The display screen on the receiver or the pump shows blood-glucose values and also indicates trend lines predictive of the direction the blood glucose is headed as well as the rate of change. You can see whether your blood glucose is stable, rising, or falling and how fast.

One brand sends glucose data wirelessly to a compatible smart device, and the data can be shared in real time with caregivers, family, or medical providers. Other brands are compatible with specific insulin pumps. Certain pumps automatically suspend insulin delivery for two hours if blood-glucose values drop below a preset low threshold.

The benefits of CGM include alarms that can be set at lower and higher ranges to audibly warn you that your blood glucose is heading out of bounds. You are then able to respond and adjust food or insulin to rectify the problem. Data can be downloaded to the computer and reports can be generated that you can review with your diabetes specialist. Daily data lines can be superimposed one over the other, and the results can uncover trends that can be used to adjust insulin regimens or drive management decisions related to diet and exercise. You still need to check blood-glucose levels with a traditional monitor to calibrate the CGM and to confirm blood-glucose levels when making insulin dosing decisions.

WARNING

The CGM device and ongoing supplies are expensive. Check with your insurance company to see whether you qualify for coverage.

Chapter **24**

Ten Tips for Controlling Carbs

Controlling blood-glucose levels requires having a handle on carb intake. It helps to problem-solve situations in advance and go into the day with a plan for how to best manage meals and snacks. The tips in this chapter may help you strategize.

Saving a Step with a Measuring Cup

Measuring cups can be used to dish up a serving from the stovetop to your plate. The stackable versions come in various portion sizes. Scoop up the desired amount of food with the appropriate cup, level off the top, and put it on your plate. Precision at home also trains your eye so you can be a better guesser when it isn't possible to measure, such as in a restaurant.

TIP

If you frequently have rice at home, buy a rice bowl that holds an appropriate amount, such as a cup. If you fill it to the correct level (not mounded), you automatically know you are having a cup each time you eat from that bowl. Use a measuring cup to find out how much your cereal bowls, cups, and glasses hold. Then whenever you use those dishes, your portion will be a known quantity. If you have a hard time controlling how much fruit you consume in one sitting, purchase a bowl that holds one cup and use it to regulate fruit servings. Use a small, festive-looking dish that holds a half cup for pudding or ice cream. Let's face it — the tendency is to fill up any dish. A smaller dish that looks full is psychologically more satisfying than a big dish that looks half empty.

Check out Chapter 8 for more tips on using weights and measures to count carbs.

Weighing Fruits in Advance

The Exchange Lists (see Appendix A) say a small apple or a medium peach each count as one fruit exchange equaling 15 grams of carb. Estimating is okay, especially if you have type 2 diabetes; just keep in mind that a small fruit is the size of a tennis ball and a medium fruit is the size of a baseball.

If you have type 1 diabetes, it pays to weigh. At least weigh enough examples to hone your eyeballing skills. If you weigh a few bananas, you'll be able to estimate more accurately in the future. I'm going to walk you through an example, and I agree it seems tedious, but it isn't as tough as it sounds. You'll need a food scale (some models cost under $10). Multiple apps and websites provide nutrient details for foods by weight. I use Calorie King for this example, as it is easily accessible online (www.calorieking.com) or via their app (see Chapter 9 for more about Calorie King).

Once you access Calorie King, use the search box to look up "apple." Then click on "Apples, with Skin, raw." The default size displayed says "extra small [4 oz. with refuse, 2.5" dia] (3.6 oz)." Scroll to change the measurement; choose "oz (1 oz)." Next, weigh your apple on your food scale. Say it weighs 6.5 ounces. You type the actual weight into the serving size box on the app. Calorie King does the math for a 6.5-ounce apple and displays the result in the familiar Nutrition Facts food label format. In this example, the Total Carbohydrate is 25.4 grams and the fiber is 4.4 grams. You can subtract the fiber because it doesn't digest. The revised count is 21 grams of carb.

Once you are set up with a food scale, weigh all the fruits in your fruit bowl. Use a permanent marker to write the number of grams of carb directly onto the banana peel or orange peel, or onto a sticker if the fruit has an edible skin. Later in the week when you grab a piece of fruit, the carb count is already done. Periodic use of a food scale hones your ability to be a better guesser. This is also something family members can do for the person with diabetes to help out with carb counting. See Chapter 8 for more information on using a food scale.

Another reliable nutrient database can be found in the USDA Food Composition Databases at https://ndb.nal.usda.gov/. They provide the details per 100 grams of the food's weight. When converting the weight of your food, keep in mind that there are 28 grams to an ounce.

Having a Carb-Counting Contest

When a child, teen, or young adult has diabetes, transferring the carb-counting skill set from adult to offspring is a worthwhile teaching process. Otherwise, when kids take off for college and parental support isn't readily available, they may be in for a rude awakening.

One strategy to get everyone involved in carb counting is to make a game out of it. Why not have a carb-counting contest? For example, each person at the family meal serves up his own starch portion such as pasta or rice, and then everyone eyeballs his plate and announces his guess. After all estimates are announced, the carb foods are scooped into a measuring cup to assess the actual carb count. Set up a reward in advance, such as "Whoever guesses closest doesn't have to do the dishes or take out the garbage." I'll tell you what; everyone improves carb-counting skills real fast.

Making Better Breakfast Choices

Start your day right by choosing wisely for the morning meal. Steer clear of breakfast options that are loaded with sugar and fat. Try the following ideas (and see Chapter 19 for some breakfast menus):

>> Check Nutrition Facts labels on cereal boxes (see Chapter 7 for help) and choose brands with less sugar. Deep down inside I think most of us realize that a neon-colored cereal probably isn't the best choice. Try to limit the sugar in cereal to less than 6 grams per serving (the lower the better). Choose cereals with 3 or more grams of fiber.

>> Opt for the oats you cook yourself rather than the instant varieties, but if you do buy instant, choose plain instead of sweetened.

>> Skip the Danish, sticky buns, and anything frosted. Try whole-grain toast with jam instead.

>> Have a carton of yogurt; compare labels to assess carb counts, fat content, and calories.

>> Whole-grain toaster waffles aren't bad, but skip the syrup. There are nearly 60 grams of sugar per ¼ cup of syrup. You can limit the carbs in the toppings to 15 grams or less if you top waffles or pancakes with ½ cup of applesauce or yogurt, or a cup of strawberries and a little whipped topping.

>> As for the meats, limit bacon and sausage, which are full of saturated fat, and choose lean ham, Canadian bacon, or vegetarian links instead.

>> Replace juices and smoothies with a cup of fresh fruit. Sweeten coffee and tea with a nonnutritive sweetener rather than sugar.

Packing Your Own Lunch

Packing your own lunch from home to bring to work or school makes it so much easier to control your carb intake. You can measure it all out at home and count carbs precisely. Use ice packs for perishable foods and keep hot foods hot in a thermos. If you want to keep it easy, check your local supermarket for prepared salads, or healthy fresh or frozen meals that can be microwaved (many have Nutrition Facts labels). Head to Chapter 20 for a number of lunch menu ideas.

Choosing Wisely at the Deli

Perhaps you want to grab lunch at your local deli. No problem! Here are some tips for eating at the deli while watching your carb intake:

>> Delis have food scales. Ask them to weigh your roll before making your sandwich. Bread has about 14 grams of carb per ounce. Many deli-sized rolls used for sandwiches weigh about 4 ounces, which would count as 56 grams of carb (14 grams of carb multiplied by 4).

>> The meat, cheese, mustard, mayo, and crunchy veggies don't really contribute much carb. Skip fatty meats like salami and bacon and choose chicken, turkey, ham, or lean roast beef. Or make it a veggie sandwich with avocado.

>> If you find yourself reaching for a bag of chips, opt for a small bag of baked chips. If you want a side dish, consider a green salad or a piece of fresh fruit.

>> Choose diet drinks or unsweetened iced tea rather than sugary beverages.

Considering the Condiments

All too often the carb content of condiments and sauces is ignored when it should be counted. While a swipe of ketchup across a bun is insignificant, having ¼ cup of ketchup with your fries is not; it contributes about 15 grams of carb. Two table-spoons of barbeque sauce can pack in 20–25 grams of carb. Don't forget to count the spaghetti sauce; it varies, but has roughly 15 grams of carb per ½ cup.

REMEMBER

When using insulin-to-carb ratios (see Chapter 6), you should be as accurate as possible with your carb counting; otherwise, your dose may be incorrect. Nothing is as frustrating as doing 95 percent of the work and not achieving the blood-glucose result you were hoping for. Don't be sabotaged by the sauces! Check the Nutrition Facts food labels or use your computer's search engine to do a search for the carb count. You can also download an app that provides carb counts so you can make an educated guess. (Check out Chapter 9 for more about online resources and apps. See Chapter 8 for tips on creating a carb-counting cheat sheet where you can keep track of the carbs in sauces for future reference.)

Fitting in a Favorite Dessert

Sugar-free gelatin is a freebie that you can have anytime you want. Add a dollop of whipped topping and decorate with a sliced strawberry if desired. There are other desserts that may satisfy your sweet tooth with just 15 grams of carb or less. Read labels on packaged puddings, cookies, and frozen desserts. The trick is to limit yourself to a small serving and not go back for more.

REMEMBER

On special occasions, you may want something more carb intense. If you know you want to fit in a dessert with 30–45 grams of carb, it makes sense to have it after a low-carb meal. Tolerating a small piece of cake is much easier after a meal that's low in carbs such as a chicken Caesar salad or a couple of tacos. Controlling blood-glucose levels is not so easy if you have tiramisu after a plate of pasta and garlic bread. If chocolate is calling your name, limit yourself to just one or two pieces from the box of chocolates, or buy the fun-size treats and don't go back for seconds. See Chapter 13 for more tips on fitting in reasonable desserts.

Planning and Portioning Snacks

If you don't pre-plan snacks and bring appropriate options with you, you place yourself at the mercy of whatever you can grab while you're out. Snacks can end up being too high in calories, carbs, fat, and sodium if you aren't careful. Finding a healthy snack isn't always easy when you're choosing from vending machines, convenience stores, and coffee shops.

TIP

Some snack foods come in single-serve packages, such as small packets of almonds, mini boxes of raisins, or individual bags of baked chips. Buying family-sized bags offers cost-savings benefits. The downside is that it may be hard to control how much you end up eating, especially if you're snacking directly from the bag. Use small zip-lock baggies to separate the multi-serve packages into single servings. Use a permanent marker to write the carb count on each baggie. Pack your pantry with pre-portioned snacks. Keep carrots, other raw vegetables, and fruits handy for snacking. Other items you can bring with you include yogurt, string cheese, hard-boiled eggs, and crackers. Flip to Chapter 22 for more snack ideas.

Curbing Late-Night Snacking

WARNING

Late dinners and evening snacking can raise blood-glucose levels unless you walk it off or fit in some exercise. Glucose levels may remain elevated throughout the evening and even overnight and into the next day. Evenings are often times of relaxation. Snacking in front of the television or simply out of boredom can derail diabetes and weight-control efforts.

Eat dinner at least three to four hours before going to bed and limit evening snacking to something small. Popcorn isn't a bad choice. A three-cup portion has only 15 grams of carb.

Chapter **25**

Ten Worthwhile Websites to Help You Manage Diabetes

S ifting through the vast amount of information about diabetes available on the Internet can be hard. The first step is finding reputable resources. The ten websites in this chapter are especially relevant to managing diabetes and related health conditions.

American Diabetes Association

www.diabetes.org

The mission of the American Diabetes Association (ADA) is to prevent and cure diabetes and to improve the lives of all people affected by diabetes. The website is an amazing resource. You'll find countless links that delve into every aspect of diabetes, from getting a grasp of the basics at diagnosis to managing food, fitness, and medications as well as keeping abreast of the latest research and diabetes events.

TECHNICAL STUFF

If you want to go deeper and can handle the medical jargon, you can find a wealth of information in the Professional section. Click the "Diabetes Pro" tab and check out the Standards of Care to read the annually updated, evidenced-based diabetes management guidelines published in the January edition of the journal *Diabetes Care*.

American Association of Diabetes Educators

www.diabeteseducator.org

Certified Diabetes Educators (CDEs) are trained experts that can help you learn to manage your diabetes. Their organization — the American Association of Diabetes Educators (AADE) — has a website dedicated to diabetes education. From the home page, navigate to the "Patient Resources" tab because most of the rest of the site is geared toward healthcare providers.

Under the Patient Resources tab, you will find valuable information related to seven key areas (click on "AADE7 Self-Care Behaviors"): healthy eating, being active, monitoring blood glucose, taking medications, problem-solving, reducing risks, and healthy coping. Information is available in English and Spanish as printable handouts. Several audio files are provided for the visually impaired. Check out the Diabetes Goal Tracker Mobile App (also under the "Patient Resources" tab), which you can download for free. You can also search for accredited diabetes education programs in your area.

Academy of Nutrition and Dietetics

www.eatright.org

If you want nutrition information, seek out the experts. The Academy of Nutrition and Dietetics (AND) is the world's largest organization of food and nutrition professionals. Their website provides sound nutritional advice with sections geared to the particular needs of kids, parents, men, women, and seniors. If you want information on the hottest nutrition topics or the nuts and bolts of eating a balanced diet, you'll find it here. There are countless articles, recipes, and interesting videos. You can search for a registered dietitian (RD) in your area; just provide your zip code.

There is also a section geared toward nutrition professionals, but you can access it from the home page by clicking on the "eatright PRO" tab. Type "position papers" in the search box to link to nutrition information that is based in science rather than hearsay. Read about nonnutritive sweeteners; functional foods; fiber; vegetarian diets; exercise; and nutrition for pregnancy, children, older adults, and much more.

U.S. Food and Drug Administration

www.fda.gov

The site of the U.S. Food and Drug Administration (FDA) has an overwhelming amount of information and a broad range of topics. From the home page, click the "Food" tab. You will find links to navigate to information on ingredients, packaging, food labeling, food safety, and emergency preparedness. Check out the link called "Resources for You" and then click the "Consumers" link. From there you can click on "Education Resource Library" or "Food Facts for Consumers." Resources include nutritional information on fruits, vegetables, and more. Get up-to-date on the latest hot topics including genetically modified foods and dietary supplements. The website also provides tabs linking you to information on drugs and medical devices.

American Heart Association

www.heart.org

The website of the American Heart Association (AHA) provides relevant information for improving heart health. Diabetes is a risk factor for heart disease, so an entire section is devoted to diabetes management strategies. Click on the "Conditions" tab and then "More"; then click on "Diabetes" under the heading "Cardiovascular Conditions" along the right side of the page. If you have problems with your cholesterol or you have high blood pressure (hypertension), you can click on links to those conditions too.

The "Healthy Living" tab on the home page is also worth investigating. You'll find tips for good nutrition and a collection of recipes. Physical activity and stress management strategies are also addressed.

UCSF Diabetes Education Online

https://dtc.ucsf.edu/

The Diabetes Teaching Center at the University of California San Francisco Medical Center has been dedicated to providing diabetes self-care education workshops since 1977. This accredited program is a true pioneer in providing education to assist clients in understanding how to self-manage their diabetes.

The award-winning Diabetes Education Online website was developed in an effort to reach and educate as many people as possible. Chinese and Spanish translations are available. Whether you are newly diagnosed and don't know where to begin or you've had diabetes for many years, this site has in-depth information for everyone and is easy to navigate. Follow links to discover more about living with and managing your diabetes. Be sure to visit the Learning Library to view videos and download educational materials.

Mayo Clinic

www.mayoclinic.org

The Mayo Clinic has locations in Minnesota, Arizona, and Florida. Their informative website is far reaching. From the home page, click the link to "Patient Care and Health Info." Choose from the following options: symptoms, diseases and conditions, tests and procedures, and drugs and supplements. From there, choose the letter of the alphabet that corresponds to your inquiry. Click "D" and scroll to diabetes, or "T" and scroll to Type 1 or Type 2 diabetes.

Joslin Diabetes Center

www.joslin.org

The Joslin Diabetes Center in Boston, Massachusetts, is internationally recognized for their efforts and advances in diabetes treatment, education, and research. Their website provides information to help you understand and manage your diabetes.

The "Managing Diabetes" tab under "Diabetes Information" is a great place to start. Scroll through their abundant list of links to access information pertinent to you. They also have a section devoted to addressing the unique needs of children with diabetes.

TIP

Registration is free if you would like to access their Learning Center to take advantage of their online diabetes courses. Several of the classes utilize sound and animation. From the home page, click on the "Diabetes Information" tab and then the "Online Diabetes Classes" tab.

U.S. Department of Agriculture Food Composition Databases

https://ndb.nal.usda.gov/

The USDA's Food Composition Databases website is the go-to site if you want to find out nutrition information details on just about any food. Search for the food after clicking "Start your search here." Be very specific; for example, specify cooked or raw. A search for boiled potatoes generates a list of ten choices. Click on the appropriate option (such as boiled without skin and without salt). In this example, you can indicate the portion size by weight or measuring cup, or you can pick from small, medium, or large. Search results will provide the nutrient info to the umpteenth detail: carbs, fiber, protein, vitamins, minerals, caffeine, and even specific types of fat: monounsaturated, polyunsaturated, or saturated.

WebMD

www.webMD.com

WebMD compiles credible news, reference materials, and advice from over 100 doctors and health experts nationwide. The website provides easy-to-understand explanations on health conditions, which can be accessed in their "Health A-Z" compilation. The "Living Healthy" tab provides tips on food and fitness. Under "Popular Tools" on the "Living Healthy" page, you can also access a "Food and Fitness" planner section. Calculate your BMI and calorie needs. Log your foods and activity and track your progress. You can even monitor calories and carbs. The "Portion Size Plate Tool" on the "Living Healthy" page has pictures that help you visualize and estimate serving sizes.

7

Appendixes

Use Exchange Lists to count your carbs.

Make the most out of measuring by identifying conversions for weights and volumes.

Appendix A

Diabetes Exchange Lists

Diabetes Exchange Lists were originally developed as a menu planning tool. Foods are grouped by their nutritional composition into various Exchange Lists. The exchange concept means you can exchange any food within a given list for any other food in that same list. Each item on the list has a similar amount of carbohydrate, protein, fat, and calories.

TECHNICAL STUFF

For many years dietitians provided set meal plans based on various calorie levels. People with diabetes were instructed to choose a certain number of exchanges from the food groups. For example, the plan for lunch might call for two starch exchanges, one fruit exchange, two nonstarchy vegetable exchanges, three lean meat exchanges, and one fat exchange. On the plus side, the meal plans encouraged a variety of foods from the various groups. Another benefit of following the meal plans precisely was that the calorie intake was controlled. But many people found these plans to be cumbersome and confusing, and compliance wasn't that great. Not many people could be that regimented from one day to the next.

Nowadays, the Exchange Lists can be used for a wide variety of purposes. The starch, fruit, milk, and vegetable lists are used for counting carbs. The lists can also be used to count calories. Meats are separated into lean, medium-fat, and high-fat selections, making it easier to choose wisely. Fats are separated into monounsaturated (the heart healthiest), polyunsaturated (the next best thing), and saturated (limited intake suggested).

TIP

You may actually eat more than the exchange portion shown on the list. For example, the starch exchange list indicates that the serving size of rice is ⅓ cup cooked. That doesn't mean that you're allowed to eat only ⅓ cup of rice at a time. It just means that ⅓ cup of rice counts as "one starch exchange," which is 80 calories, 15 grams of carb, 3 grams of protein, and 0–1 gram of fat. If you eat one full cup of cooked rice, that counts as 45 grams of carb, or three starch exchanges.

As you familiarize yourself with the lists in this appendix, you will notice that starchy vegetables and the dried bean family are housed in the starch exchange list, not the vegetable list. Some veggies, such as potatoes, have carb counts similar to grains, while others, such as broccoli, are far lower in carb, so they are on different lists. Not all dairy products are the same, either. Milk and yogurt have carbohydrate, but cheese and butter don't. Cheese is listed with the meats, and butter is in the saturated fats list. Avocados and nuts are also in the fat group.

REMEMBER Spend some time looking through the lists to identify foods that you typically eat. When counting carbs, use standardized measuring cups to ensure accuracy (see Chapter 8 for more information and Appendix B for measurement conversion tables).

Starches

The starch list includes breads, grains, tortillas, rice, noodles, starchy vegetables, and legumes (dried beans). Each item in the starch list contains approximately 15 grams carbohydrate, 3 grams protein, 0–1 gram fat, and 80 calories. (The foods in the Legumes section provide 7 grams of protein in addition to 15 grams of carbohydrate.) Table A-1 shows starch exchange serving sizes.

TABLE A-1 **Starches**

Type	Food	Portion Size
Breads		
	Bagel, large (4 ounces)	¼ bagel (1 ounce)
	Biscuit (2½ inches across)	1
	Bread	1 slice (1 ounce)
	Bread (reduced calorie)	2 slices (1½ ounces)
	Bun (hamburger or hot dog)	½ bun (1 ounce)
	Challah	1 slice (1 ounce)
	Chapati (6 inches across)	1 (1½ ounces)
	Cornbread (2-inch cube)	1 (1½ ounces)
	English muffin	½ muffin (1 ounce)
	Pancake (4 inches across by ¼ inch thick)	1 pancake
	Pita bread (6 inches across)	½ pita
	Roll, small	1 (1 ounce)
	Stuffing, prepared	⅓ cup
	Tortilla (6 inches across, corn or flour)	1 tortilla
	Tortilla, large (10 inches across)	⅓ tortilla

Type	Food	Portion Size
Rice, noodles, and grains		
	Amaranth, cooked	1/3 cup
	Arrowroot, dry	2 tablespoons
	Barley, cooked	1/3 cup
	Buckwheat groats, cooked	1/2 cup
	Bulgur wheat, cooked	1/2 cup
	Cornstarch, dry	2 tablespoons
	Couscous, cooked	1/3 cup
	Farro, cooked	1/3 cup
	Flour (wheat, dry)	3 tablespoons
	Grits, cooked	1/2 cup
	Kasha, cooked	1/2 cup
	Maize, cooked	2 tablespoons
	Matzo meal, dry	2½ tablespoons
	Millet, cooked	1/3 cup
	Oatmeal, cooked	1/2 cup
	Pasta or noodles, cooked	1/3 cup
	Polenta, cooked	1/3 cup
	Popcorn	3 cups (popped)
	Quinoa, cooked	1/3 cup
	Rice, cooked, brown or white	1/3 cup
	Sorghum, cooked	1/3 cup
	Tabbouleh, prepared	1/2 cup
	Teff, cooked	1/3 cup
	Wild rice, cooked	1/2 cup

(continued)

Type	Food	Portion Size
Starchy vegetables		
	Cassava	⅓ cup
	Corn	½ cup
	Corn on the cob, large	½ cob (5 ounces)
	Hominy, canned	¾ cup
	Parsnips	½ cup
	Peas, green	½ cup
	Plantain, cooked	⅓ cup
	Potato, baked, with skin	1 small (3 ounces)
	Potato, boiled, mashed	½ cup (3 ounces)
	Pumpkin, canned	1 cup
	Squash, acorn or butternut	1 cup
	Succotash	½ cup
	Yam or sweet potato, plain	½ cup
	Yucca, cooked	¼ cup
Legumes		
	Baked beans	⅓ cup
	Beans: black, garbanzo, kidney, lima, navy, pinto, white (cooked)	½ cup
	Lentils, cooked	½ cup
	Peas: black-eyed, split-peas (cooked)	½ cup
	Refried beans, canned	½ cup

Fruits

Each item in the fruit list contains approximately 15 grams carbohydrate, 0 grams protein, 0 grams fat, and 60 calories. Table A-2 shows fruit exchange serving sizes.

TABLE A-2   **Fruits**

Type	Food	Portion Size
Fresh		
	Apple, small, 2 inches across	1 (4 ounces)
	Apricots	4 (5½ ounces)
	Banana, extra small, ½ large	1 (4 ounces)
	Blackberries, blueberries	¾ cup
	Cherries	12 (3 ounces)
	Figs, fresh, medium	2 (3½ ounces)
	Grapefruit, large	½ (11 ounces)
	Grapes, small	17 (3 ounces)
	Kiwi	1 (3½ ounces)
	Mango, cubed	½ cup
	Melon: cantaloupe, honeydew, cubed	1 cup
	Nectarine, small	1 (5 ounces)
	Orange, small	1 (6½ ounces)
	Papaya, cubed	1 cup
	Peach, medium	1 (6 ounces)
	Pear, large	½ (4 ounces)
	Persimmon (2½ inches across)	½
	Pineapple, cubed	¾ cup
	Plums, small	2 (5 ounces)
	Raspberries	1 cup
	Strawberries	1¼ cups
	Watermelon, cubed	1¼ cups (13½ ounces)
Dried fruit		
	Apples	4 rings (1 ounce)
	Apricots	8 halves (1 ounce)
	Dates, small	3 (1 ounce, including pits)

(continued)

TABLE A-2 *(continued)*

Type	Food	Portion Size
	Dried fruits (blueberries, cherries, cranberries, and mixed fruits)	2 tablespoons (¾ ounce)
	Figs	3 (1 ounce)
	Prunes	3 (1 ounce)
	Raisins	2 tablespoons (¾ ounce)
Canned fruit, unsweetened		
	Applesauce, unsweetened	½ cup
	Fruit cocktail	½ cup
	Grapefruit sections	¾ cup
	Mandarin oranges	¾ cup
	Peaches	½ cup
	Pears	½ cup
Fruit juice		
	Unsweetened apple, grapefruit, orange, pineapple	½ cup
	Fruit juice blends of 100% juice, grape, prune	⅓ cup

Milk and Yogurt

Each item in the milk and yogurt list contains approximately 12 grams carbohydrate and 8 grams protein. Fat content and calories vary:

Type of Milk	Fat (Grams)	Calories
Nonfat, 1 percent	0–3	100
Reduced fat, 2 percent	5	120
Whole	8	160

Table A-3 shows exchange serving sizes for milk and yogurt. Chapter 12 has the scoop on nonnutritive sweeteners that you may find in yogurts. For soy milk, rice milk, almond milk, and all other milk substitutes, read the Nutrition Facts food labels as products vary (see Chapter 7 if you need guidance).

TABLE A-3　　**Milk and Yogurt**

Type	Food	Portion Size
Nonfat, skim, and low-fat milk and yogurt		
	Buttermilk	1 cup
	Evaporated skim milk	½ cup
	Milk, nonfat, skim, or 1%	1 cup
	Yogurt, nonfat or 1%, plain or flavored with a nonnutritive sweetener	⅔ cup
Reduced-fat milk and yogurt		
	Milk, 2%	1 cup
	Yogurt, 2%, plain or flavored with a nonnutritive sweetener	⅔ cup
Whole milk and yogurt		
	Evaporated whole milk	½ cup
	Milk, whole	1 cup
	Yogurt, plain, whole	1 cup

Nonstarchy Vegetables

As I mention earlier in this appendix, some vegetables (including potatoes, corn, peas, and legumes) are similar to starches in terms of carbohydrate counts, so you will find them grouped on the starch list. Each item in the following nonstarchy vegetable list contains approximately 5 grams carbohydrate, 2 grams protein, 0 grams fat, and 25 calories:

- » Amaranth
- » Artichoke
- » Asparagus
- » Baby corn
- » Bamboo shoots
- » Bean sprouts
- » Beets
- » Bitter melon

- » Bok choy
- » Broccoli
- » Brussels sprouts
- » Cabbage
- » Carrots
- » Cauliflower
- » Celery
- » Chayote

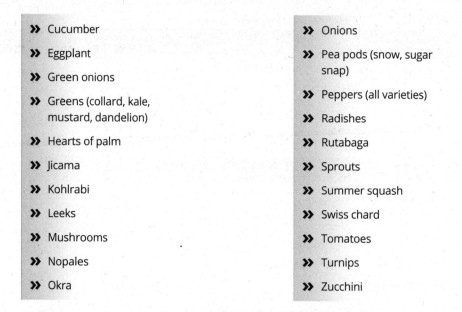

» Cucumber	» Onions
» Eggplant	» Pea pods (snow, sugar snap)
» Green onions	» Peppers (all varieties)
» Greens (collard, kale, mustard, dandelion)	» Radishes
» Hearts of palm	» Rutabaga
» Jicama	» Sprouts
» Kohlrabi	» Summer squash
» Leeks	» Swiss chard
» Mushrooms	» Tomatoes
» Nopales	» Turnips
» Okra	» Zucchini

TIP

Salad greens such as arugula, chicory, endive, escarole, lettuce, radicchio, spinach, and watercress have minimal impact on blood-glucose levels due to their very low carb count. Salad greens are included in the "free foods" list later in the chapter.

Table A-4 shows nonstarchy vegetable exchange serving sizes, which depend on the preparation method.

TABLE A-4   ## Nonstarchy Vegetables

Food	Portion Size
Vegetables, all, raw	1 cup
Vegetables, all, cooked	½ cup
Vegetables, all, juiced	½ cup

Meats and Meat Substitutes

A meat or meat substitute exchange is carbohydrate free (has negligible carbohydrate) and contains 7 grams of protein. The different Exchange Lists in the following sections are based on the fat and calories in a portion that gives you 7 grams of protein.

Lean meats and meat substitutes

Each item in the lean meats and meat substitutes list contains approximately 0 grams carbohydrate, 7 grams protein, 0–3 grams fat, and 45 calories. Table A–5 lists serving sizes equivalent to an ounce. Any 4-ounce serving of protein from this list provides 28 grams of protein and about 180 calories.

TABLE A-5 ## Lean Meats and Meat Substitutes

Food	Portion Size (Cooked)
Beef, Select or Choice, trimmed of fat: ground round, chuck roast, round, sirloin, tenderloin, jerky	1 ounce
Cheeses with 3 grams of fat or less per ounce, low-fat	1 ounce
Cottage cheese, fat-free or low-fat	¼ cup
Egg substitute, plain	¼ cup
Egg whites	2
Fish, fresh or frozen: catfish, cod, flounder, haddock, halibut, orange roughy, salmon, tilapia, trout, tuna	1 ounce
Game: buffalo, ostrich, rabbit, venison	1 ounce
Hot dog, only those with 3 grams of fat or less per ounce	1
Lamb: roast, chop, leg	1 ounce
Lunch meat, 3 grams or less of fat per ounce: chipped beef, deli thin-sliced meats, turkey ham, turkey kielbasa, turkey pastrami	1 ounce
Oysters, medium, fresh, or frozen	6
Pork, lean: Canadian bacon, chop, ham, tenderloin	1 ounce
Poultry without skin: Cornish hen, chicken, domestic duck or goose (drained of fat), turkey	1 ounce
Sardines, canned	2 medium
Shellfish: clams, crab, imitation crab, lobster, scallops, shrimp	1 ounce
Tuna, canned in water or oil, drained	1 ounce
Veal: loin chop, roast	1 ounce

Medium-fat meats and meat substitutes

Each item in the medium-fat meats and meat substitutes list contains approximately 0 grams carbohydrate, 7 grams protein, 4–7 grams fat, and 75 calories. Table A-6 lists serving sizes equivalent to an ounce. Any 4-ounce serving of protein from this list provides 28 grams of protein and about 300 calories.

TABLE A-6   ## Medium-Fat Meats and Meat Substitutes

Food	Portion Size (Cooked)
Beef, Prime grades, trimmed of fat: corned beef, ground beef, meatloaf, prime rib, short ribs, tongue	1 ounce
Cheeses with 4–7 grams of fat per ounce: feta, mozzarella, pasteurized processed cheese spread, reduced-fat cheeses, string	1 ounce
Eggs	1
Fish, fried	1 ounce
Lamb: ground, rib roast	1 ounce
Pork: cutlet, shoulder roast	1 ounce
Poultry: chicken with skin, fried chicken, dove, ground turkey, pheasant, squab, wild duck or goose	1 ounce
Ricotta cheese	¼ cup (2 ounces)
Sausages with 4–7 grams of fat per ounce	1 ounce
Veal cutlet, no breading	1 ounce

High-fat meats and meat substitutes

Each item in the high-fat meats and meat substitutes list contains approximately 0 grams carbohydrate, 7 grams protein, 8 or more grams of fat, and 100 calories. Table A-7 lists serving sizes equivalent to an ounce. Any 4-ounce serving of protein from this list provides 28 grams of protein and about 400 calories.

TABLE A-7   ## High-Fat Meats and Meat Substitutes

Food	Portion Size
Bacon, pork	2 slices (1 ounce each before cooking)
Bacon, turkey	3 slices (½ ounce each prior to cooking)
Cheeses, all regular (full-fat, not reduced-fat): American, bleu, brie, cheddar, hard goat, Monterey jack, queso fresco, Swiss	1 ounce
Hot dog, regular (full-fat, not reduced-fat): beef, chicken, pork, turkey	1
Lunch meat, 8 or more grams of fat per ounce: bologna, pastrami, hard salami	1 ounce
Pork: ground, sausage, spareribs	1 ounce
Sausage with 8 or more grams of fat per ounce: bratwurst, chorizo, Italian, knockwurst, Polish, smoked, summer sausage	1 ounce

Fats

Fats are divided into three groups based on the type of fat they contain: monounsaturated, polyunsaturated, or saturated. Each item in the fats list contains approximately 0 grams carbohydrate, 0 grams protein, 5 grams fat, and 45 calories. Nuts contain small amounts of carbohydrate and protein but are predominately fat. Table A–8 shows the exchange serving sizes for fats.

TABLE A-8   ## Monounsaturated, Polyunsaturated, and Saturated Fats

Type	Food	Portion Size
Monounsaturated fats		
	Almonds	6
	Avocado	2 tablespoons (1 ounce)
	Brazil nuts	2
	Cashews	6
	Filberts (hazelnuts)	5
	Macadamia nuts	3
	Nut butters: almond butter, cashew butter	1½ teaspoons

(continued)

TABLE A-8 *(continued)*

Type	Food	Portion Size
	Oil: canola, olive, peanut	1 teaspoon
	Olives, black	8 large
	Olives, green with pimento	10 large
	Peanuts	10
	Peanut butter	1½ teaspoons
	Pecans	4 halves
	Pistachios	16
Polyunsaturated fats		
	Margarine, trans fat–free	1 tablespoon
	Margarine, trans fat–free: squeeze, stick, tub	1 teaspoon
	Mayonnaise, reduced-fat	1 tablespoon
	Mayonnaise, regular	1 teaspoon
	Oil: corn, cottonseed, flaxseed, grape seed, safflower, soybean, sunflower	1 teaspoon
	Pine nuts	1 tablespoon
	Salad dressing, regular	1 tablespoon
	Seeds: flax, pumpkin, sesame, sunflower	1 tablespoon
	Tahini or sesame paste	2 teaspoons
	Walnuts	4 halves
Saturated fats		
	Butter, reduced-fat	1 tablespoon
	Butter, stick	1 teaspoon
	Butter, whipped	2 teaspoons
	Chitterlings, boiled	2 tablespoons (½ ounce)
	Coconut, shredded	2 tablespoons
	Coconut milk	1½ tablespoons
	Cream, half-and-half	2 tablespoons
	Cream, heavy	1 tablespoon

Type	Food	Portion Size
	Cream, light	1½ tablespoons
	Cream, whipped	2 tablespoons
	Cream cheese, reduced-fat	1½ tablespoons
	Cream cheese, regular	1 tablespoon
	Oil: coconut, palm, palm kernel	1 teaspoon
	Salt pork	¼ ounce
	Shortening or lard	1 teaspoon
	Sour cream, reduced-fat	3 tablespoons
	Sour cream, regular	2 tablespoons

Free Foods

These items have few or no calories, carbohydrates, protein, or fat:

>> Bouillon, broth, consommé

>> Carbonated water, club soda, diet soft drinks, diet drink mixes

>> Coffee, tea, herbal tea

>> Flavoring extracts (such as vanilla, almond, peppermint)

>> Herbs, spices, garlic, hot-pepper sauce

>> Lemons, limes

>> Mustard, horseradish

>> Nonnutritive sweeteners (sugar substitutes; see Chapter 12 for more information)

>> Salad greens (arugula, chicory, endive, escarole, lettuce, radicchio, spinach, and watercress)

>> Sugar-free gelatin

>> Vinegar

Appendix B

Conversion Guide

Measuring foods increases carb-counting accuracy. The Nutrition Facts food label correlates serving sizes and product weights to carbohydrate amounts (see Chapter 7). To count carbs in fresh or bulk foods, refer to Chapter 8 and Appendix A, where foods are organized by serving size and carbohydrate content. At the minimum you need standardized measuring cups, but a food scale comes in handy for items that don't fit neatly into a cup. The following tables show equivalent measures in various units.

Liquid Measurement Conversions: Ounces to Milliliters, Deciliters, and Liters

1 fluid ounce	=	30 ml	=	0.3 deciliters
8 fluid ounces	=	240 ml	=	2.4 deciliters
33.8 fluid ounces	=	1,000 ml	=	1 liter

Volume Conversions: U.S. Units to Metric Units

1 cup	=	16 tablespoons	=	240 ml
¾ cup	=	12 tablespoons	=	180 ml
⅔ cup	=	10⅔ tablespoons	=	160 ml
½ cup	=	8 tablespoons	=	120 ml
⅓ cup	=	5⅓ tablespoons	=	80 ml
¼ cup	=	4 tablespoons	=	60 ml
2⅛ cup	=	2 tablespoons	=	30 ml
1 tablespoon	=	3 teaspoons	=	15 ml
1 teaspoon	=	⅓ tablespoon	=	5 ml
½ pint	=	1 cup	=	8 fluid ounces
1 pint	=	2 cups	=	16 fluid ounces
1 quart	=	2 pints	=	32 fluid ounces
1 gallon	=	4 quarts	=	128 fluid ounces

Weight Conversions: Metric to U.S. Units

28 grams	=	1 ounce	=	$\frac{1}{16}$ pound
0.45 kilograms	=	16 ounces	=	1 pound
1 kilogram	=	35.3 ounces	=	2.2 pounds

Length Conversions: Basic

12 inches	=	1 foot
3 feet	=	1 yard
100 centimeters	=	1 meter

Length Conversions: Metric to U.S. Units

2.54 centimeters	=	0.0254 meters	=	1 inch
30.45 centimeters	=	0.3045 meters	=	1 foot
91.44 centimeters	=	0.9144 meters	=	1 yard

Index

Symbols and Numerics

%DV (%Daily Value), 98–99, 103
70/30 insulin, 91–92
100% whole grain stamp, 114
504 plan, 270

A

A1C test
  average blood glucose, 60–61
  diagnostic criteria, 35
  estimated Average Glucose, 61–62
  overview, 334–335
AADE (American Association of Diabetes Educators), 142, 344
AADE Diabetes Goal Tracker app, 142
absorption rates. *See* digestion
Academy of Nutrition and Dietetics (AND), 187, 344–345
acanthosis nigricans, 34, 272
Acceptable Daily Intake (ADI), 185
Acceptable Macronutrient Distribution Range (AMDR), 69
accuracy (blood glucose monitors), 331
acesulfame potassium, 186
ADA (American Diabetes Association)
  A1C calculator, 62
  alcohol consumption, 234
  blood-glucose targets during pregnancy, 275–276
  diabetes app, 142
  diet guidelines, 68
  lifestyle modifications to improve heart health, 252
  Standards of Medical Care in Diabetes, 168–169, 273
  substitutes for refined carbs and added sugars, 150
  sugar consumption recommendations, 176
  website, 343–344
added sugars
  calculating sugar content, 110
  consumption of in U. S., 185
  digestion rate and, 149
  food labels, 103
  in soda, 176
ADI (Acceptable Daily Intake), 185
adipose, 228
adolescents with diabetes, 270–271
adrenaline, 240
adult-onset diabetes, 30. *See also* type 2 diabetes
Advantame, 186
aerobic activity, 212
Afrezza, 87
agave nectar, 13, 181
age
  adjusting carb intake for, 76
  caloric needs based on, 70
  type 2 diabetes and, 33
AHA (American Heart Association)
  exercise recommendations, 264
  fat consumption, 256
  sugar consumption recommendations, 176, 185
  website, 345
ALA omega-3 fatty acid, 255
alcohol
  carbs and calories, 171–173
  effect on body, 170–171
  hypoglycemia and, 24, 233–234
  monitoring blood glucose levels, 173–174
  recommended limits and portions, 173
  risk factors, 169–170
allergens (listed on food labels), 111–112
AMDR (Acceptable Macronutrient Distribution Range), 69
American Association of Diabetes Educators (AADE), 142, 344
American Diabetes Association. *See* ADA
American Heart Association. *See* AHA
amino acids, 55, 63–64
amylase, 54
AND (Academy of Nutrition and Dietetics), 187, 344–345

animal foods. *See also* dairy foods; meat

  fats, 41, 51, 106, 124

  fiber, 41

anti-tissue transglutaminase (tTG) test, 284

apps

  diabetes apps, 141–142

  importance of using, 20

  integrating with food scale, 142

  overview, 140–141

aspartame, 184, 186, 188

autoimmune diseases, 29–30. *See also* celiac disease;
     type 1 diabetes

autonomic neuropathy, 216

avocados, 43, 120

B

baking, 188

balanced diet. *See also* meals

  caloric intake, 69–72

  carb intake, 72–77

  heart health, 251–259

  managing diabetes and, 36

  official diet guidelines, 68–69

  overview, 14, 67

  for seniors with diabetes, 279–280

Barbados sugar, 179

barley, 288

basal rate (insulin pump), 87, 156

bedtime lows (hypoglycemia), 244

beer

  calories, 172

  carb content, 171, 172

  gluten-free diet, 290

beta-cells (islet cells), 27

beverages. *See* liquids

bicarbonate, 55

biguanides (Metformin), 94, 274

bile, 252, 257

blended insulin, 86–87, 91–93, 232–233

blood glucose. *See also* hyperglycemia; hypoglycemia;
     monitoring blood glucose levels

  alcohol and, 173–174

  basing injection timing on pre-meal blood-glucose
     levels, 91

  hyperglycemia, 12

  hypoglycemia, 12

  measuring, 2

  preventing complications and, 9

  reducing fluctuations, 152–154

  stabilizing, 82–84

  target levels during pregnancy, 275–276, 333

  type 1 diabetes and exercise and, 221

blood glucose monitors, 22, 210, 236, 244, 329–330

blood pressure

  exercise and, 216, 224

  hypertension, 24

  preventing complications and, 9

  type 2 diabetes and, 33, 34

blood samples, 330–331

blood sugar. *See* blood glucose

blood tests

  A1C test, 35, 60–62, 334–335

  C-peptide, 30

  fasting blood glucose, 35

  oral glucose tolerance test, 35

blood-ketone testing, 65

bloodstream (circulatory system), 56

blue agave plant, 181

blurred vision, as symptom of diabetes, 29

body fat. *See* fat (body)

body mass index (BMI), 71–72, 265, 272

bolus rate (insulin pump), 87, 156

bones

  calcium and, 198, 296

  exercise and, 215

  vitamin D and, 296

bran (whole grain), 46

breakfast

  healthy options, 339–340

  importance of during pregnancy, 277

  menus, 300–302

  overview, 299–300

  personalizing meal plan, 303–304

  stabilizing blood glucose levels, 83

breastfeeding

  adjusting carb intake during, 75

  blood glucose levels during, 276

  type 1 diabetes and, 32

brown rice, 148

brown sugar, 13, 178–179

C

caffeine, 54

calcium
- dairy foods, 198–199
- gluten-free diet, 296
- milk, 163–164

Calorie King app, 338

Calorie King website, 131, 140, 142

calories
- adjusting intake for weight target, 71–72
- alcohol, 171–173
- estimating caloric needs, 69–71
- food labels, 102–103, 105
- liquids, 167–169
- in snacks, 321

canned goods, 262

carbohydrate cheat sheet, 126–127

carbohydrates. *See also* tracking carbs
- alcohol, 171–173
- balanced meals and, 14
- in breakfasts, 300–302
- carb-free foods, 49–52
- carb-glucose connection, 11–12
- chemical structure of, 40–42
- complex, 45–48
- counting, 15–18
- in dinners, 314–317
- Grams of Carb per Ounce of Food list, 130
- how body processes, 26–27
- hypoglycemia and, 231–233
- liquid carbs, 52, 133, 146
- listed on food labels, 107–110
- in lunches, 306–309
- nutrition in carb food groups, 13–14
- overview, 12–13, 39–40
- regulating intake, 18–19
- simple, 42–45
- in snacks, 321

carbon atoms, 253–254

cardiovascular disease, 34, 224–225. *See also* heart health

CDC (Centers for Disease Control and Prevention), 25–26

CDE (certified diabetes educator), 10, 344

celiac disease, 21, 283, 284–285, 295

Centers for Disease Control and Prevention (CDC), 25–26

cereals, 113, 339

certified diabetes educator (CDE), 10, 344

CFRD (cystic fibrosis–related diabetes), 31

CGM (continuous glucose monitor), 236, 244, 336

chain restaurant food facts, 139

cheese, 44, 49. *See also* dairy foods

chemical structure of carbohydrates, 40–42

children with diabetes
- adolescents, 270–271
- fitting in treats, 269–270
- nutritional needs, 269
- overview, 267–268
- supervising, 270
- type 2 diabetes, 271–273
- viewing glucose results as data, 269

chili recipe, 126

chocolate, 147

chocolate shakes, 168

cholesterol
- exercise and, 224
- food labels, 106–107
- HDL, 51
- heart healthy diet, 252–253
- LDL, 50–51
- saturated fat and, 106
- trans fat and, 106
- type 2 diabetes and, 34

Choose MyPlate image, 134–135

chronic disease, 215

circulatory system (bloodstream), 56

coconut palm sugar, 179

coffee, 163

combo bolus (insulin pump), 157

Commission on Dietetic Registration, 36

communion wafers, 291

complex carbohydrates
- digestion, 148
- fiber, 46–48
- overview, 13
- shopping for, 48
- starches, 45–46

complications, preventing, 9, 24

concentrated insulin
  Degludec (Tresiba), 86
  Humulin Regular, 85
  Lispro (Humalog), 86
  Toujeo U300, 86

condiments, 318, 341

confectioners' sugar (powdered sugar), 178

continuous glucose monitor (CGM), 236, 244, 336

convenience foods, 262

conversion guide
  length conversions, 365
  liquid measurement conversions, 365
  volume conversions, 365
  weight conversions, 365

cookbooks, 138

cooking
  digestion and level of cooking, 150
  heart healthy diet, 259
  lower-fat cooking methods, 204–205
  overview, 203–204
  portion control, 205
  using sugar substitutes, 188

cooling down (exercise), 213

corn syrup, 179

cornbread, 126

cortisol, 217, 218

cottage cheese, 49

counter-regulatory hormones
  cortisol, 217, 218
  digestion, 83
  epinephrine, 217, 218
  glucagon, 217–218, 240–241
  growth hormone, 217, 218

counting carbohydrates
  increasing accuracy, 20
  portion control, 17–18
  reading food labels, 19
  resources for, 19–20
  set insulin doses and, 16, 17
  type 1 diabetes, 15, 16
  type 2 diabetes, 15
  weight management, 17–18

C-peptide test, 30

cross-contamination (gluten), 292–293

crystalline fructose, 180, 181

cyclamates, 186

cystic fibrosis–related diabetes (CFRD), 31

D

dairy foods
  calcium, 198–199
  fat, 198, 254
  low-carb, 121
  non-dairy substitutes, 164, 199–200
  overview, 197
  protein, 198

DASH diet, 260–261

dawn phenomenon, 92

DCCT (Diabetes Control and Complication Trial), 9

Degludec (Tresiba), 86

dehydration
  cycle of, 160
  in seniors with diabetes, 281
  thirst, 28

delayed hypoglycemia, 220, 233

dentist, 10

dessert/sweets, 201–203
  fruit, 202
  homemade, 201
  including in diet, 341
  including in diet of child with diabetes, 269–270
  portion control, 202–203

DHA omega-3 fatty acid, 195, 196

diabetes. *See also* managing diabetes; type 1 diabetes; type 2 diabetes
  causes of, 27–28
  cystic fibrosis–related diabetes, 31
  defined, 8
  diabetes team, 9–10
  diagnosing, 34–35
  gestational diabetes, 30–31, 34, 274–275
  improving outcomes, 8–9
  maturity-onset diabetes of the young, 31
  neonatal diabetes, 31
  overview, 25–26
  prediabetes, 8, 30
  preventing complications, 9
  risk factors, 32–34

symptoms of, 28–29

trends in diabetes epidemic, 8

diabetes apps, 141–142

Diabetes Control and Complication Trial (DCCT), 9

Diabetes Education Online website, 346

Diabetes Medical Management Plan, 270

Diabetes Mellitus, 28. *See also* diabetes

diabetes nurse educator, 10

diabetes team

  certified diabetes educator, 10

  dentist, 10

  diabetes nurse educator, 10

  endocrinologist, 9

  eye doctor, 10

  managing diabetes and, 36–37

  mental-health specialist, 10

  pharmacist, 10

  podiatrist, 10

  primary care provider, 9

  registered dietitian, 10

  self-care, 37

  support group, 10

diabetic ketoacidosis (DKA), 65, 66

diagnosing diabetes, 34–35

diet drinks, 163, 185

dietary fat. *See* fat (dietary)

Dietary Guidelines for Americans, 252

Dietary Reference Intake (DRI), 69, 72, 164

digestion

  aligning insulin and digestion rates, 154–157

  blood-glucose control and, 52

  complex carbs, 148

  extracting glucose via, 55–56

  fat, 149

  fiber and, 40, 46, 148

  food processing and, 149

  fruit, 147–148

  glycemic index, 150–151

  glycemic load, 151

  grains, 150

  insulin timing and, 19

  level of cooking and, 150

  liquid carbs, 146

  overview, 145–146

  particle size and, 149

  reducing blood glucose fluctuations, 152–154

  ripeness and, 150

  starches and, 40

  sugars, 147

digestive enzymes, 40

dinner

  menus, 313–318

  stabilizing blood glucose levels, 83–84

disaccharides, 13, 40–41, 182. *See also* simple carbohydrates

distilled spirits (hard alcohol), 171, 172, 233

distributing carb intake

  eating three meals per day, 80–81

  smaller meals more often, 81–82

DKA (diabetic ketoacidosis), 65, 66

double sugar molecules, 13, 40–41, 182. *See also* simple carbohydrates

DRI (Dietary Reference Intake), 69, 72, 164

drinks. *See* liquids

duodenum, 55

duration of exercise, 214

duration times (insulin action), 85

durum, 288

dyslipidemia, 30

E

eAG (estimated Average Glucose), 61–62

eating out

  lunch menus, 310–311

  portion control, 132–133

Educational apps, 142

eggs

  cholesterol, 252

  as source of protein, 49

electrolyte-replacement drink, 168

elevated glucose. *See also* hyperglycemia

  adjusting carb intake for, 76

  glucose in urine, 58–59

  glycosylation, 60–62

emotional health, 271

endocrinologist, 9

endorphins, 264

endosperm (whole grain), 46

energy drinks, 168

EPA omega-3 fatty acid, 195, 196

epi pen, 286

epinephrine, 217, 218

error issues (blood glucose monitors), 331

erythritol, 183

esophagus, 54

estimated Average Glucose (eAG), 61–62

estimating carb counts for foods without labels, 118–127. *See also* Exchange Lists

  food composition lists, 118–124

  mixed dishes and ethnic foods, 124–126

  preparing carbohydrate cheat sheet, 126–127

  in recipes, 126

ethnic foods, 124–126

ethnicity, type 2 diabetes and, 33

Exchange Lists

  as carb counting resource, 19

  fats, 124, 361–363

  free foods, 363

  fruit, 120, 354–356

  meat and protein, 122–123, 358–361

  milk and yogurt, 120–121, 356–357

  nonstarchy vegetables, 121–122, 357–358

  origin of, 125

  overview, 118–119, 351–352

  starches, 119, 352–354

exercise

  adjusting carb intake for activity level, 76

  aerobic activity, 212

  benefits of, 214–215

  caloric needs based on, 70

  cooling down, 213

  duration, 214

  exercising safely, 208–211

  frequency, 213

  fruit juice and, 167

  glycogen storage capacity and, 58

  heart health and, 264

  how diabetes alters, 218–219

  hypoglycemia, 219–220, 247

  importance of, 21

  intensity, 213–214

  medical limitations, 215–217

  overview, 207–208, 211–212

  reducing blood glucose fluctuations, 153

  resistance training, 212–213

  role of hormones in, 217–218

  for seniors with diabetes, 281

  stress management and, 23

  stretching, 213

  sugary liquids and, 146

  talk-sing test, 213

  tapping into fuels, 219

  type 1 diabetes, 220–223

  type 2 diabetes, 223–226

  walking, 212

  warming up, 213

eye disease, 9

eye doctor, 10

F

family history

  cholesterol production, 252

  type 1 diabetes, 32

  type 2 diabetes, 33

fast foods, 262

fasting blood glucose, 35, 333

fat (body)

  as fuel source, 219

  ketones and, 65

  type 2 diabetes and, 33

fat (dietary)

  byproducts of metabolism, 64

  dairy foods, 198

  digestion of, 149

  Exchange List, 124, 361–363

  food labels, 105–106

  hand model portions, 136

  healthy, 200

  heart healthy diet, 253–257

  heartburn and, 54

  milk, 164

  overview, 50

  as part of balanced diet, 74

  rapid-acting insulin, 155–156

  role of, 11

  saturated fats, 50, 105, 253–254

  trans fats, 50–51, 105, 254

  unsaturated fats, 50, 106, 253–254

fatigue, 29

fatty acids, 55

FDA (Food and Drug Administration)

  Cyclamate, 188

  food labels, 97

gluten-free label, 288
low calorie sweeteners, 185
mercury in fish and seafood, 196
MiniMed 670G, 88
restaurant food labeling, 138
website, 345
feet friendly activities, 216
fiber
as complex carbs, 13
digestion and, 40, 56, 148
heart healthy diet, 257–258
insoluble, 47, 257
lack of in animal foods, 41
listed on food labels, 108–109
overview, 46
recommended intake, 47–48
in snacks, 321
soluble, 46, 47, 257
fillers, 291
fine sugar crystals, 178
fish and seafood
Exchange List, 123
food labels, 111
mercury risk, 196
omega-3 fatty acids, 195, 196, 255
as source of protein, 49
fitness. *See* exercise
504 plan, 270
folate (folic acid), 295
Food Allergen Labeling and Consumer Protection
    Act of 2006, 111
food allergies, 286
Food and Drug Administration. *See* FDA
food composition lists. *See* Exchange Lists
food databases, 20, 140
food intolerances (food sensitivities), 287
food labels
%Daily Value, 98–99, 103
added sugars, 103
allergens, 111–112
amounts, 98–99
calcium, 164
calories, 102–103, 105
carbohydrates, 107–110
cholesterol, 106–107
counting carbs and, 19
dietary fat, 105–106

fat, 256
fish and seafood, 111
food labeling regulations, 138–139
gluten-free, 288
ingredients, 111
label claims, 112–115
nutrition facts, 104–112
overview, 97–98
potassium, 103
pre-packaged snacks, 325
protein, 110–111
saturated fat, 105
serving sizes, 102, 105
servings per container, 102, 105
simple carbohydrates on, 45
sodium, 107
traditional version, 100–101
trans fats, 51
updated version, 101–104
using to prepare carbohydrate cheat sheet, 115
vitamins and minerals, 103–104
food processing, digestion and, 149
Food Pyramid, 134
food scales
importance of using, 20
integrating apps and, 142
overview, 128–131
weighing fruit, 338
food sensitivities (food intolerances), 287
free foods, 363
fried foods, 51, 80, 259
fructose
crystalline fructose, 180–181
high-fructose corn syrup, 43, 44, 179, 181
as simple carbohydrate, 43
fruit. *See also* plant foods
as dessert, 202
digestion and, 147–148
Exchange List, 120, 354–356
grams of carb per ounce, 130
hand model portions, 136
nutrients, 42
overview, 191–193
portion control, 14
sugars, 13, 43
weighing, 338–339

fruit juice
  carb and calorie counts, 168
  exercise and, 167
  hypoglycemia and, 166
  overview, 165–166
fueling cells, 56–57
fueling exercise
  hormones and, 217–218
  how diabetes alters fuel use, 218–219
  hypoglycemia, 219–220
  tapping into fuels, 219
fungal infections, 29

G

gastroparesis, 9, 47–48
GDM (gestational diabetes mellitus), 30–31, 34, 274–275
gender
  caloric needs based on, 69–70
  establishing mealtime carb targets, 81
  recommended fiber intake, 47
  type 2 diabetes and, 34
Generally Regarded As Safe (GRAS) list, 187
genetics
  cholesterol production, 252
  type 1 diabetes, 32
  type 2 diabetes, 33
germ (whole grain), 46
gestational diabetes mellitus (GDM), 30–31, 34, 274–275
GI (glycemic index)
  agave nectar, 181
  defined, 17
  digestion and, 150–151
GL (glycemic load), 151
glass measuring cups, 127–128
glucagon, 217–218, 240–241
gluconeogenesis, 63–64
glucose
  extracting via digestion, 55–56
  in fruit, 43
  importance of, 18, 42
  insulin and, 26–27
  molecular structure, 180
  movement though body, 55
glucose gel, 239
glucose monitors, 22, 210, 236, 244, 329–330

gluten-free diet
  celiac disease and, 21, 284–285
  cross-contamination, 292–293
  following for personal reasons, 287
  food allergies, 286
  food intolerances, 287
  gluten-containing foods, 290–291
  grains that contain gluten, 288–289
  hidden gluten in foods, 291
  nutritional needs, 293–296
  oats, 289
  overview, 283–284
  type 1 diabetes and, 21
glyburide, 274
glycemia, 152
glycemic control, 224
glycemic index. *See* GI
glycemic load (GL), 151
glycogen
  controlling blood glucose levels, 217–218
  defined, 11
  exercise and, 219
  in liver, 57–58
  in muscles, 58
glycosylation, 35, 60–62
Go Meals app, 141
grains. *See also* plant foods
  containing gluten, 288–289
  digestion, 150
  malted grains, 44
  refined grains, 46, 193–194
  whole grains, 42, 46, 113–114, 193–194
GRAS (Generally Regarded As Safe) list, 187
growth hormone, 217, 218
guesstimating portions
  hand model, 136
  overview, 133–134
  plate model, 134–135

H

hand model, 136
hard alcohol (distilled spirits), 171, 172, 233
HDL cholesterol, 51
Health and Human Services (HHS), 68
healthy diet

cooking process and, 203–205

dairy foods, 197–200

dessert/sweets, 201–203

fat, 200

fruit, 191–193

importance of, 20–21

protein, 194–197

vegetables, 191–193

whole grains, 193–194

heart, 56

heart health

diet, 251–259

exercise and, 264

hypertension, 260–263

stress management, 264

tobacco and secondhand smoke, 264

weight management, 265

heartburn, 54

hemoglobin A protein, 35

hexose, 180

HHS (Health and Human Services), 68

high blood glucose. *See* hyperglycemia

high blood pressure. *See* hypertension

high blood sugar. *See* hyperglycemia

high-carb meals, 75

high-fat meats Exchange List, 360–361

high-fructose corn syrup, 43, 44, 179, 181

homemade dessert, 201

honey, 13, 44, 179

hormones. *See also* insulin

cortisol, 217, 218

epinephrine, 217, 218

glucagon, 217–218, 240–241

growth hormone, 217, 218

insulin-to-carb ratios and, 89

regulating blood glucose, 217–218

HSH (hydrogenated starch hydrolysates), 183

Humalog (Lispro), 86

Humulin Regular, 85

hunger, as symptom of diabetes, 28

hybrid closed-loop system, 88

hydration, 159–161, 211. *See also* liquids

hydrochloric acid, 54

hydrogen atoms, 253

hydrogenated fat, 254

hydrogenated starch hydrolysates (HSH), 183

hydrogenation, 51, 254

hyperglycemia. *See also* elevated glucose

defined, 228

in evening, 80

gestational diabetes and, 274

insulin and, 76

pregnancy and, 275

rebounds, 240

variables affecting, 12

hypertension. *See also* blood pressure

DASH diet, 260–261

exercise and, 216

importance of controlling, 24

sodium, 261–263

hypoglycemia

alcohol and, 169–170

bedtime lows, 244

blood-glucose logs, 248–249

candy and, 147

causes, 229–234

defining low blood glucose level, 229

exercise and, 219–220

fruit juice and, 166

general discussion, 227–229

hypoglycemia unawareness, 236–237

insulin action, 244–245

mealtime lows, 242–243

oral diabetes medication and, 94

preventing, 246–247

sugary liquids and, 146

symptoms, 235

treating, 237–241

undereating carbs and, 62–63

variables affecting, 12

hypoglycemia unawareness, 235, 236–237

I

ICR (insulin-to-carb ratios)

calculating mealtime doses, 123

fiber and, 109

flexibility of, 89–90

IgE (immunoglobin E) antibody, 286

illness, managing diabetes during, 76–77

immunoglobin E (IgE) antibody, 286

infusing water, 162

infusion set (insulin), 87

ingredients (food labels), 111

inhaled insulin, 87

insoluble fiber, 47, 257

insulin
  aligning digestion rates and, 154–157
  blended insulin, 86–87, 91–93, 232–233
  blood-glucose targets, 333
  comparing options, 85
  concentrated insulins, 85–86
  coordinating with meals, 88–92
  dosing mistakes, 230
  glucose and, 26–27
  hybrid closed-loop system, 88
  hypoglycemia, 244–245
  insulin pump, 87
  insulin resistance, 27–28, 30
  matching insulin timing to digestion timing, 19
  overview, 84
  set insulin dosing, 16, 17
  sliding-scale insulin dosing, 16, 90
  stacking doses, 230–231
  type 1 diabetes, 8, 221–222
  type 2 diabetes, 8

insulin pump
  basal delivery, 87, 156
  bolus delivery, 87, 156
  combo bolus, 157
  "low glucose suspend" feature, 244

insulin-dependent diabetes mellitus(IDDM), 30. See also type 1 diabetes

insulin-to-carb ratios. See ICR

intensity of exercise, 213–214

intermediate-acting insulin, 85, 92

International Food Information Council Foundation, 187

interval training, 214

intestinal villi (celiac disease), 285

invert sugar, 179

iron
  %Daily Value, 111
  gluten-free diet, 296
  vitamin C and, 192

islet cells (beta-cells), 27

isomalt, 183

J

Joslin Diabetes Center website, 346–347

juicing, 165–166

juvenile diabetes, 30. See also type 1 diabetes

K

ketones, 64–66, 223

kidney disease, 9

kidneys
  elevated glucose and, 58–59
  increased urination and, 28
  sugary liquids and, 160

L

label claims
  net carbs, 112–113
  no sugar added, 114
  rules for, 98
  sodium-related, 263
  sugar-free, 115
  whole grains, 113–114
  zero trans fat, 113

lactitol, 183

lactose, 13, 43–44, 121

lactose intolerance, 44, 287

lactose-free milk, 44, 164, 287

lancets
  disposing of, 332
  setting depth, 330

late night snacking, 342

LDL cholesterol, 50

lean body mass, losing, 63–64

lean meat Exchange List, 359

legumes, 42, 46

lemonade, 162–163

length conversions, 365

life cycle, adjusting diet during, 75–76

Light/lite sodium label claim, 263

lipid levels, 224. See also cholesterol

liquid sugar, 179

liquids
  alcohol, 169–174
  with breakfast, 304, 340

calories, 167–169

fruit juice, 165–167

importance of hydration, 159–161

liquid carbs, 52, 133, 146

liquid measurement conversions, 365

low carb beverages, 162–163

measuring, 129

milk, 163–164

non-dairy milk substitute, 164, 199–200

water, 162

Lispro (Humalog), 86

liver

cholesterol production, 252

glycogen in, 55, 57–58

processing alcohol, 170–171

processing fructose, 180

rebounds, 240

logbook (blood glucose levels), 333–334

long-acting insulin, 85

low blood glucose (low blood sugar). *See* hypoglycemia

low carb beverages, 162–163

"low glucose suspend" feature (insulin pump), 244

Low sodium label claim, 263

lower-fat cooking methods, 204–205, 259

lunches

eating out, 340

menu options, 305–309

packing your own, 340

personalizing, 310–311

vegetarian lunch options, 310

lungs, ketones and, 64

M

macronutrients. *See also* carbohydrates

defined, 11, 39–40

fats and oils, 40

in milk, 121

proteins, 40

magnesium, 296

malabsorption of nutrients, 285, 295

malt vinegar, 291

malted grains, 44

maltitol, 183

maltitol syrup, 183

maltodextrin, 180

maltose, 43, 44

managing diabetes

balanced diet and, 36

diabetes team and, 36–37

exercise, 21

healthy diet, 20–21

medication, 22

monitoring blood glucose levels, 22–23

overview, 35–36

preventing complications, 24

problem-solving, 23–24

stress management, 23

mannitol, 182, 183

maple syrup, 44, 179

margarine, 254

maternal glucose control, 273–274

maturity-onset diabetes of the young (MODY), 31

Mayo Clinic, 187, 346

meals. *See also* balanced diet

breakfast, 83, 277, 299–304, 339–340

coordinating insulin action with, 88–92

dinner, 83–84, 313–318

eating three meals per day, 80–81

lunches, 305–311

mealtime lows, 242–243

smaller meals more often, 81–82

measuring tools

food scales, 128–131

measuring cups, 19, 337–338

standardized cups and spoons, 127–128

meat

Exchange List, 122–123, 358–361

fats, 254

as source of protein, 49

meatless protein, 197

medical alert ID, 209–210, 230

medical limitations (exercise)

autonomic neuropathy, 216

exercising while seated, 216

feet friendly activities, 216

high blood pressure, 216

medical exam before planning exercise, 208–209

nephropathy, 217

overview, 215–216

peripheral vascular disease, 217

retinopathy, 217

medical nutrition therapy, 9

medication

  hypoglycemia and, 230–231, 232–233

  importance of, 22

medium-fat meat Exchange List, 360

meglitinides, 94

men

  caloric needs, 69–70

  establishing mealtime carb targets, 81

  recommended fiber intake, 47

mental health, 215

mental-health specialist, 10, 36

menus

  breakfast, 300–302

  dinner, 313–318

  lunch, 305–311

  snacks, 320–326

mercury, in fish and seafood, 196

metabolic rate, 225

metabolic syndrome, 32, 272

Metformin (biguanides), 94, 274

metric measurement system

  volume conversions to U. S. units, 365

  weight conversions to U.S. units, 365

micronutrients, 11, 39

milk and yogurt

  benefits of, 163–164

  Exchange List, 120–121, 356–357

  lactose-free milk, 44

  macronutrients in, 121

  nutrients, 42

MiniMed 670G, 88

mixed dishes, 124–126

mixed meals, 51–52

MODY (maturity-onset diabetes of the young), 31

molasses, 178

monitoring blood glucose levels

  A1C lab test, 334–335

  accuracy, 331

  continuous glucose monitor, 236, 244, 336

  disposing of lancets and needles, 332

  error issues, 331

  glucose monitors, 329–330

  knowing blood glucose targets, 333

  logbook, 333–334

  obtaining blood samples, 330–331

  overview, 22–23

  varying test times, 332

monosaccharides, 13, 40–41, 182. *See also* simple carbohydrates

monounsaturated fat, 50, 253

muscles

  effect of undereating carbs on, 63

  exercise and, 215

  glycogen in, 55, 58

Muscovado sugar, 179

MyFitnessPal app, 142

MyPlate method, 134–135

N

National Cancer Institute, 187

National Health and Nutrition Examination Survey (NHANES), 185

National Institutes of Health, 18

National Weight Control Registry, 226

naturally occurring sugars, 110

needles, disposing of, 332

neonatal diabetes, 31

Neotame, 186

nephrons, 58

nephropathy, 217

nerve disease, 9

Net carbs label claim, 112–113

neuropathy, 216

NHANES (National Health and Nutrition Examination Survey), 185

NIDDM (non-insulin-dependent diabetes mellitus), 30. *See also* type 2 diabetes

No sugar added label claim, 114

non-dairy milk substitutes, 164, 199–200

non-insulin-dependent diabetes mellitus (NIDDM), 30. *See also* type 2 diabetes

nonnutritive sweeteners. *See* sugar substitutes

nonstarchy vegetables Exchange List, 121–122, 357–358

numbness, as symptom of diabetes, 29

Nutrition Facts food labels. *See also* food labels

  allergens, 111–112

  calories, 105

  carbohydrates, 107–110

  cholesterol, 106–107

  dietary fat, 105–106

ingredients, 111
other nutrient content, 111
overview, 19
protein, 110–111
serving sizes, 105
servings per container, 105
sodium, 107
nutritional needs
children with diabetes, 269
gluten-free diet, 293–296
managing diabetes during pregnancy, 277–278
seniors with diabetes, 279–281
nutritionists, 36
nuts and nut butters, 254

O

oats, 258, 289, 339
obesity. *See also* weight management
BMI, 72
breakfast and, 83
obesity-related diseases, 25
sugar consumption and, 185
type 2 diabetes and, 33
OGTT (oral glucose tolerance test), 35
oils. *See also* fat (dietary)
oligosaccharides, 44
omega-3 fatty acids
ALA, 255
EPA and DHA, 195, 196
online resources
Academy of Nutrition and Dietetics, 344–345
American Association of Diabetes Educators, 344
American Diabetes Association, 343–344
American Heart Association, 345
Certified Diabetes Educators, 344
chain restaurant food facts, 139
Diabetes Education Online, 346
Food and Drug Administration, 345
food databases, 140
Joslin Diabetes Center, 346–347
Mayo Clinic, 346
search engines, 140
USDA's Food Composition Databases, 347
WebMD, 347
onset times (insulin action), 85

oral diabetes medication
limitations of, 94
meglitinides, 92
sulfonylureas, 93–94
oral glucose tolerance test (OGTT), 35
osteoporosis, 215, 285
outcomes, improving, 8–9
overweight. *See also* weight management
BMI, 72
overweight children, 272
type 2 diabetes and, 33

P

pancreas, 26, 28, 55, 84, 217–218
particle size, digestion and, 149
PCOS (polycystic ovarian syndrome), 34
peak times (insulin action), 85
pediatric diabetes
adolescents, 270–271
fitting in treats, 269–270
nutritional needs, 269
overview, 267–268
supervising, 270
type 2 diabetes, 271–273
viewing glucose results as data, 269
pentose, 180
peripheral vascular disease, 217
pharmacists, 10
phenylalanine, 188
physical activity. *See* exercise
pillars of diabetes management
exercise, 21
healthy diet, 20–21
medication, 22
monitoring blood glucose levels, 22–23
preventing complications, 24
problem-solving, 23–24
stress management, 23
plant foods. *See also* fruit; grains; vegetables
cholesterol, 252
fiber, 41
nutrients, 42
oils, 254, 255
plant-based fats, 124
saturated fat, 41

plate model, 52, 134–135

podiatrist, 10

polycystic ovarian syndrome (PCOS), 34

polysaccharides, 40–41, 44, 183. *See also* complex carbohydrates

polyunsaturated fat, 50, 254

portion control (portioning)

  cooking process and, 205

  counting carbohydrates and, 17–18

  dessert/sweets, 202–203

  estimating carb counts for foods without labels, 118–127

  guesstimating, 133–136

  liquid carbs, 133

  measuring tools, 127–131

  overview, 117–118

  portioning guidelines, 68–69

  reducing blood glucose fluctuations, 152–153

  snacks, 342

  when eating out, 132–133

potassium, 103, 261

powdered sugar (confectioners' sugar), 178

preconception counseling, 31

prediabetes, 8, 30

preeclampsia, 276

pregnancy

  adjusting carb intake during, 75

  blood-glucose target levels, 333

  gestational diabetes mellitus, 30–31, 274–275

  managing diabetes during, 273–278, 333

primary care provider, 9

printed resources

  cookbooks, 138

  Exchange Lists, 138

  food labeling regulations, 138–139

  food labels, 138

  overview, 137

problem-solving

  hypoglycemia, 246–247

  importance of, 23–24

protein. *See also* meat

  cheese, 49

  dairy foods, 49, 163, 198

  defined, 49

  fish and seafood, 196

  food labels, 110–111

  hand model portions, 136

  healthiest options, 195–196

  meatless, 197

  milk, 163

  overview, 194–195

  as part of balanced diet, 74

  portion control, 17, 318

  role of, 11

pumping insulin, 87

pure-sugar candies, 147

R

rapid-acting insulin

  action profile, 85

  balanced meal and, 155

  fatty meal and, 156

  70/30 insulin, 92

  treating mealtime hypoglycemia, 242–243

RBCs. *See* red blood cells

RDA (Recommended Dietary Allowances), 69

RDNs (registered dietitian nutritionists). *See* registered dietitians

RDs. *See* registered dietitians

rebounds, 240

recipes, estimating carb counts in, 126

Recommended Dietary Allowances (RDA), 69

red blood cells (RBCs)

  circulatory system, 56

  glycosylation, 60

  hemoglobin A protein, 35

Reduced/less sodium label claim, 263

refined grains

  fiber, 46

  whole grains versus, 193–194

registered dietitian nutritionists (RDNs). *See* registered dietitians

registered dietitians (RDs)

  defined, 36

  medical nutrition therapy, 9

  as part of diabetes team, 10

regular (short-acting) insulin, 85

Remember icon, 4

resistance training (strength training), 212–213

resources

  Academy of Nutrition and Dietetics, 344–345

  American Association of Diabetes Educators, 344

  American Diabetes Association, 343–344

American Heart Association, 345

Certified Diabetes Educators, 344

chain restaurant food facts, 139

cookbooks, 138

for counting carbohydrates, 19–20

Diabetes Education Online, 346

Exchange Lists, 138

Food and Drug Administration, 345

food databases, 140

food labeling regulations, 138–139

Joslin Diabetes Center, 346–347

Mayo Clinic, 346

search engines, 140

USDA's Food Composition Databases, 347

WebMD, 347

retinopathy, 216, 217

rice syrup, 179

ripeness, digestion and, 150

risk factors

  type 1 diabetes, 32–33

  type 2 diabetes, 33–34, 272

Rule of 15, 166

rye, 288

S

saccharin, 186, 187

saliva, 54

salt, 107, 261–262

satiety, 51–52

saturated fat, 50, 105, 253–254

screening, importance of, 9

search engines, 140

seasonings, 261–262, 318

secondhand smoke, 264

sedentary lifestyle, 34, 69, 218

seeds, 254

seizures, 241

self-care, 37

self-talk, 23

seniors with diabetes

  exercise and, 281

  nutritional needs, 279–281

service dogs, 244

serving sizes (food label), 102, 105

servings per container (food label), 102, 105

set insulin dosing, 16, 17

70/30 insulin, 91–92

severe hypoglycemia, 240

short-acting (regular) insulin, 85

shrimp, 252

sickness, managing diabetes during, 76–77

simple carbohydrates

  on food labels, 45

  fructose, 43

  glucose, 43

  honey, 44

  lactose, 43–44

  maltose, 44

  overview, 13, 42–43

  shopping for, 45

  sucrose, 44

  syrups, 44

single sugars, 13, 40–41, 182. *See also* simple carbohydrates

skipping meals, 14, 226

sleep, exercise and, 215

sliding-scale insulin (SSI) dosing, 16, 90

smoking, 264

smoothies, 168

snacks

  carb-controlled, 320–325

  controlling late night snacking, 342

  overview, 319–320

  portion control, 342

  pre-packaged, 325–326

soda, 168, 185

sodium

  food labels, 107

  hypertension, 261–263

Sodium free label claim, 263

soluble fiber, 46, 47, 257

sorbitol, 182, 183

soups, 262

soy sauce, 262, 290

specialty coffee drink, 168

sphincter (stomach), 54

SSI (sliding-scale insulin) dosing, 16, 90

stabilizing blood glucose

  breakfast, 83

  dinner, 83–84

stackable measuring cups, 127–128

starch fragments, 40–41, 44, 183. *See also* complex carbohydrates

starches
  as complex carbs, 13
  digestion, 148
  digestion and, 40
  Exchange List, 119, 352–354
  grams of carb per ounce, 130
  hand model portions, 136

stevia, 184, 186

stomach, 54–55

strength training (resistance training), 212–213

stress management
  exercise and, 215
  heart health and, 264
  importance of, 23
  stress hormones, 76–77

stretching (exercise), 213

sucralose, 184, 186

sucrose (white sugar), 13, 43–44, 168, 178

sugar alcohols, 182–184

sugar beets, 178

sugar substitutes
  overview, 184–185
  saccharin, 187
  safety records, 186–188
  using in cooking and baking, 188

sugarcane, 178

sugar-free drink mixes, 163

sugar-free gelatin, 341

Sugar-free label claim, 115

sugar-free syrup, 304

sugars
  added sugars, 110
  agave nectar, 181
  Barbados sugar, 179
  brown sugar, 178–179
  coconut palm sugar, 179
  corn syrup, 179
  digestion, 147
  fructose, 180–181
  high-fructose corn syrup, 43, 44, 179, 181
  honey, 179
  liquid sugar, 179
  listed on food labels, 110

maltodextrin, 180

maple syrup, 179

molasses, 178

Muscovado sugar, 179

naturally occurring, 110

no sugar added label claim, 114

overview, 175–177

rice syrup, 179

sugar consumption in U.S., 185

sugar-free label claim, 115

white sugar (sucrose), 13, 43–44, 168, 178

sulfonylureas, 93–94

support group, 10

sweeteners. *See also* sugars
  sugar alcohols, 182–184
  sugar consumption in U.S., 185
  sugar substitutes, 184–188

syrups, 13, 44, 340

T

T1D/T1DM. *See* type 1 diabetes

T2D/T2DM. *See* type 2 diabetes

talk-sing test (exercise), 213

tea, 163

Technical Stuff icon, 4

test strips, 331

test times (blood glucose levels), 332

thirst
  dehydration cycle, 160
  seniors with diabetes and, 281
  as symptom of diabetes, 28

timing carb intake
  distributing carb intake, 80–82
  insulin and, 84–93
  oral diabetes medication and, 93–94
  overview, 18–19, 79
  stabilizing blood glucose levels, 82–84

Tip icon, 3

toaster waffles, 181

tobacco use, 264

tomatoes, 43, 120

tools
  apps, 140–142
  online resources, 140, 343–347
  printed resources, 137–139

Toujeo U300, 86
tracking carbs
  in bloodstream, 56
  elevated glucose, 58–62
  extracting glucose via digestion, 55–56
  fueling cells, 56–57
  glycogen, 57–58
  overview, 53–54
  stomach, 54–55
  undereating carbs, 62–65
traditional food labels, 100–101
trans fat
  food labels, 105
  hydrogenation and, 254
  overview, 50–51
  zero trans fat label claim, 113
Tresiba (Degludec), 86
triticale, 288
tropical fats, 254
tTG (anti-tissue transglutaminase) test, 284
type 1 diabetes (T1D/T1DM)
  celiac disease and, 21, 284
  counting carbohydrates and, 15, 16
  exercise and, 220–223
  insulin, 22
  ketones and, 66
  managing during pregnancy, 273–274
  maternal glucose levels, 276
  overview, 29–30
type 2 diabetes (T2D/T2DM)
  in children, 271–273
  counting carbohydrates and, 15
  exercise and, 223–226
  insulin and, 22
  managing during pregnancy, 273–274
  maternal glucose levels, 276
  overview, 30

U

U. S. measurement system
  volume conversions to metric units, 365
  weight conversions to metric units, 365
UKPDS (United Kingdom Prospective Diabetes Study), 9

undereating carbs
  hypoglycemia, 62–63
  ketones, 64–66
  losing lean body mass, 63–64
United Kingdom Prospective Diabetes Study
    (UKPDS), 9
unsaturated fat, 50, 106, 253–254
updated food labels, 101–104
urination
  glucose in urine, 58–59
  as symptom of diabetes, 28
USDA (U.S. Department of Agriculture), 68, 70
USDA Food Composition Database, 140,
    338, 347
USDA National Nutrient Database, 131

V

vegans, 14
vegetable shortening, 51, 254
vegetables. See also plant foods
  compared to fruit, 166
  fructose, 180
  hand model portions, 136
  nonstarchy, 121–122, 357–358
  nutrients, 42
  overview, 191–193
  starchy, 45–46
  sugars, 43
vegetarian lunch options, 310
vegetarian meat replacements, 49
vegetarians, 14
Very low sodium label claim, 263
viral triggers (type 1 diabetes), 32
vitamins and minerals
  food labels, 103–104
  gluten-free supplements, 291
  role of, 11
  vitamin A, 296
  vitamin B12, 14, 279, 295
  vitamin D, 103, 296
  vitamin E, 296
  vitamin K, 296
volume conversions, 365

W

waffles, 181, 340
walking, 212
warming up (exercise), 213
Warning icon, 4
water, 162
WebMD website, 347
websites
  Academy of Nutrition and Dietetics, 344–345
  American Association of Diabetes Educators, 344
  American Diabetes Association, 343–344
  American Heart Association, 345
  Certified Diabetes Educators, 344
  Diabetes Education Online, 346
  Food and Drug Administration, 345
  Joslin Diabetes Center, 346–347
  Mayo Clinic, 346
  USDA's Food Composition Databases, 347
  WebMD, 347
weighing food, 128–131, 338–339
weight conversions, 365
weight management
  adjusting caloric intake for, 71–72
  counting carbohydrates and, 17–18
  estimating caloric needs, 69–70
  heart health and, 265
  type 2 diabetes and exercise and, 225–226

wheat allergy, 283
white rice, 148
white sugar (sucrose), 13, 43–44, 168, 178
white whole-wheat bread, 114
whole grains
  fiber and, 46
  food label claims, 113–114
  nutrients, 42
  options, 194
  refined grains versus, 193–194
Whole Grains Council, 114
wine, 171, 172, 233
women
  caloric needs, 69–70
  establishing mealtime carb targets, 81
  recommended fiber intake, 47

X

xylitol, 183

Y

yeast infections, 29

Z

Zero trans fat label claim, 113

About the Author

Sherri Shafer, RD, CDE, received her degree in nutrition and dietetics from the University of California at Berkeley. She has spent the last 25 years dedicated to diabetes education in the outpatient diabetes specialty clinics at the University of California San Francisco (UCSF) Medical Center. As a senior registered dietitian and certified diabetes educator, Sherri has counseled thousands of individuals, both adults and children. She is an instructor for diabetes self-management workshops held at the UCSF Diabetes Teaching Center and also provides individual and group instruction on managing diabetes and pregnancy. She has lectured extensively to medical professionals as well as public audiences. Sherri has contributed to healthcare websites and professional publications, and developed dozens of diabetes educational materials. In 2016 Sherri was honored with the prestigious PRIDE award for demonstrating professionalism, respect, integrity, diversity, and excellence in her career. She is the author of *Diabetes Type 2: Complete Food Management Program* (Random House).

Dedication

This book is dedicated to all the people with diabetes who have shared their personal stories with me and have entrusted me to help them navigate through a portion of their diabetes journey. I also dedicate this book to my family: my husband, Rich, and my children, Carter and Coral. They have made my life complete. To my mother, Janet Flodquist, for being a role model and teaching me her work ethic; to my father, Ronald Flodquist, for "loving his family"; and to my siblings, Cyndi, Michael, and Pat.

Author's Acknowledgments

I want to thank Wiley for their commitment to diabetes education and for publishing this book. Special thanks and gratitude goes to my acquisitions editor, Tracy Boggier, for being so amazing both professionally and personally. Thanks to my project manager, Michelle Hacker, for her responsiveness and oversight; to my development editor, Georgette Beatty, for her organization and vision; to my copy editor, Christy Pingleton, for her keen eye to detail; to my illustrator, Kathryn Born, for quality visuals; and to my technical editor, Patricia Booth, for her dedication to quality and accuracy.

I want to acknowledge my many colleagues and mentors at UCSF; Claudia Lutz, who initially hired me and grew to be one of my dearest friends; and Pat Booth, who has been influential in so many aspects of my career.

Publisher's Acknowledgments

Senior Acquisitions Editor: Tracy Boggier

Project Manager: Michelle Hacker

Development Editor: Georgette Beatty

Copy Editor: Christine Pingleton

Technical Editor: Patricia Booth, MS, RD, FADA

Art Coordinator: Alicia B. South-Hurt

Production Editor: Antony Sami

Illustrator: Kathryn Born, MA

Cover Photo: © Tetra Images/Getty Images, Inc.

Apple & Mac

iPad For Dummies,
6th Edition
978-1-118-72306-7

iPhone For Dummies,
7th Edition
978-1-118-69083-3

Macs All-in-One
For Dummies, 4th Edition
978-1-118-82210-4

OS X Mavericks
For Dummies
978-1-118-69188-5

Blogging & Social Media

Facebook For Dummies,
5th Edition
978-1-118-63312-0

Social Media Engagement
For Dummies
978-1-118-53019-1

WordPress For Dummies,
6th Edition
978-1-118-79161-5

Business

Stock Investing
For Dummies, 4th Edition
978-1-118-37678-2

Investing For Dummies,
6th Edition
978-0-470-90545-6

Personal Finance
For Dummies, 7th Edition
978-1-118-11785-9

QuickBooks 2014
For Dummies
978-1-118-72005-9

Small Business Marketing
Kit For Dummies,
3rd Edition
978-1-118-31183-7

Careers

Job Interviews
For Dummies, 4th Edition
978-1-118-11290-8

Job Searching with Social
Media For Dummies,
2nd Edition
978-1-118-67856-5

Personal Branding
For Dummies
978-1-118-11792-7

Resumes For Dummies,
6th Edition
978-0-470-87361-8

Starting an Etsy Business
For Dummies, 2nd Edition
978-1-118-59024-9

Diet & Nutrition

Belly Fat Diet For Dummies
978-1-118-34585-6

Mediterranean Diet
For Dummies
978-1-118-71525-3

Nutrition For Dummies,
5th Edition
978-0-470-93231-5

Digital Photography

Digital SLR Photography
All-in-One For Dummies,
2nd Edition
978-1-118-59082-9

Digital SLR Video &
Filmmaking For Dummies
978-1-118-36598-4

Photoshop Elements 12
For Dummies
978-1-118-72714-0

Gardening

Herb Gardening
For Dummies, 2nd Edition
978-0-470-61778-6

Gardening with Free-Range
Chickens For Dummies
978-1-118-54754-0

Health

Boosting Your Immunity
For Dummies
978-1-118-40200-9

Diabetes For Dummies,
4th Edition
978-1-118-29447-5

Living Paleo For Dummies
978-1-118-29405-5

Big Data

Big Data For Dummies
978-1-118-50422-2

Data Visualization
For Dummies
978-1-118-50289-1

Hadoop For Dummies
978-1-118-60755-8

Language & Foreign Language

500 Spanish Verbs
For Dummies
978-1-118-02382-2

English Grammar
For Dummies, 2nd Edition
978-0-470-54664-2

French All-in-One
For Dummies
978-1-118-22815-9

German Essentials
For Dummies
978-1-118-18422-6

Italian For Dummies,
2nd Edition
978-1-118-00465-4

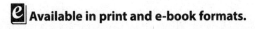 **Available in print and e-book formats.**

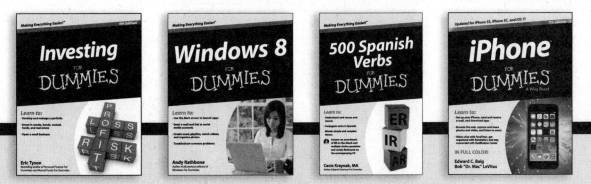

Available wherever books are sold. **For more information or to order direct visit www.dummies.com**

Math & Science

Algebra I For Dummies, 2nd Edition
978-0-470-55964-2

Anatomy and Physiology For Dummies, 2nd Edition
978-0-470-92326-9

Astronomy For Dummies, 3rd Edition
978-1-118-37697-3

Biology For Dummies, 2nd Edition
978-0-470-59875-7

Chemistry For Dummies, 2nd Edition
978 1 118 00730 3

1001 Algebra II Practice Problems For Dummies
978-1-118-44662-1

Microsoft Office

Excel 2013 For Dummies
978-1-118-51012-4

Office 2013 All-in-One For Dummies
978-1-118-51636-2

PowerPoint 2013 For Dummies
978-1-118-50253-2

Word 2013 For Dummies
978-1-118-49123-2

Music

Blues Harmonica For Dummies
978-1-118-25269-7

Guitar For Dummies, 3rd Edition
978-1-118-11554-1

iPod & iTunes For Dummies, 10th Edition
978-1-118-50864-0

Programming

Beginning Programming with C For Dummies
978-1-118-73763-7

Excel VBA Programming For Dummies, 3rd Edition
978-1-118-49037-2

Java For Dummies, 6th Edition
978-1-118-40780-6

Religion & Inspiration

The Bible For Dummies
978-0-7645-5296-0

Buddhism For Dummies, 2nd Edition
978-1-118-02379-2

Catholicism For Dummies, 2nd Edition
978-1-118-07778-8

Self-Help & Relationships

Beating Sugar Addiction For Dummies
978-1-118-54645-1

Meditation For Dummies, 3rd Edition
978-1-118-29144-3

Seniors

Laptops For Seniors For Dummies, 3rd Edition
978-1-118-71105-7

Computers For Seniors For Dummies, 3rd Edition
978-1-118-11553-4

iPad For Seniors For Dummies, 6th Edition
978-1-118-72826-0

Social Security For Dummies
978-1-118-20573-0

Smartphones & Tablets

Android Phones For Dummies, 2nd Edition
978-1-118-72030-1

Nexus Tablets For Dummies
978-1-118-77243-0

Samsung Galaxy S 4 For Dummies
978-1-118-64222-1

Samsung Galaxy Tabs For Dummies
978-1-118-77294-2

Test Prep

ACT For Dummies, 5th Edition
978-1-118-01259-8

ASVAB For Dummies, 3rd Edition
978-0-470-63760-9

GRE For Dummies, 7th Edition
978-0-470-88921-3

Officer Candidate Tests For Dummies
978-0-470-59876-4

Physician's Assistant Exam For Dummies
978-1-118-11556-5

Series 7 Exam For Dummies
978-0-470-09932-2

Windows 8

Windows 8.1 All-in-One For Dummies
978-1-118-82087-2

Windows 8.1 For Dummies
978-1-118-82121-3

Windows 8.1 For Dummies, Book + DVD Bundle
978-1-118-82107-7

Available in print and e-book formats.

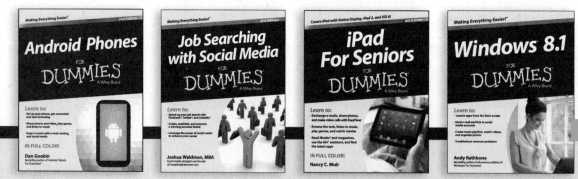

Available wherever books are sold. **For more information or to order direct visit www.dummies.com**

Take Dummies with you everywhere you go!

Whether you are excited about e-books, want more from the web, must have your mobile apps, or are swept up in social media, Dummies makes everything easier.

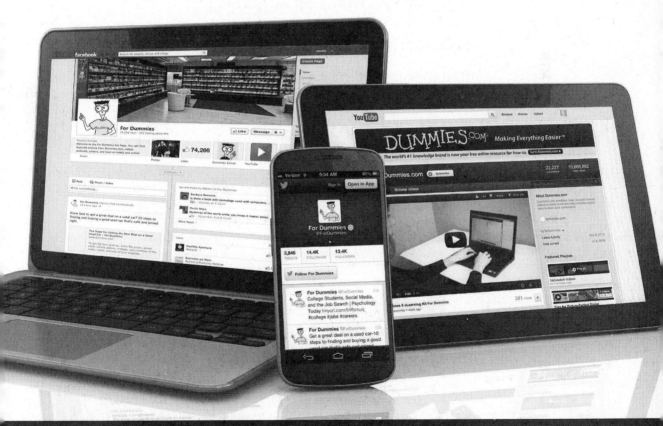

Leverage the Power

For Dummies is the global leader in the reference category and one of the most trusted and highly regarded brands in the world. No longer just focused on books, customers now have access to the For Dummies content they need in the format they want. Let us help you develop a solution that will fit your brand and help you connect with your customers.

Advertising & Sponsorships

Connect with an engaged audience on a powerful multimedia site, and position your message alongside expert how-to content.

Targeted ads • Video • Email marketing • Microsites • Sweepstakes sponsorship

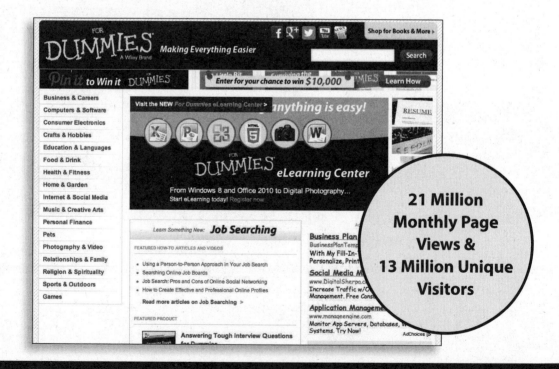

21 Million Monthly Page Views & 13 Million Unique Visitors